GERIATRIC MENTAL HEALTH CARE

Geriatric Mental Health Care
A Treatment Guide for Health Professionals

GARY J. KENNEDY

THE GUILFORD PRESS
New York   London

© 2000 The Guilford Press
A Division of Guilford Publications, Inc.
72 Spring Street, New York, NY 10012
www.guilford.com

Printed in the United States of America

This book is printed on acid-free paper.

Last digit is print: 9   8   7   6   5   4   3   2   1

Library of Congress Cataloging-in-Publication Data

Kennedy, Gary J., 1948–
    Geriatric mental health care : a treatment guide for health
professionals / Gary J. Kennedy.
        p. cm.
    Includes bibliographical references and index.
    ISBN 1-57230-592-4 (hardcover)
        1. Geriatric psychology. 2. Primary care (Medical care).
    3. Aged—Mental health services. 4. Aged—Mental health. I. Title.

    RC451.4.A5 K46 2000
    618.97′689—dc21   00-042231

To my wife, Jenny,
who remains my first and favorite editor

About the Author

Gary J. Kennedy, MD, is Professor of Psychiatry and Behavioral Science at Albert Einstein College of Medicine and Director of the Division of Geriatric Psychiatry and the Psychogeriatric Fellowship Training Program at Montefiore Medical Center in Bronx, New York. He is also Supervising Psychiatrist of the Geriatric Unit at Bronx Psychiatric Center. More than 30 psychiatrists have completed geriatric training under his direction. His research and teaching have focused on cardiac arrhythmias, the epidemiology of depression and dementia, and mental health care in nursing homes and in the community.

Dr. Kennedy has served as a consultant to the New York State Commission on Life and the Law regarding physician-assisted suicide and was also a member of the New York State Department of Health Advisory Work Group on Human Subject Research Involving Protected Classes. He has been a member of the American Psychiatric Association's Council on Aging and the Mental Disorders of Aging Initial Review Group of the National Institute of Mental Health. He also chaired the Education Committee of the American Association for Geriatric Psychiatry, is presently psychiatric liaison to the Education Committee of the American Geriatrics Society, and chairs the Education Committee of the Geriatric Mental Health Foundation.

Dr. Kennedy's work has been supported by the National Heart, Lung and Blood Institute, the National Institute on Aging, the Forchheimer Foundation, the Resnick Gerontology Center, the New York State Department of Health, the United Jewish Appeal, the University Place Foundation, and the Irving Weinstein Foundation. He has received a New Investigator Award from the National Institutes of Health and a travel study fellowship from the United States–World Health Organization, and is a fellow of the Brookdale Center on Aging at Hunter College. Since 1992, he has been listed in Woodward/White, Inc., *The Best Doctors in America.*

Preface

Although there are a number of excellent geriatric mental health texts, none is written expressly for generalists in primary care and mental health, who represent the majority of practitioners providing care for older Americans with mental illness. With the increasing proportion of older adults in the population, general care will take on more of the attributes of geriatric care. For complex cases, generalists may consult colleagues who have specialized in geriatrics. But more often they will rely on reference texts to augment their care of senior patients. Given the pressures to contain costs, this practical guide to geriatric psychiatry can help the generalist to be efficient, without sacrificing quality or consumer satisfaction.

Geriatric Mental Health Care presents a concise approach to geriatric conditions for the clinician already familiar with basic diagnosis and treatment of mental illness. It is meant to serve the needs of the widest possible audience, from students and trainees in nursing, social work, psychology, and medicine, to practicing clinicians, managed care administrators, elder care managers, ethicists, and elder lawyers. It should also serve as an introductory text for psychiatric residents and fellows in geriatric medicine and geriatric psychiatry. Throughout, the challenges of geriatric care are balanced by the rewards. There is considerable coverage of the misfortune of illness and the need to negotiate good care in difficult circumstances. But there are also chapters (Chapters 1, 5, 9, and 15) written with healthy elders in mind, emphasizing health promotion and illness prevention.

Beyond instruction on diagnosis and treatment, my goal is to show how one works with seniors, their families, and the rest of the care team. I have sought to emphasize the differences between age, illness, and inactivity and to counter myths and misapprehensions about them.

The text is evidence-based wherever possible, but its focus is on practice rather than research. Where legal and ethical issues are addressed, I have added scientific and historical background to approach value-based decisions. I have also tried to avoid psychiatric terminology where commonsense language expressed the ideas just as well. The reader might find it helpful to sample parts of several chapters for a specific problem, rather than read one chapter from start to finish.

In some instances I have linked topics that are traditionally separated because I felt the connection would be more informative. For example, the diagnosis and pharmacotherapy of anxiety and depression are combined in a single chapter (Chapter 2), reflecting the frequency with which they co-occur as well as the growing routine of prescribing antidepressants for both. The psychotherapies, which have been individually tailored to fit either depression or anxiety, are discussed in Chapter 7, along with a discussion of caregiver counseling and work with the family. (This same discussion, pertaining to group and couple psychotherapy, appears in Chapter 8.) This separation is not meant to imply that generalists need not provide counseling and psychotherapy. Indeed, I believe the best practitioners develop an intuitive approach similar to that which is reflected in the research literature.

I also discuss late-life mania and psychosis in one chapter (Chapter 4) because of the similarities in the approach to their pharmacotherapy as well as the special problems posed by forging a relationship with patients for whom collaboration is difficult. Chapter 3 addresses the diagnosis and treatment of dementia. The assessment of decisional capacity and the ethics of end-of-life care are the focus of Chapter 14.

Because care provided in nursing homes and by home care agencies is so rarely taught to physicians yet is so prevalent among seniors, Chapter 13 is dedicated to these underserved care sites. The inclusion of material on how to make a house call, conduct a therapeutic family meeting, perform a bioethics consultation, and deal with cases of elder abuse may seem beyond the scope of practice for some readers. However, knowledge of these topics is invaluable when a crisis occurs.

These are contradictory times in health care. We can afford care for all but lack the resolve to do so. The autonomy of the physician has declined, yet the authority with which diagnosis and treatment can be provided is more compelling than ever. Scientific advances are accelerating, pressing health care providers both to be technical experts and to see volumes of new patients. Yet the public expects the comfortable, compassionate service that emerges from a long-standing relationship

with a generalist. The considerable benefits of our sophisticated technology cannot be realized without the personal touch and more equitable access. Too often we focus on the challenge and cost of working
with older people and lose sight of the satisfactions. Indeed, those
lucky enough or motivated enough to have aged successfully need little that we have to offer, but they have much to teach. It is my hope
that the inspiration I have drawn from both the sick and the well is obvious.

Acknowledgments

First, I thank my patients and their families for their generosity of spirit. Time and limits on space did not permit me to include more of the comedy, tragedy, and everyday heroism they have shared with me. What I know about seniors is what they and their physicians have taught me. This is not to say that my mother, at 85, has run out of lessons for me. "You have to break in a new doctor," she says, and I am delighted to add that she has "broken" many herself.

Regarding colleagues and mentors, I thank Byram Karasu, Chairman and Silverman Professor of Psychiatry and Behavioral Science at the Albert Einstein College of Medicine. I am reminded of his early practical geriatric text, written with the now deceased, but distinguished Dr. Leopold Bellak. Herman van Praag, the former Chairman, appointed me to my current position and urged me to write. I also thank Donna Cohen and Carl Eisdorfer, whose enthusiasm for geriatric care added fuel to the fire of my ambition. The humanism and bedside manners of David Hamerman and Nancy Dubler continue to inspire me, as they did from my first days at Montefiore Medical Center. Nancy's review of Chapter 14, on bioethics, particularly her generosity with material on the bioethics consultation, is warmly acknowledged. I thank Howard Kelman, Cynthia Thomas, and Dan Blazer, whose devotion to research was critical to my academic development. I thank as well Jim Spikes for the opportunity to come to Montefiore.

The leadership, staff, and residents of the Margaret Tietz Center for Nursing Care have taught me the meaning of quality in long-term care. I also acknowledge contributions from the staff and administration of Bronx Psychiatric Center. The nobility of their commitment to the sickest and most disadvantaged of the mentally ill at "Bronx State" is too often unappreciated. To the students, trainees, and fellows with whom I have worked, their success is a gratifying reminder that one teaches in order to learn. And finally, I acknowledge my colleagues in the Divisions of Geriatric Medicine and Geriatric Psychiatry at Montefiore Medical Center—the physicians, nurses, and social workers whose work I so admire.

Contents

1

Introduction to the Geriatric Imperative

Competence in geriatric care has become imperative. The number of older persons is increasing, their average age is advancing, and the costs of their health needs, both personal and societal, pose substantial economic and policy challenges. Even if the incidence of an illness such as Alzheimer's disease with a late onset declines, the absolute increase in the number of older persons means an increase in the number of cases the average practitioner will see. Of the present $1 trillion health care bill, the federal share is 25%. By 2012, when the health expenditures are projected to reach $1.6 to $2.3 trillion, the federal share will be 50%. Cost containment through increased efficiency and reduced fees for service may already have reached maximum savings. Rowe (1999), among others (e.g., Hazzard, 1995), has called for a new preventive approach to illness in late life, one that would require a remodeling of Medicare. Thus the need to rapidly incorporate research advances into the practices of generalist practitioners cannot be ignored (Pardes et al., 1999). Patients, their families, managed care entities, and practitioners have divergent views and motivations about what is desirable in health care. Extensive technical information necessary for quality care must be integrated into a matrix of individual needs and preferences, family and social resources, financial and legal determinants, and caregiving systems. What follows are data and concepts to guide the generalist practitioner through common psychogeriatric problems. The goals are to expand the practitioner's therapeutic vantage while making prognosis more realistic and care more efficient. In this way the challenge of working with seniors will be equaled if not surpassed by the reward. Subsequent chapters provide specifics on diagnosis and treatment.

CORE CONCEPTS FROM SOCIOLOGY
AND CLINICAL SCIENCES

Myths about Aging

There are a number of myths about aging shared by many patients, practitioners, and policymakers that need to be countered (Busse, 1989). These include the following:

1. Age is an illness.
2. Genetics determines illness and disability.
3. Disability is inevitable and increasing among seniors.
4. Loss of social ties leaves the older adult alone and isolated.
5. Most elderly are depressed, demented, or dependent.
6. Because of accumulated chronic illness, social factors are less salient in late life.
7. Old age leads to physiological and social homogeneity (i.e., seniors generally have the same needs and potentials).
8. Advances in biotechnology and pharmacology are the most important elements in reducing late-life dependency.
9. Projections based on present data are sufficient for social policy planning over the next decades.
10. Aging and mortality are synonymous.
11. The older the patient, the greater the cost.

These misconceptions are examined next.

Aging and Mental Illness

The interplay of mental and physical illness, social factors, and the accumulation of years make comorbidity the rule rather than the exception in geriatric practice. For both causality and course of illness, mental and physical health are inseparable in aged persons (Katz 1996). Primary care practitioners rather than mental health specialists provide the diagnosis and pharmacological treatment of mental illness among most Americans (Pincus et al., 1998). This is even more the case for older adults. Despite an increase in subspecialty geriatric training in internal medicine, family practice, and psychiatry, instruction in the recognition and treatment of mental illness in seniors remains less than ideal in the health professions (Kennedy et al., 1999). Moreover, the prevalence of both mental and physical disability increases with advanced age because illnesses that occur late in life are persistent and less lethal, and thus accumulate. The fastest growing segment is the 85 and older group in whom the prevalence of dementia approaches 50%.

Nonetheless, although depressive symptoms and complaints of impaired cognition increase with age, the majority of older persons are neither demented nor seriously depressed. Physically healthy seniors have the lowest rates of anxiety, depression, and substance abuse among the adult population (Kennedy et al., 1990).

Biological Theories of Aging

A number of biological theories have been advanced to explain why and how we age. These include genetic, metabolic, autoimmune, and endocrine explanations. Genetic factors are represented by programmed cell death (apoptosis) and accumulation of genetic errors occurring during repeated cell replication. As the genetic material is copied, the integrity of the chromosomes (telomerase failure) or gene products (stochastic "hits") is eroded. In the metabolic theory, activity essential to the respiratory cycle causes oxidative stress and the production of free radicals which "rust out" subcellular processes. Alternatively, nonenzymatic processes between proteins and glucose cause haphazard, irreversible peptide cross-links by glycosylation, "cooking down" or aging body tissue and degrading DNA. In the autoimmune theory of aging, the lifelong assault of antigens on the immune system leads either to exhaustion or misidentification of the host. The result is malignancy from failure to check unwanted growth or autoimmune disease. In the endocrine theory, age-related changes in body composition and hypothalamic function are paralleled by endocrine fatigue. As muscle mass declines, body fat increases by roughly 35% and is distributed away from the surface into and around the viscera. Elders paradoxically are fatter but less well insulated and more cold intolerant than younger adults. Melatonin, testosterone, growth hormone, insulin-like growth factor-I, and dehydroepiandrosterone all decline. Although estrogen replacement has clear benefits in reducing death and disability among women, in the absence of large-scale human trials the National Institute on Aging (1997) cautions against the use of other hormones in any routine way. In the biological clock theory, critical systems unwind losing speed, accuracy, and integration with the whole. Taste, smell, peripheral vision, proprioception, and the sensation of pain are blunted with age. Even in the absence of disease the kidney, lung, and skin age more rapidly than do the heart and liver. The musculoskeletal system and gonads atrophy at different times in men and women. If there is a biological clock, different organ systems keep different time (Leventhal, 1996).

     None of the aging theories adequately explains the determinants of the older person's level of independence or productivity. Martin

(1998) argues that at age 45, humans escape the pressure of natural selection and the capacity of biological theories of adaptation to explain
what is most important to the older person, that is, independence and
well-being. Indeed psychosocial factors, lifestyle, and behavioral patterns may play a greater role in the effects of aging than does biology.

Demography of Advanced Age

From 1900 to the 1990s, the number of older Americans tripled from 4%
to 13.5% (Treas, 1995). From 1980 to the year 2000, the number of individuals over the age of 80 increased by 67% (Eustis et al., 1984). The expo-
nential growth in this age group will extend to the middle of the 21st century. By the year 2030, the percentage of persons older than 65 in the
United States will have doubled from 11% to 22%, ultimately representing 55 million individuals (U.S. Bureau of the Census, 1992). Although
the average age of older Americans will continue to increase well into
the century, close to half of all the people who ever lived to the age of 65
are alive today. From 1982 to 1994 the percentage of older persons in
nursing homes declined from 6.3% to 5.2%. In 1994 nearly three quarters
of those between 75 and 84 reported no disability. Of those age 85 or
older, 40% were fully functional (Manton et al., 1997). At age 65, life expectancy for women is 84 years, 14 of which can be expected to be active,
5 years dependent. Men at 65 can expect 15 years more of life, 12 years of
which will be fully independent. Nonetheless at age 85 nearly half the remaining years will be dependent (Rowe & Kahn, 1998).

Although the increase in life expectancy has slowed, the decline in
death rates has accelerated. And trends in death rates and maximum
age at death show no signs of approaching the oft-assumed 85 year
limit (Wilmoth, 1998). Obviously the emergence of unexpected infectious disease such as AIDS can alter any extrapolation about morbidity
and mortality as seen so tragically in Africa. And advances in biotechnology such as manipulation of a gene that halts the age-related short-
ening of telomers during *in vitro* cell replication show promise of extending the lifespan (Bodnar, 1998). Changes in mortality or morbidity
at the end of life show less impact than those that occur earlier in life
when the cumulative change will have a larger statistical contribution.
The greatest uncertainties regarding active lifespan lie in social and
political developments rather than the technological (Wilmoth, 1998).

Changing Patterns of Disability

The present older generation is healthier, more active, and in better financial condition than any previous cohort of persons age 65 or older.
Only 5% require institutional care and only 10% require assistance in

the community. Two-thirds of older adults rate themselves in good to excellent health. Three-quarters report no more than minor if any limitations in activities of daily living (Jette, 1996). Sunderland (1998a, 1998b) speculates that if the onset of dementia could be forestalled by 10 years, the number of persons disabled by dementia would not increase much beyond the present numbers despite the increased proportion of older Americans. In short, delaying the incidence to the point at which natural mortality thins the ranks of the susceptible cohort would reduce the prevalence rates despite greater numbers of at-risk individuals. The implications are even more important in light of the fact that dementia is the major cause of functional dependence in the elderly (Agüero-Torres et al., 1998).

Ultimately the goal of good geriatric practice is to maximize the active lifespan. Advances in the control and prevention of infection and accidents, as well as improved economic and environmental well-being, have substantially reduced death rates in late life. The mortality curve increasingly takes on a squared rather than sinusoidal shape. More and more seniors will thus approach their maximum lifespan. More recent data suggest that the morbidity curve is also squaring off. More seniors will remain functionally intact to the end.

And if the increasing proportion of older adults who are employed continues to grow, it will reverse the downward trend noticed from the 1980s (Treas, 1995). Revocation of mandatory retirement policies and smaller birth cohorts of younger persons competing in the job market are only two factors favoring increased numbers of older workers. Older adults are increasing their expectations of health and productivity in old age (Pardes et al., 1999). Thus the dependency ratio (number of employed supporting those not employed) may not rise as dramatically as expected as the baby boomers born between 1946 and 1963 reach the formal age of retirement at 65 (Zarit & Zarit, 1998). Both the direct and indirect contributions that healthy, active seniors will make to their families and communities may be much greater than expected.

Comorbidity and the Geriatric Syndromes

Comorbidity, meaning the coexistence of more than one illness or condition, is the rule rather than the exception among mentally or physically impaired older persons. For a younger person a single disease is likely to be the sole cause of disability. Cure the disease and you eliminate the disability. However, in late life the presence of comorbidity, chronic conditions, and frailty requires an approach less preoccupied with curative interventions. It is more focused on rehabilitation and return to optimum function. This is the "functional approach" and re-

quires a range of interventions that include not only diagnosis and definitive treatment but also supportive and restorative measures. The
goal is to eliminate "excess (avoidable) disability" which is a major focus of the chapters on dementia and depression. The "geriatric syndromes" include frailty, failure to thrive, osteopenia and sarcopenia
(wasting of bone and muscle), falls and gait disturbance, incontinence,
cognitive impairment, and depression. All are examples in which a
host of diagnoses and age-related impairments must be countered for
the individual to benefit. A "comprehensive geriatric assessment" will
use geriatric syndromes, the functional approach to treatment, and the
theory of excess disability to help clarify what may seem to be a bewil-
dering array of etiologies and treatment options.

Beyond Diagnosis to Functional Assessment

Functional assessment entails an evaluation of the person's capacity to
perform activities of daily living (ADL). These include personal components such as the maintenance of physical hygiene and grooming as
well as more instrumental tasks such as the management of finances
and property. Clearly the distinction between personal and instrumental ADL is important but can be exaggerated. And emotional support
has a significant role to play in sustaining levels of physical performance associated with lesser need for ADL assistance (Seeman et al.,
1995). There are ADL scales for the scientific study of populations.
However, on an individual basis a commonsense approach to determining what the person is capable of managing is more than adequate.
Simply knowing the presence of impaired ADL skills tells the evaluator little about the cause, persistence, or progression of the impairments. For example, marked physical disability due to stroke may not
mean the affected person is mentally impaired. Even when the brain's
motor programs are damaged, preventing the manipulation of objects
in space (apraxia), patients may be able to direct others to assist them
in personal and instrumental ADL.

Nevertheless if the disability is accompanied by aphasia—an impairment in language and communication—the person may be fully aware
of needs but unable to meet them either personally or through the direction of others. A speech pathologist can be invaluable in characterizing the nature and density of aphasia and assisting the practitioner to
find the most effective means of communicating with the patient. Similarly an occupational or physical therapist can provide a formal assessment of ADL problems as well as suggest exercises or assistive devices
to maximize function despite weakness and apraxia. But to be fully
meaningful, the assessment should be a multifaceted measure of the

person's strengths, weaknesses, and resources—not just the mental and physical but also financial, social, and interpersonal.

Adaptive Capacity and Successful Aging

The capacity to adapt to the stress and strain of daily life changes with age. Adaptive reserves are inevitably diminished. For example, the extent of third-degree burns that prove lethal to half of burn victims less than 60 years of age is 35%. Over the age of 60 it is 15%. At age 75, 10% total body burned is lethal to 50%. However, the majority of the diminishment in cardiac and pulmonary function is the result of diminished physical activity rather than age (Rowe & Kahn, 1998). Some persons of advanced age may be independent but are nonetheless catastrophically vulnerable to physical, emotional, or social disruptions that would have been minor stressors earlier in life. Such frailty implies an age-related risk of becoming partially or wholly dependent on others. However, many individuals (those who have been lucky enough to have aged successfully) remain robust to their last days. Happily, luck in the terms of inheritance has less to do with desirable aging than many think. With advancing age, genetic risk factors become less important as lifestyle elements play an increasing role in modifying susceptibility as well as resilience.

Only recently has the older person's capacity to slow age-related decline in physical and mental function been fully appreciated. Research indicates that a major part of the physical decline experienced by older adults is caused by lack of health promotion and disease prevention rather than aging as such. Simple interventions focused on factors that contribute to the most prevalent chronic disease exist but are not widely recognized or practiced. For all the attention to diet, it appears that weight reduction in late life is more important than the optimal mix of dietary elements. Rowe and Kahn (1998) describe the predictors of successful aging as (1) avoiding disease and disability, (2) maintaining physical and mental function, and (3) continued engagement with other persons in productive activities.

Indeed preventive gerontology encompasses the promise of maximizing function (reducing morbidity) without the illusion of extending the maximum lifespan. As a result, even greater heterogeneity in seniors should be expected. Recognizing this heterogeneity, both medicine and the law have adopted a functional rather than a categorical orientation. Thus the older person can no longer be deprived of civil liberties through guardianship proceedings without a determination of functional impairment. Old age may predict but does not define decline and disability.

Gender, Race, and Ethnicity

The fastest growing group of ethnic elders are Hispanics who are also among the most underserved of the elderly. In contrast, most older Americans at present are white women of European heritage. While women enjoy a survival advantage over men, men are less likely than women to be disabled late in life. On average, women marry men who are 4 years their senior. Men are more likely to remarry than women. Forty-two percent of older women are married compared to 77% of older men (U.S. Bureau of the Census, 1992). Because men are less frequently widowed than older women, they are also more likely to be cared for in the community rather than placed in a nursing home once they have lost their independence. However, community care is often a euphemism for "daughter care" such that any presumed cost offset of "community care" is, rather, a cost transfer.

At present African Americans' life expectancies at birth in the United States compared to that of whites are 8 years fewer for men and 6 years fewer for women due largely to differences in early life mortality rates. However, at age 65 life expectancy is still 2 years less than that observed among whites. African American seniors lived through an era of segregated care that Medicare requirements ended in the 1960s. Nonetheless, *de facto* segregation in housing and thereby access to care remains a reality. Ethnic elders may not be in the minority in their home community. But when admitted to a nursing facility, their minority status may be painfully obvious. Their attitude toward medical research as a result of the now infamous Tuskegee study is also less than favorable. Not surprisingly, trust in the institution or provider may not be automatic. Conversely, some older persons from disadvantaged minorities may be excessively deferential. The practitioner should be aware that deference is not synonymous with compliance.

Older patients are less diverse ethnically than their younger health care providers. Differences in age, ethnicity, or gender should neither be emphasized nor ignored. Indeed, it may be important to acknowledge the need to develop trust and express a willingness to discuss difficulties openly should they arise. Apologies for being different, defensive denials, or clichés about fundamental similarities will not be taken as genuine. Differences in language and culture may be bridged by family or other caregivers but not always with full fidelity to the patient's expressions. Practitioners should be wary of dismissing mental symptoms as a cultural expression when the patient is clearly disabled. Knowing the appropriate greeting and farewell in the patient's language helps achieve rapport.

Issues of Assimilation and Identity among Older Émigrés

Immigration is another factor affecting the presentation of illness and use of health care services among older adults. Recently arrived older immigrants experience the disadvantage of cultural shock and role loss within the family. The younger family members upon whom the elders rely for cultural liaison take on an authority and independence that may not have been characteristic of their culture of origin. Through work, education, and child rearing they have greater opportunities to assimilate the new language and culture. In contrast, their elders may be socially isolated and cut off from traditional roles of seniority within the family. The mental health services in their homeland may be even less available and more stigmatized than that which exists in the United States today. Furthermore the mind–body duality of physical and mental illness may be more sharply realized. Preventive measures may also have been lacking (American Psychiatric Association Task Force on Ethnic Minority Elderly, 1993).

Differing expectations regarding individuality, autonomy, and decision making also affect care. The vaulted individualism of the West often dictates that presentation of therapeutic choices be placed before the individual who will then mediate the family's influence. In other cultures major personal decisions are forged through family consensus. Choices presented to the individual in absence of the family may be seen as insensitive and even manipulative. Advanced health directives, do-not-resuscitate orders, and durable power of attorney for health care are only some of the examples that traditional, extended family cultures would see as shared rather than individual choices.

Religion and the Older Adult

Religious institutions are the most common and widely accessible source of social support for older Americans. Senior citizens profess greater religious belief and more frequent religious practice than do younger persons. Yet religious institutions and religious leaders have only recently been seen as pivotal sources of referral for depressed or suicidal older adults and for family caregivers of persons with dementia (Gwyther, 1995). Restrictions on diet, alcohol, and tobacco are obvious examples of how religious affiliation may influence health. However, more subtle influences from beliefs and practices are also thought to be operative, more so in the aftermath of illness than in etiology (Kennedy 1998).

Because religious holidays are often milestones in the older person's life, they offer a ready assessment of social connections and physical restrictions. A simple inquiry as to with whom the elder spent the holiday is both a sociable greeting ("ice breaker") and a powerful yet inoffensive probe. Adjustment to loss, hope for the future, and a sense of meaning despite declining capacity may emerge. The question also identifies the younger practitioner as interested in the patient as a person and sets the stage for exploration of more sensitive areas if needed. Moralizing is avoided by emphasizing the social aspect of religious affiliation and asking what has kept the person from returning to devotional activities if he or she once strongly valued them. Many older persons who may have out-of-date ideas about the treatment of mental symptoms may be directed to their clergy to gain a more modern perspective (and permission) to follow through with diagnosis and treatment.

Shrinking Social Networks, Increasing Need for Social Support

Although the size of one's social network declines late in life, close relationships remain. The smaller networks are characterized by emotional closeness and strong feelings of embeddedness. Lang et al. (1998) suggest that elders become more selective of their relationships, seeking shorter-term emotionally gratifying goals rather than longer-range material objectives associated with advancement in work, career, or marriage. The loss of casual acquaintances and distant relatives may be less significant when close friends or close family remains. Indeed, family status rather than personality predicts close relationships. Older adults may make compensatory investments in a few close relationships that promote and sustain their adaptation to advanced age. Thus there are many avenues to a socially adaptive old age.

THE NEW PSYCHOPHARMACOLOGY: BURDENS AND BENEFITS

The development of psychotropic medications has progressed from empiricism to theory-driven "designer drugs" which manipulate mechanisms of monoamine and cholinergic neurotransmission. This has led to a virtual golden era of psychotropics, which can leave the generalist bewildered by the expanding array of highly touted pharmaceuticals. Direct marketing of prescription drugs to the public is also a relatively recent phenomenon, reflecting the considerable profits to be made. Indeed, the fastest growing cost in health care may be new prescription drugs. However, more often than not, what promises to be a breakthrough turns out not to live up to expectations (Drachman & Leber, 1997). For both better and for worse, every professional working with older adults needs a new orientation to psychopharmacology.

Precautions When Prescribing

Before one prescribes it is necessary to consider the patient's risk of suicide and the potential toxicity of a given agent. The selective serotonin reuptake inhibitors (SSRIs) are relatively free of life-threatening side effects. However, polypharmacy can endanger even the most cautious approach. As the number of medications increases, the risk of adverse reactions and drug interactions multiplies. Human factors must also be taken into account. The more complex the regimen, the greater the error rate for even the most compliant, compulsive patient. Social isolation means that the patient may not have a concerned party to reinforce the regimen, pick up a forgotten dose, or be vigilant for dangerous side effects. Costs of the more recently introduced agents are substantially greater than the drugs that have become available generically. Indeed, those best suited to the older patient may not be available as generics. Due to the expense, the older person on a fixed or otherwise limited income may conserve medications by reducing the dose, in effect stretching out the number of pills to reduce the cost of treatment. In addition to a rough awareness of the relative costs, it is helpful to inquire whether the patient has a prescription plan or concerns about costs. Herbal alternatives are not necessarily less expensive than generic medications. Physical illnesses, frailty, and cognitive impairment further argue for conservatism.

However, clinical indications for the use of antidepressants have expanded in recent years to include anxiety disorders, posttraumatic stress disorder, sleep disturbance, and chronic pain syndromes, as well as depressive disorders (Ereshefsky et al., 1995). With the introduction of medications without life-threatening side effects and the focus on the need to prevent recurrence as well as to induce remission, controversy has arisen regarding the duration of antidepressant treatment. Clearly, for recurrent depression, treatment may well need to be life long. The risks of undesirable side effects are overshadowed by the potentially permanent loss of capacity occasioned by recurrence. Risk can be minimized but not eliminated. Most prescription medications given in excessive amounts over a prolonged period will lead to a change in mental status. The older antidepressants and antianxiety agents as well as some of the antihypertensives are the most frequent offenders. Antipsychotic medications may also have a disabling effect through their propensity to cause Parkinson's disease-like rigidity. However, in low doses and when used singly rather than in combination, antidepressants and antipsychotics are remarkably safe and effective.

Lessening Problems with Therapeutic Adherence

When the older adult takes a number of medications with a complex dosing schedule, noncompliance becomes the norm. Both the number of medications and the frequency of doses should be assessed. Age or illness-related decrements in metabolism often allow reductions in either the dose or the frequency of administration. Can any of the medications be eliminated? Are there alternative medications more appropriate for the aged? This usually means "clean" medications, which are short-lived, free of active metabolites, and selective in activity. However, a side effect such as sedation may be a desirable therapeutic element for the sleep-deprived depressed patient. If the patient needs reminding, a longer half-life medication or extended release preparation could be prescribed so that family, day-care staff, and home health aides can monitor ingestion on a once-daily or every-other-day schedule. Lithium (Eskalith CR), bupropion (Wellbutrin SR), and venlafaxine (Effexor XR) are examples that may be considered. Citalopram or fluoxetine (10–60 mg) are longer lived SSRIs. Clonazepam is a longer half-life antianxiety agent. The depot antipsychotics (Haldol decanoate, Prolixin enanthate) are given as deep intramuscular injections with half-lives ranging from 28 to 14 days. However, these agents should follow stabilization with oral medication, usually on an inpatient basis. Most often they are given to individuals who are too suspicious to take oral medications or those for whom a court order was secured for treatment over objection.

Added to one's appreciation for costs and dosing problems are models that can minimize medication compliance problems. The health beliefs model posits four critical elements to a person's acceptance of a medication or any other medical intervention (Mirotznik et al., 1998). First, persons must perceive that they are either at risk or affected by the condition (or its recurrence) under consideration. The perception of the chronicity of the illness is also important. Does the person view the condition as temporary and episodic or chronic and recurring? Second, are the consequences of the condition undesirable, a serious threat to health, independence, or well-being? Do symptoms merit treatment? Third, is treatment effective and not overly burdensome and are the side effects only an inconvenience or, if serious, acceptable given the alternative? Fourth, and particularly important for older adults on a fixed income, is the cost of treatment reasonable in light of the probability that symptoms will be reduced and function re-stored? Unrecognized differences across these four elements between the prescriber and the patient or the patient and family may help ex-plain why medications are not taken as recommended or not refilled. More important, these elements serve as negotiating points which can clarify expectations for patient and practitioner alike.

Pharmacokinetics and Dynamics

Minimizing the risk of adverse reactions depends in part on recogni-tion of age-related changes in pharmacokinetics and dynamics of med-ication. Pharmacokinetics are the effects the body has on the drug. Pharmacodynamics are the effects the drug has on the person. Of the pharmacokinetic properties, absorption is the least salient consider-ation in advanced age followed by excretion, distribution, and metabo-lism in order of importance. Absorption may be affected when medica-tions are taken in combination or when antacids or soluble fiber preparations sit in the stomach. For agents such as lithium, gaba-pentin, and mirtazepine, which are cleared by the kidneys rather than the liver, the age-related decline in renal excretion should be kept in mind. Slowed excretion should be countered by reducing the fre-quency of the dose. Also, lean body mass declines with age so that there is a relatively greater volume of fat into which lipophilic psycho-tropic agents will deposit. However, loading doses are not recom-mended in the aged due to slowed hepatic metabolism. The greater fat storage of medications means that adverse reactions may be persistent and the washout period may be prolonged. Drug metabolism may be as rapid in robust seniors as it is in younger adults. Indeed, advanced age is associated with greater physiological diversity. However, dis-eases that congest the liver and drugs that are enzyme inducers or competitors will add to the usual age-related slowing in hepatic drug detoxification or predispose the person to drug–drug interactions.

Regarding pharmacodynamics, it is important to be aware of the dose–response relationship. For agents with hypotensive, arrhythmic, amnestic, or extrapyramidal side effects, risk of an adverse reaction may be negligible at low doses. Highly selective agents may become less so as the dose is increased. Both efficacy and adverse reactions are more likely as well. Because interindividual variability increases with age, an adequate trial of medication may take longer for an older adult than for a younger person. Regarding antidepressants, including St. John's wort, patients should be made aware of the latency of effect on mood. However, the beneficial effects of the more sedative antidepressants on sleep disturbance and anxiety may be realized within the first days of treatment. Similarly, most adverse reactions occur in the early stage of treatment. Thus it is essential to counsel patients as to which side effects should be seen as tolerable and which are not. Dry mouth, constipation, vivid dreams, gastrointestinal upset, and temporary increases in anxiety or tremor are not cause for alarm. In contrast, lowered blood pressure, syncope, or cardiac arrhythmias are warning signs of potentially dangerous adverse reactions.

SSRIs Are Not the Panacea

The SSRIs are the most frequently prescribed antidepressants in primary care. However, they are hardly a panacea and they present exemplary problems for practitioners caring for older adults. They may directly induce bradycardia, easy bruising, and the syndrome of inappropriate antidiuretic hormone—particularly in patients taking diuretics (Druckenbrod & Mulsant, 1994). As the dose increases, the SSRIs also exert effects on dopamine reuptake, which may lead to movement disorders more often encountered with typical neuroleptics such as haloperidol. These extrapyramidal symptoms include Parkinsonism, akathisia, dystonia, and acute and tardive dyskinesia. Of the SSRIs, sertraline appears least likely to cause movement disorders (Gerber & Lynd, 1998). However, it is their activity on the drug-metabolizing hepatic enzyme cytochrome P450 that has drawn concern when prescribed for older adults and other persons with complex medical regimens. Inhibition of the P450 system will elevate the levels of beta-blockers, type 1C antiarrhythmics, benzodiazepines, and anticoagulants (Nemeroff et al., 1996). Alterations in the P450 system may also affect estrogen and its metabolites and the anticholinesterases. Nonetheless, Mourilhe and Stokes (1998) found a relatively low incidence of serious drug interactions with these agents. Thus it is not so much the age of the patient but the number, kind, and dosing regimen of medications prescribed that becomes the overriding concern.

Symptoms following abrupt withdrawal of tricyclic antidepressants have been attributed to anticholinergic rebound. With the introduction of SSRIs, reports have emerged of a serotonergic withdrawal syndrome lasting 2 to 3 weeks and characterized by light-headedness, insomnia, agitation, nausea, headache, and sensory disturbances. Mood disturbance may also occur. The shorter-acting SSRIs (sertraline, paroxetine) are more often reported, but venlafaxine and other SSRIs have also been implicated. These agents should not be stopped abruptly for fear of inducing a hyposerotonergic state (Zajeca et al., 1997).

Botanicals

Medicinal preparations derived from plants are more properly referred to as botanicals, a category that includes the true herbs. Practitioners should be aware of herbal and other botanical preparations with reputed sedative, antianxiety or antidepressant properties, not because there is compelling evidence of their efficacy but because a significant minority of patients purchase them and need advice as to safety. These include black cohosh (*Cimicifuga recemosa Nutt*), valerian (*Valeriana officinalis*), German chamomile (*Matricaria recutita*), hops (*Humulus lupulus*), kava (*Piper methysticum*), rosemary, oat straw, lavender, lemon balm (*Melissa officinalis*), skullcap (*Scutellaria laterifolia*), passion flower (*Passiflora incarnata*), chocolate, and jasmine (Wong et al., 1998). They are more safely ingested as weak infusions (chocolate excluded, of course) after being steeped in boiled water. Powdered herbals in capsules or extracts dissolved in oil or alcohol may be more potent and potentially less safe. None are subject to Food and Drug Administration (FDA) approval or quality control. St. John's wort (*Hypericum perforatum*) is the most prominent herbal antidepressant (Zeuss, 1997). Controlled trials sponsored by the National Institute of Mental Health and early reports suggest a serotonergic profile with a latency effect of 2 to 6 weeks. None of these agents are proven effective for major depression; neither is their safety known at high doses or in combination with other medications. I ask patients prescribed a psychotropic to discontinue St. John's wort and kava but not necessarily to stop valerian or chamomile. More information is available regarding valerian and chamomile for sleep (Chapter 5), *Ginkgo biloba* for dementia (Chapter 3), and black cohosh for menopausal symptoms (Chapter 9). Greater detail is available from the American Botanical Council (512-962-4900; *www.herbalgram.org*) and the U.S. Pharmacopeia (800-822-8772, *www.usp.org*). In summary, the new psychopharmacology, including botanicals, is of interest to every professional working for the older person—not just those who prescribe.

ATTRIBUTES OF SUCCESSFUL GERIATRIC PRACTICE

From our examination of the myths associated with aging, it is clear that older Americans are not easily categorized. Their needs and preferences are varied and becoming more so. An established clinical relationship with a generalist primary care provider is the best insurance that older adults will get the care they deserve. In addition there are a number of personal attributes (adapted from Spar & LaRue, 1997) that the practitioner should either amplify or adopt for success with seniors:

- Comfort with broad-based rather than narrowly focused interventions.
- Appreciation for the social factors in older people's health and well-being.
- Remaining an activist in the face of degenerative or terminal disease.
- Patience for the time required and complexity encountered with seniors.
- Lack of embarrassment when confronted with one's youth and inexperience.
- Comfort in teamwork with family and other providers (shared authority).
- Focus on function, rehabilitation, and quality of life rather than on survival.
- Capacity to anticipate the older adult's needs and advocate for care.
- A "sort out" rather than "rule out" view of illness and disability causality.
- Appreciation for cultural as well as physiological diversity.
- Awareness of greater heterogeneity among the aged; flexibility.
- Willingness to physically interact (touch) and give concrete health advice.
- Capacity to tolerate dependency yet press for optimum autonomy.
- Ability to lead as well as follow in the person's care and decisions.
- Ongoing commitment to clinical education.

REFERENCES

Agüero-Torres, H., Fratiglioni, L., Guo, Z., et al. (1998). Dementia is the major cause of functional dependence in the elderly: 3-year follow-up data from a population-based study. *American Journal of Public Health, 88*, 1452–1456.

American Psychiatric Association Task Force on Ethnic Minority Elderly. (1993). *Ethnic minority elderly: A task force report of the American Psychiatric Association.* Washington, DC: American Psychiatric Press.

Bodnar, A. G., Ouellette, M., Frolkis, M., et al. (1998). Extension of life-span by introduction of telomerase into normal human cells. *Science, 279*, 349–352.

Busse, E. W. (1989). The myth, history and science of aging. In E. W. Busse & D. G.

Blazer (Eds.), *Geriatric psychiatry* (pp. 3–34). Washington, DC: American Psychiatric Press.

Drachman, D. A., Leber, P. (1997). Treatment of Alzheimer's disease: Searching for a breakthrough, settling for less. *New England Journal of Medicine 336*, 1245–1247.

Druckenbrod, R., Mulsant, B. H. (1994). Fluoxetine-induced syndrome of inappropriate antidiuretic hormone secretion: A geriatric case report and a review of the literature. *Journal of Geriatric Psychiatry and Neurology, 7*, 255–258.

Ereshefsky, L., Overman, G., Karp, J. (1995). Current psychotropic dosing and monitoring guidelines. *Primary Psychiatry, 5*, 42–53.

Eustis, N., Greenberg, J., Palten, A. (1984). *Long-term care for older persons: A policy perspective.* Monterey, CA: Brooks/Cole.

Gerber, P. E., Lynd, L. D. (1998). Selective serotonergic reuptake inhibitor-induced movement disorders. *Annals of Pharmacotherapy, 32*, 692–698.

Gwyther, L. (1995). *You are one of us: Successful clergy/church connections to Alzheimer's families.* Durham, NC: Duke University Medical Center.

Hazzard, W. R. (1995). Weight control and exercise: Cardinal features of successful preventive gerontology. *Journal of the American Medical Association, 274*, 1964–1965.

Jette, A. M. (1996). Disability trends and transitions. In R. H. Binstock & L. K. George (Eds.), *Handbook of aging and the social sciences* (pp. 94–114). San Diego: Academic Press.

Katz, I. R. (1996). On the inseparability of mental and physical health in aged persons. *American Journal of Geriatric Psychiatry, 4*, 1–6.

Kennedy, G. J. (1998). Religion and depression. In H. G. Koenig (Ed.), *Handbook of religion and mental health* (pp. 129–146). San Diego: Academic Press.

Kennedy, G. J., Goldstein, M. Z., Northcott, C. J., et al. (1999). The evolution of geriatric curriculum in general residency training: Recommendations for the coming decade. *Academic Psychiatry, 23*, 1–11.

Kennedy, G. J., Kelman, H. R., Thomas, C. (1990). Emergence of depressive symptoms in late life: The importance of declining health and increasing disability. *Journal of Community Health, 15*, 93–104.

Lang, F. R., Staudinger, U. M., Cartensen, L. L. (1998). Perspectives on socioeconomic selectivity in late life: How personality and social context do (and do not) make a difference. *Journals of Gerontology: Psychological Sciences, 53B*, 21–30.

Leventhal, E. A. (1996). Biology of aging. In J. Sadavoy, L. W. Lazarus, L. F. Jarvik, et al. (Eds.), *Comprehensive review of geriatric psychiatry—II* (2nd ed., pp. 81–112). Washington, DC: American Psychiatric Press.

Manton, K. G., et al. (1997). Chronic disability trends in elderly United States population, 1982–1994. *Proceedings of National Academy of Sciences*, 2593–2598.

Martin, G. M. (1998). Aging theories. *European Archives of Psychiatry and Clinical Neuroscience, 248*, S2.

Mirotznik, J., Ginzler, E., Zagon, G., et al. (1998). Using the health belief model to explain clinic appointment-keeping for the management of a chronic disease condition. *Journal of Community Health, 23*, 195–210.

Mourilhe, P., Stokes, P. E. (1998). Risks and benefits of selective serotonergic reuptake inhibitors in the treatment of depression. *Drug Safety, 18,* 57–82.

National Institute on Aging. (1997). *Pills, patches, and shots: Can hormones prevent aging?* Bethesda, MD: Author.

Nemeroff, C. B., DeVamne, C. L., Pollock, B. G. (1996). Newer antidepressants and the cytochrome P450 system. *American Journal of Psychiatry, 153,* 311–320.

Pardes, H., Manton, K. G., Lander, E. S., et al. (1999). Effects of medical research on health care and the economy. *Science, 283,* 36–37.

Pincus, H. A., Taniellan, T. L., Marcus, S. C., et al. (1998). Prescribing trends in psychotropic medications: Primary care, psychiatry, and medical specialties. *Journal of the American Medical Association, 279,* 525–531.

Rowe, J. W. (1999). Geriatrics, prevention and the remodeling of Medicare. *New England Journal of Medicine, 340,* 720–721.

Rowe, J. W., Kahn, R. L. (1987). Human aging: Usual and successful. *Science, 237,* 143–149.

Rowe, J. W., Kahn, R. L. (1998). *Successful aging.* New York: Pantheon.

Seeman, T. E., Berkman, L. F., Charpentier, P. A., et al. (1995). Behavioral and psychosocial predictors of physical performance: MacArthur Studies of Successful Aging. *Journals of Gerontology: Biological Sciences and Medical Sciences, 50,* 177–183.

Spar, J. E., LaRue, A. (1997). *Concise guide to geriatric psychiatry* (2nd ed.). Washington, DC: American Psychiatric Press.

Sunderland, T. (1998a). Alzheimer's disease: Cholinergic therapy and beyond. *Journal of the American Association for Geriatric Psychiatry* (Suppl. 1), S56–S63.

Sunderland, T. (1998b, April 9). *Cognitive enhancers and other anti-dementia agents on the horizon.* Paper presented at the Geriatric Psychopathology and Treatment Symposium, New York.

Treas, J. (1995). Older Americans in the 1990's and beyond. *Population Bulletin, 50,* 1–45.

U.S. Bureau of the Census. (1992). *Sixty-five plus in America* (Current Population Reports, Special Studies, Series No. P23–178). Washington, DC: U.S. Government Printing Office.

Wilmoth, J. R. (1998). The future of human longevity: A demographer's perspective. *Science, 280,* 395–397.

Wong, A. H. C., Smith, M., Boon, H. S. (1998). Herbal remedies in psychiatric practice. *Archives of General Psychiatry, 55,* 1033–1044.

Zajecka, J., et al. (1997). Discontinuation symptoms after treatment with serotonergic reuptake inhibitors: A literature review. *Journal of Clinical Psychiatry 58,* 291–297.

Zarit, S. H., Zarit, J. M. (1998). Normal processes of aging. In *Mental disorders in older adults* (pp. 9–30). New York: Guilford Press.

Zeuss, J. (1997). *The natural prozac: How to use St. John's wort, the antidepressant herb.* New York: Three Rivers Press.

2

Depression and Anxiety

Symptoms of depression and anxiety are frequently seen together in late life, making the disorders more difficult to distinguish, diagnose, and treat than in younger persons. Although the psychotherapeutic techniques for anxiety and depressive disorders are different, the choice of medications (antidepressants for either condition) and the approach to the course of illness are quite similar. Given the frequency with which depression and anxiety disorders go untreated in comparison to the safety and efficacy of present interventions, practitioners are urged to lower the threshold for offering treatment. Yet late-life depression, and to some extent late-life anxiety, should be considered geriatric syndromes due to the multiple, interacting factors that contribute to the disability associated with either. A comprehensive rather than narrow focus on interventions and outcomes is justified and will lead to greater satisfaction for the patient, family, and practitioner.

ASSESSMENT

Because late-life mental illness is so closely associated with functional disability, the functionally oriented comprehensive geriatric assessment (Winograd, 1992) is most likely to lead to optimum treatment. The assessment identifies therapeutic avenues, obstacles, and goals. The end point is the most independent level of function attainable given the person's capacities, support, and setting. The assessment need not be exhausting to be comprehensive. Most older adults are brought to the attention of mental health specialists by family, a primary care provider, or a social service agency. Thus physical examination and laboratory procedures have often been performed prior to referring the patient. An interview with a collateral informant is usually acceptable to the patient, may be essential both for assessment and maintenance of a therapeutic regimen, and makes the work more efficient for the therapist and less burdensome for the patient.

A review of medications (and botanicals) both prescribed and otherwise may reveal unfavorable interactions or regimens that the patient has difficulty following. Reduction in polypharmacy and switching to other medications may improve the older person's mental status and quality of life (Testa et al., 1993). Nutritional assessment may also be indicated when the patient is frail, when dentition is in disrepair, and when weight loss is a problem. Functional assessment of activities of daily living includes a review of the person's capacity to manage personal hygiene, ambulating, shopping, finances, the extent to which assistance is required in these areas, and whether there are disabilities that might be remedied with physical or occupational therapy.

An assessment of social rhythms (Reynolds et al., 1992b), the day-to-day flow of both formal and informal socially supportive activities, will indicate the extent to which the patient is isolated or has abandoned social sources of self-esteem while identifying socially meaningful points of intervention and measures of recovery. Finally, elective procedures may be indicated when the patient fails to respond to interventions or when a latent dementia or another central nervous system disorder is suspected. These include neuropsychological evaluation, brain imaging, and electroencephalogram.

SYMPTOM IDENTIFICATION, SCREENING FOR THE DISORDERS

Although screening older adults in primary care for cognitive disorders (dementia, delirium) is recommended, routine queries about other mental illnesses remain controversial. The Geriatric Depression Scale (Sheikh & Yesavage, 1986), the Center for Epidemiologic Studies Depression Scale (Radloff, 1977), the Beck Depression Inventory (Beck et al., 1961), the Zung Depression Scale (Zung, 1990), the Zung Anxiety Scale (Zung, 1986), the Hamilton Rating Scale for Depression (Williams, 1988), the Hamilton Rating Scale for Anxiety (Hamilton, 1959), the Beck Anxiety Inventory (Beck et al., 1988), and the Agoraphobia Cognition Questionnaire (Chambless et al., 1984) are each screening rather than diagnostic instruments for anxiety and depressive disorders. The Primary Care Evaluation of Mental Disorder Procedure (PRIME-MD) is lengthier than the previously mentioned screens yet not as long as structured research interviews. It provides a brief set of questions designed for rapid diagnosis. Wooley et al. (1997) found that a positive response to either of two questions from the PRIME-MD may be as effective as the longer screening instruments to detect depression. Both questions begin with the following, "During the last month have you often been bothered by . . . , " and end with either "feeling down, depressed, or hopeless?" or "little interest or pleasure in doing things?" The practitioner may choose to forego a formal screening instrument but a screening question or two for depression seems warranted in high-risk older adults who have experienced recent disability due to cardiovascular episode, stroke, fracture, or hospitalization.

The depression screens are sensitive to major depression yet not so specific that they exclude individuals with diagnosable anxiety disorder. Minor depression (only two criteria symptoms continuously present for 2 weeks) and dysthymia (two symptoms for 2 years running) may be missed. And because diagnostic criteria for depressive disorders require the presence of either depressed mood or loss of interest (apathy, irritability), one need not be depressed to have a depressive disorder. The diagnosis is made more difficult because the sleep disturbances, somatic preoccupation, loss of concentration and energy, appetite disturbance, and thoughts of death (but not suicide) are frequently part of physical illness in late life. Similarly, the sudden, catastrophic sensations of shortness of breath, palpitations, and dizziness are frequently interpreted as signs of physical disorder rather than panic attack. A brief review of systems is likely to uncover key symptoms in panic disorder patients or those whose agoraphobia is associated with panic attacks.

However, unexplained decline in motor function (slow movements, gait), dress, grooming, hygiene, and interest in leisure or family, as well as denial of depressed expression and irritability despite their obvious presence should alert the clinician to possible depression. Psychotic depression may be missed because the somatic, nihilistic or paranoid delusions seem to be plausible exaggerations of everyday fears. Delusional depressed patients may argue that treatment is futile because their condition is hopeless or that they are impoverished despite ample "rainy-day" savings. Others will have the conviction that vital organs are missing or that the "doctors know it's cancer but refuse to tell." Some feel they are being punished for past indiscretions or unjustified family resentments. Suspicious inferences ("they want my apartment; they watch me when I go out") are also encountered. A discussion with a collateral informant is usually sufficient to establish reality.

GERIATRIC SYNDROMES, DEPRESSION, AND ANXIETY

The geriatric syndrome terminology encompasses frequent conditions of old age in which the conventions of etiology and diagnostic nomenclature are an insufficient guide to treatment. Cognitive impairment, incontinence, deficits in hearing or vision, osteopenia (osteoporosis and fractures), falls, impaired mobility, pressure ulcers, malnutrition, and polypharmacy are the most frequently cited geriatric syndromes (Beck, 1989). The syndrome terminology reflects the multifactorial etiology typical of these conditions and the requirement for multidimensional treatment to return the older person to optimum function.

A major change in the clinical approach to old-age depression occurred in the 1990s (Karasu et al., 1993; National Institutes of Health Consensus Development Panel, 1992), resulting in an expanse of therapeutic indications, treatments, outcomes, and end points that is best captured by the geriatric syndrome concept. The syndromal approach also resolves much of the conflict between epidemiological (Myers et al., 1984b) and clinical (Kermis, 1986) studies of depression in old age. Epidemiological studies find depressive symptoms pervasive but depressive disorders infrequent in older community residents. In medical clinic populations, both symptoms and disorders are frequent. The symptoms may arise from bereavement, the despondency associated with recent-onset disability, a perception of failing health, loss of hope as a result of confinement from agoraphobia, or a major depressive episode. As argued later, when symptoms do not conform to diagnostic criteria for a major mental disorder, they may yet be associated with genuine disability, which is in turn a legitimate focus of clinical attention.

COMORBIDITY OF MENTAL
AND PHYSICAL DISORDERS

As many as 30% of elderly primary care patients demonstrate significant depressive symptomatology (Katz et al., 1988). Close to half that number meet criteria for a depressive disorder (Rapp et al., 1988). Hypnotics and antianxiety agents are more often prescribed for older adults with depressive symptoms than are antidepressants. Not surprisingly, depressive symptoms tend to persist in the routine care context (Kennedy et al., 1991). Depressive symptoms among older adults lead to utilization of outpatient services and nursing facilities (Kelman & Thomas, 1990) beyond that expected for the level of disability associated with their medical conditions. Depression amplifies physical disability, and even minor depression may be more disabling than most chronic physical conditions (Wells et al., 1989). As many as one quarter of those with minor depression experience a major depressive disorder within 24 months (Wells et al., 1992). More important, the disability of depression may be avoidable (Strain et al., 1991).

Major depression occurs in more than half of patients within 6 months following stroke (Parikh et al., 1987). Generalized anxiety disorder is also common in the poststroke period, with close to one-quarter of patients meeting diagnostic criteria. Of those, three-quarters will also meet criteria of major or minor depression (Schultz et al., 1997). Both anxiety and depression substantially interfere with rehabilitation. Twenty percent of Parkinson patients develop a major depressive episode and 20% experience dysthymia frequently combined with anxiety (Menza et al., 1993). Depressive symptoms are also common in dementia patients (Rovner et al., 1989) and their caregiving family members in the community (Gallagher et al., 1989). Dementia is the most prevalent mental illness in nursing homes, but depression and dementia complicated by depression are also frequently encountered (Rovner et al., 1990).

Although older adults are more likely to develop a major depressive episode following bereavement than are younger adults (Zisook et al., 1994), physical illness and disability explain substantially more of the variance in the prevalence and course of depressive symptoms than do sociodemographic, life event, and interpersonal factors (Kennedy et al., 1989). Katz (1996) summarizes two general theories regarding the biological origins of depression in late life. First, subclinical cerebrovascular disease may induce depressive symptoms through neurohumoral or structural brain changes. Indeed the profile of depressive symptoms in depression of vascular disease is characterized by motor retardation, lack of insight, and impaired executive (planning) function suggesting frontal brain system dysfunction (Lebowitz et al., 1997). Second, systemic illness may induce depression through cytokine-mediated changes in behavior which allow the sick individual time to recover physiological equilibrium by reducing conative (sex and aggression) activity.

ANXIETY DISORDERS

The fourth edition of the *Diagnostic and Statistical Manual of Mental Disorders* (DSM-IV; American Psychiatric Association, 1994) lists several anxiety disorders. They include panic disorder with and without agoraphobia, agoraphobia without history of panic, social phobia (social anxiety disorder), specific (simple) phobia, obsessive–compulsive disorder, generalized anxiety disorder, anxiety disorder due to a general medical condition, posttraumatic stress disorder (chronic, acute or delayed onset), and acute stress disorder. Duration of symptoms and their temporal relation to the traumatic event distinguishes posttraumatic from acute stress disorder. Posttraumatic stress disorder may arise at some distance from the event but lasts at least 1 month. Acute Stress Disorder arises within one month of the event and lasts from 2 days to one month. In either disorder the patient experiences intrusive recollections or images of the traumatic event, emotional numbing, recurrent nightmares, avoidance of stimuli associated with the traumatic event, hypervigilance, sleep disturbance, and irritability. These individuals relive the trauma and are substantially disabled as a result.

Among physically healthy older community residents without cognitive disorders, agoraphobia may be more common than depression, affecting 6% of women and 3.6% of men. Panic disorder and obsessive–compulsive disorder affect less than 1% each. Considering all anxiety disorders combined, women experience a 6.8% prevalence and men, 3.6%. Minor depression and the mixed syndrome of depression with anxiety affect more than 1% of older community residents (Blazer et al., 1989b). There is considerable comorbidity of depression with generalized anxiety disorder and phobias in older persons (Flint, 1994). Subsyndromal anxiety and anxiety comorbid with psychiatric and medical disorders are also significant (Smith et al., 1995). Anxiety may be evidence of poor recovery from a previous episode of depression (Blazer et al., 1989a).

The symptom profiles of anxiety disorders in late life are similar to those seen at younger ages with the exception of obsessive–compulsive disorder in which "fear of having sinned" is more frequent in seniors (Kohn et al., 1997). Anxious persons are apprehensive and tense and have a sense of dread. They may be irritable, startle easily, feel restless or on edge, and find it difficult to fall asleep. As with depression, they have physical symptoms. They have difficulties with gastrointestinal function, including trouble swallowing, indigestion, excessive flatulence, and either too frequent or too few bowel movements. They may worry excessively about their health, their memory, their money, the safety of the neighborhood and falling or being mugged while out of the house. Hyperthyroidism, congestive heart failure, and chronic diseases cause anxiety, as do steroids, thyroid hormone, caffeine, and ephedra.

Most older patients with panic disorder have experienced the onset early in life and have received little or no treatment (Sheikh et al., 1991). Not surprisingly, panic disorder tends to become chronic. Simple phobias, generalized anxiety disorder, and obsessive–compulsive disorder are commonly associated with panic disorder (American Psychiatric Association, 1994). Untreated panic attacks may lead to agoraphobia (Klein, 1981), depression (Katon et al., 1987), alcohol abuse (Kushner et al., 1990), and suicide (Weissman et al., 1989). Of those who are treated, the mainstay anxiolytic has been a benzodiazepine. Benzodazepines are sedative, impair cognition, put the person at risk for a fall, and are difficult to withdraw. Notably, 11% of men and 25% of women ages 60 to 74 use anxiolytics; individuals ages 65 and older consume 21% of all benzodiazepine prescriptions. Older adults taking long-acting benzodiazepines experience excess numbers of motor vehicle accidents (Hemmelgram et al., 1997). In summary, the bulk of evidence indicates that when generalized anxiety and depression are concurrent, the primary diagnosis in late life is a depressive disorder whether encountered in the community, clinic (Blazer et al., 1989a), or nursing home (Parmalee et al., 1993).

SUICIDE

Although a depressive episode is present in the majority (Conwell et al., 1990) of older adults who commit suicide, physical illness plays a critical role (Mackensie & Popkin, 1987). Twenty percent of older suicides have seen a physician within 24 hours of death. Although the physicians recall only vague physical complaints and denial of mental symptoms, the patients' families recall difficulties with depression, alcohol, and prescription drugs (Clark, 1992). The profile of suicidal risk (see Chapter 12) indirectly indicates the components of treatment. Mental illness, suicidal intent, physical disability, social isolation, alcohol abuse, and firearms in the home all need attention. Suicidal intent should be distinguished from the older person's preparations for death which may be age appropriate (e.g., burial arrangements, last will and testament, and end of a terminal illness). However, the older person who describes acts that will lead to death should be considered depressed until proven otherwise. Conversely, once depression is recognized, the practitioner should always inquire about suicidal ideas. Because completed suicide is usually planned rather than impulsive, the practitioner should not hesitate to question suicidal intent for fear of "planting the seed."

COMPREHENSIVE TREATMENT OF DEPRESSION AND ANXIETY DISORDERS

As shown in Tables 2.1 and 2.2 the treatment of late-life depression and anxiety requires an approach composed of definitive, rehabilitative, and supportive components. In the case of depressive illness, the approach spans the course of treatment including the acute, continua-

TABLE 2.1. Treatment of Anxiety Disorders

- First, sort out related conditions, social setting, medications.
- If anxiety is secondary to medication, social isolation, somatic illness, disability or depression, treatment should be:
  - Definitive, restorative (e.g., correction of hyperthyroidism and treatment for major depression)
  - Rehabilitative (e.g., physical or occupational therapy, exercise, and home care services)
  - Supportive (e.g., family/caregiver counseling and psychoeducation)
- When anxiety arises *de novo* offer psychotherapy plus medication.
- When psychotherapy alone is preferred (relief not immediate, requires 6–12 sessions):
  - Focused cognitive-behavioral (panic disorder, agoraphobia, obsessive–compulsive) or eclectic (generalized anxiety disorder)
- When medication is preferred or required as adjunctive therapy:
  - Sertraline (not sedative, no cardiovascular or cognitive risks)
  - Venlafaxine (few drug interactions, anorexic, elevates blood pressure)
  - Paroxetine (more drug interactions than sertraline, mild sedative)
  - Fluvoxamine (obsessive–compulsive disorder)
  - Nefazodone (theoretically appealing, little data to support use)
  - Buspirone (less effective, safe, will not displace a benzodiazepine, delayed relief)
  - Short-acting benzodiazepines, lorazepam, oxazepam (rapid relief for generalized anxiety, difficult to taper, sedative)
  - Long-acting benzodiazepines: alprazolam, clonazepam (effective within first week, difficult to taper, sedative)
- If medication alone is ineffective after 4 weeks, reevaluate for diagnosis, compliance, medications or alcohol, personality disorder, add psychotherapy.
- Once therapy is effective, continue for at least 6 months, recurrence rate approaches 50% once medications are withdrawn.

tion, and maintenance phases. Because late-onset mental disorders are so often associated with structural brain changes, they are more often recurrent (Krishnan et al., 1997; Alexopoulos et al., 1997). Recurrence prevention is as important as attaining an initial remission of symptoms (Frank, 1994).

The relationships between mental and physical illness and disability are reciprocal, that is, interventions must be relevant to etiology, course, and treatment of each to be fully effective (Gurland et al., 1988). For example, a physical disorder such as hypothyroidism accompanied by depression should be treated definitively with thyroid replacement. Similarly, generalized anxiety resulting from hyperthyroidism requires treatment of thyroid disease to be definitive. However, symptomatic treatment of depression or anxiety should not be withheld until the somatic disorder remits. Rather, the decision to treat should be

TABLE 2.2. Treatment of Depression as a Geriatric Syndrome

- When depression is associated with somatic illness, disability, or dementia:
  - Definitive, restorative (e.g., thyroid replacement)
  - Rehabilitative (e.g., physical or occupational therapy)
  - Supportive (e.g., family/caregiver counseling and psychoeducation)
- When depression arises *de novo* or the above approaches seem inadequate:
  - Psychotherapy
    - Interpersonal or cognitive-behavioral, marital, family, group
  - Pharmacotherapy of unipolar disorders
    - Nortriptyline (therapeutic levels, mild anticholinergic effect)
    - Sertraline (not sedative, no cardiovascular or cognitive risks)
    - Citalopram (longer acting than sertraline)
    - Paroxetine (like sertraline but somewhat sedative, more drug interactions)
    - Nefazodone (mild sedative, no cardiovascular or cognitive risks)
    - Trazodone (sedating, hypotensive but not anticholinergic)
    - Mirtazapine (sedating, not hypotensive or anticholinergic, renal clearance)
    - Bupropion (not sedating but associated with seizures, weight loss)
    - Venlafaxine (few drug interactions, anorexic, elevates blood pressure)
    - Fluoxetine (very long half life, may be taken on alternate days)
    - Buspirone (for anxiety with depression)
    - Methylphenidate (rapid onset of action, for frail, apathetic elderly)
  - Pharmacotherapy of bipolar (manic–depressive) disorder or to augment unipolar regimen; sodium valproate (therapeutic levels)
- When depression occurs with psychosis or fails to respond to combinations of the above:
  - Add haloperidol or perphenazine (extrapyramidal effect, no cardiovascular risk) to nortriptyline, trazodone, nefazodone, mirtazapine
  - Add thioridazine (no extrapyramidal effects, but hypotensive, sedative) to SSRI, venlafaxine, or bupropion
- When depression is life threatening or fails to respond to combinations of the above:
  - Electroconvulsive therapy, twice weekly, over 3–5 weeks

based on the extent to which the person's function is impaired as well as the intensity of dysphoria. The cause may be obvious, but when recovery is not spontaneous or the condition too painful, interventions are justified.

Medication and/or psychotherapy may be sufficient when depression or anxiety occurs without comorbid conditions. More often, interventions in the environment and with the caregivers will be required. Social isolation may be lessened by referral (or return) to a senior citizen or religious center, hiring a home health aide or companion, or helping family to schedule a more reliable pattern of visitation. Occupational therapy to improve hygiene and nutrition may be critical to the restoration of self-worth and pride in appearance. Physical and occupational therapy are particularly useful when apraxia complicates stroke or dementia and when a simple phobia about walking or self-care has developed. A speech pathologist may be essential if aphasia interferes with rehabilitation of mood and interpersonal skills. If the patient cannot benefit from the restorative approach, the focus turns to the caregiver to help maintain the patient's independence and well-being.

Psychotherapies

The indications for psychotherapy and psychoeducation clearly go beyond medication noncompliance, comorbidity, and social isolation. Pharmacotherapy combined with psychotherapy appears to minimize treatment attrition and disease recurrence (Reynolds et al., 1992a). Interpersonal psychotherapy (IPT) and cognitive-behavioral therapy (CBT) have been developed and manualized specifically for research in depression. Among older persons the benefits of CBT have more often been demonstrated with physically healthy, cognitively intact, community residents (Teri et al., 1994). Cognitive group therapy may be particularly appropriate for depressed geriatric patients (Yost et al., 1986).

CBT has also been systematized and may be the preferred psychotherapy for the treatment of panic and agoraphobia and obsessive–compulsive disorders. However, eclectic therapists frequently incorporate the techniques of teaching anxiety management skills, ongoing panic self-monitoring, cognitive restructuring, and graded exposure to anxiety-provoking stimuli (Workgroup on Panic Disorder, 1998). Psychoeducation for patient and family and the provision of factual material regarding the illness in written or narrative formats are central elements of the cognitive-behavioral technique but should be offered by all practitioners treating mental illness regardless of the patient's age.

Depression and anxiety may degrade marital and family relations (Coyne, 1976). Problems with intimacy, communication, and individuality common to marital therapy among younger couples may be difficult to resolve in older couples without attending to the individual's need for concrete social services or medication (Greenberg & Kennedy, 1991). Treatment of sexual dysfunction (see Chapter 9) should not be neglected. The misfortune of the recurrence of depression despite medication compliance in older patients highlights the need for a family psychoeducational approach as a multigenerational treatment modality for depression.

Although psychotherapy alone may be offered for anxiety or depressive disorders, some patients may prefer medication and most will need both (Telch & Lucas, 1993). With the exception of benzodiazepines for generalized anxiety disorder, the benefits of medications and/or psychotherapy will not be immediate. Psychotherapy may be tapered after remission of symptoms has occurred with periodic "booster" sessions added to reinforce lessons learned or to counter acute stress. However, medications will need to be sustained for a minimum of 6 months or longer for depressive disorders. When the initial episode is severe, requires hospitalization, or is complicated by psychosis or suicidal intent and when depression is recurrent, pharmacotherapy should be indefinite, just as it is with bipolar (manic–depressive) disorder. Given the ease of administration and relative safety of the antidepressants and the likelihood that repeated episodes of illness will not be followed by complete recovery, the balance between risk and benefit weighs heavily on the side of ongoing medication. A similar consensus has yet to emerge for anxiety disorders.

For patients who have recovered from depression and prefer to be free of medications, a minimum 6-month treatment following the initial episode and 12 months following a second episode are recommended (Lebowitz et al., 1997). Patients should be warned that the emergence of sleep disturbance may be the first sign of recurrence. During the treatment phase, medications should be maintained at the level that achieved remission of symptoms rather than tapered. Nonetheless, patients who wish to discontinue medication should be slowly tapered over 2 to 6 weeks. If a serotonergic agent is tapered off too fast, some patients experience a transient withdrawal syndrome, which should not be interpreted as recurrence of the anxiety disorder.

Psychopharmacological Treatment

Whether the diagnosis is depression or anxiety, physical exam and laboratory studies are indicated to exclude other sources of symptoms and to ensure the safety of treatment. Thyroid studies, electrocardiogram, complete blood count, and vitamin B_{12} and folate levels should be considered. Side effect profile, availability of therapeutic levels, and patient characteristics, rather than differences in effectiveness, dictate the choice of antidepressants whether used for depression or for anxiety. Because the antidepressant and antipanic effects may be delayed in the elderly (Perel, 1994), considerable skill is necessary to sustain the patient's and family's collaboration. However, associated anxiety, agitation, and sleep disturbance may be reduced within days of instituting therapy with the more sedative antidepressants. Regardless of class, the medication should be started at the lowest available dose and titrated upward to minimize undesirable side effects (see Tables 2.3 and 2.4). Patients need to be educated about which effects are transient nuisances (dry mouth, gastrointestinal upset) and which are signs of

TABLE 2.3. Selected Antidepressants for Older Adults

Generic name	Trade name	Initial dose (mg)	Final dose (mg)	Amnestic, arrhythmic potential	Hypotensive potential	Sedative potential	Precautions	Advantages
TCAs								
Nortriptyline	Pamelor Aventyl	10–25	25–100	Moderate	Moderate	Moderate	Lower final dose; may be fatal in overdose, glaucoma, prostatic disease	Therapeutic window 80–120 ng/ml
Desipramine	Norpramin	10–25	25–150	Moderate	Moderate	Low	May be fatal in overdose, glaucoma, prostatic disease	Therapeutic level 125–300 ng/ml; stimulant
SSRIs								
Fluoxetine	Prozac	10 A.M.	20–40	Low	Low	Low	Prolonged T½; nausea, tremor, insomnia, drug interactions	Side effects not life threatening; liquid preparation available; approved for geriatric depression
Sertraline	Zoloft	25 A.M.	100–200	Low	Low	Low	Nausea, tremor, insomnia	Few drug interactions
Paroxetine	Paxil	10 h.s.	20–40	Low	Low	Low	Nausea, tremor, drug interactions	Mild sedative effect
Citalopram	Celexa	10 A.M.	20–40	Low	Low	Low	Nausea, tremor	Few drug interactions; T½ longer than sertraline
Venlafaxine	Effexor Effexor XR	25 b.i.d.	75–225	Low	Low	Low	Mild hypertensive; headache, nausea, vomiting; do not stop abruptly; not for hypertensives	SSRI and SNRI; fewer drug interactions; sustained-release preparation

MAOIs								
Tranylcypromine	*Parnate*	10–20	30–60	Low	Moderate	Low	Life-threatening diet and drug interactions	When depression resists TCA/SSRI; stimulant; short T½
Others								
Bupropion	*Wellbutrin* *Wellbutrin SR*	75 b.i.d. 75 A.M.	150–300 150–300	Low	Low	Low	Dopaminergic, noradrenergic, agitation, insomnia, seizures; dose should be divided	Anxiolytic; for apathetic depression when TCA/SSRI fail; sustained-release preparation available
Nefazodone	*Serzone*	50 b.i.d.	200–400	Low	Moderate	Moderate	Dry mouth; give more at h.s. than A.M.; drug interactions	Sedative; anxiolytic; promotes analgesics
Trazodone	*Desyrel*	25–50	100–400	Low	High	High	Very sedative; no partial response	For sleep disturbance
Mirtazapine	*Remeron*	7.5	15–30	Low	Low	Moderate	Prolonged T½, renal clearance, dry mouth, weight gain	When depression resists TCA/SSRI; sedative
Hypericum perforatum	St. John's wort	300 b.i.d.	900 t.i.d.	Low	Low	Low	Use standardized, freeze-dried extract 0.3% hypericin, serotonergic, anticholinergic, latency of response	Low side effect profile; OTC
Stimulants								
Methylphenidate	*Ritalin*	5	20 b.i.d.	Low	Low	Low	Anorexia, insomnia, daytime use only	Quick results; for the frail and apathetic

Note. MAOI, monoamine oxidase inhibitor; OTC, over-the-counter; SNRI, selective noradrenergic reuptake inhibitor; SSRI, selective serotonin reuptake inhibitor; TCA, tricyclic antidepressant; T½, half-life; b.i.d., twice daily; t.i.d., three times daily; h.s., at bedtime.

TABLE 2.4. Selected Antianxiety Agents for Older Adults

Generic name	Trade name	Initial dose (mg)	Final dose (mg)	Amnestic potential	Hypotensive potential	Sedative potential	Precautions	Advantages
Benzodiazepines								
Lorazepam	Ativan	0.5	3 b.i.d.	Moderate	Low	High	Falls, dependence, controlled substance	Immediate relief, short T½, no active metabolite, good p.r.n.; i.m. injection available
Oxazepam	Serax	10 b.i.d.	30 b.i.d.	Moderate	Low	High	Falls, dependence, controlled substance	Immediate relief, short T½, no active metabolite, good p.r.n.
Clonazepam	Klonopin	0.5 h.s.	2 b.i.d.	Moderate	Low	Moderate	Long T½, falls, dependence, controlled substance	Immediate relief, daily dosing
Alprazolam	Xanax	0.25 b.i.d.	2 b.i.d.	Moderate	Low	Moderate	Falls, dependence, controlled substance	Immediate relief, FDA approved for panic disorder
SSRIs								
Nefazodone	Serzone	50 b.i.d.	400	Low	Moderate	Moderate	Dry mouth; give more at h.s. than A.M.; drug interactions	Sedative SSRI
Sertraline	Zoloft	25 A.M.	200	Low	Low	Low	Relief not immediate; nausea, tremor, insomnia	No sedation or dependence, fewer drug interactions, FDA approved for panic disorder, obsessive–compulsive disorder, posttraumatic stress disorder
Fluvoxamine	Luvox	25 A.M.	25–100	Low	Low	Low	Relief not immediate; nausea, tremor, insomnia, drug interactions	FDA approved for obsessive–compulsive disorder

Generic	Trade	Dose					Side effects	Comments
Paroxetine	*Paxil*	10 h.s. / 40	Low	Low	Low	Moderate	Relief not immediate; nausea, tremor, drug interactions	Mild sedation, no dependence, FDA approved for panic, obsessive–compulsive disorder, and social phobia
Venlafaxine	*Effexor* / *Effexor XR*	25 b.i.d. / 75–225	Low	Low	Low	Low	Mild hypertensive; headache, nausea, vomiting; do not stop abruptly; not for hypertensives	SSRI and SNRI, fewer drug interactions, sustained release preparation, FDA approved for generalized anxiety disorder
TCAs								
Nortriptyline	*Pamelor* / *Aventyl*	10 h.s. / 100	Moderate	Moderate	Moderate	Moderate	Life-threatening side effects	Immediate relief, no dependence, therapeutic window 50–150 ng/ml
Others								
Bupropion	*Wellbutrin*	75 b.i.d. / 300	Low	Low	Low	Low	Dopaminergic, noradrenergic, seizures; dose should be divided	No sedation or dependence
Buspirone	*Buspar*	10 b.i.d. / 60	Low	Low	Low	Low	Relief not immediate; not for benzodiazepine withdrawal	No sedation or dependence
Herbals, botanicals								
Matricaria recutita	German chamomile	As tea h.s. / t.i.d.	None	None	None	Low	Not FDA regulated, allergic reactions	OTC, no withdrawal, very mild
Valeriana officinalis	Valerian	150 b.i.d. / 300 h.s.	None	None	None	Low	Not FDA regulated; products may vary and include other ingredients; delayed onset	OTC, no withdrawal, very mild

Note. FDA, Food and Drug Administration; i.m., intramuscular; p.r.n., as needed. Other abbreviations as in Table 2.3.

danger (orthostatic hypotension, cardiac arrhythmias). Treatment maintained at acute-phase levels achieves the lowest recurrence rate for depression (Georgotas et al., 1988).

Nortriptyline is the most extensively studied antidepressant for older adults. It is both adrenergic and serotonergic, may be effective in doses as low as 10 mg daily, and is mildly sedative with a moderate to low risk of hypotension, arrhythmia, and amnesia. It has mild anticholinergic properties which can be magnified by strongly anticholinergic prescriptions such as Demerol, Lomotil, and Amantadine, or over-the-counter medications such as Sominex or Dristan (Salzman, 1994). Although not employed in controlled studies of panic disorder, nortriptyline is presumed to be equivalent to imipramine, which has shown substantial benefits (Workgroup on Panic Disorder, 1998). Nortriptyline is unique among antidepressants in that it possesses a therapeutic window (50–150 ng/ml), which can be used to determine whether lack of response is due to too little drug or whether the dose should not be increased further due to the risk of toxicity. A soluble fiber laxative may be started with the first prescription to prevent constipation.

Trazodone (25 mg initial dose) may be preferable when sleep disturbance or agitation is the most salient problem. It is an effective antidepressant, but hypotension and sedation limit its usefulness. It may be effective for panic disorder but less so than other agents (Workgroup on Panic Disorder, 1998). Nefazodone (50 mg twice daily to start) has serotonergic reuptake inhibitor properties, is free of amnestic and arrhythmic effects, and is sedative but less so than trazodone. The majority of the dose may be given at bedtime to assist with sleep as well as minimize daytime drowsiness. It has not been extensively studied for panic disorder but appears to be effective (Workgroup on Panic Disorder, 1998). Mirtazapine is a sedating antidepressant but because it is cleared almost exclusively by the kidneys, caution should be exercised in its use with older patients.

The SSRI sertraline (up to 200 mg daily) may be better for lethargic or demented, frail, or hypotensive patients. Paroxetine (up to 60 mg daily) may have more cytochrome P450 inhibiting properties than sertraline but also possesses a calming effect and may be administered at hour of sleep. Cardiac medications and anticoagulants will need to be monitored more closely until the dose of paroxetene is stabilized. Both paroxetine and sertraline may be superior antipanic agents compared to benzodiazepines and nortriptyline (Workgroup on Panic Disorder, 1998). Citalopram 10–40 mg daily is relatively free of drug interactions and has a longer half-life than sertraline. Fluoxetine has the dual advantages of being very long lived and available in liquid form. For patients whose medication can be supervised less than daily, fluoxetine may be a superior choice for depression. It is also FDA approved for geriatric depression.

For the depression of Parkinson's disease, and especially for the frail patient in whom no side effects can be tolerated, bupropion (75 mg twice daily) is a reasonable choice. Bupropion is free of cardiovascular and cognitive toxicity and drug interactions (Karasu et al., 1993). A sustained-release form is available to obviate the need for twice-daily dosing. However, bupropion may be too stimulatory for some patients, leaving them agitated and sleepless. In addition to patients with vascular dementia or Parkinson's disease, methylphenidate (5–15 mg after breakfast and lunch) may be prescribed for frail elders who are apathetic, have lost appetite, and are unable to tolerate the nuisance side effects of nortriptyline and SSRIs (Wallace et al., 1995). Methylphenidate has the advantage of rapidly elevating mood, initiative, and appetite when it is effective. It has no role in treatment of anxiety disorders. Nortriptyline may be superior to the SSRIs for depressed patients with Parkinson's disease whose cognition and cardiovascular status are intact.

Venlafaxine (25 mg twice daily) shows promise for patients who have not improved with other agents. It is unique among antidepressants in that it mildly elevates blood pressure. It should not be administered to hypertensives but has few drug interactions. It may cause nausea, vomiting, and headache if the dose is started too high or advanced too fast. It should not be stopped abruptly. Data from two studies suggest it may also be effective in panic disorder (Workgroup on Panic Disorder, 1998).

Mirtazapine (7.5 mg daily to start) is relatively new and promising for depressed patients who have not responded or do not tolerate tricyclic antidepressant (TCA) or SSRI therapy. It is neither anticholinergic nor hypotensive. However, mirtazapine has a prolonged half-life and is dependent on renal clearance for elimination, requiring caution in persons of advanced age or with reduced kidney function. Data on its use in anxiety disorders are not available.

Benzodiazepines and Others

The benzodiazepines have been the mainstay of antianxiety treatment. They are rapidly effective, particularly for situational anxiety. They also have a significant role in reversing the sleep disturbance of depression when a nonsedating antidepressant is prescribed. Dose escalation and abuse are rare among older adults. The benzodiazepines do not have the anticholinergic and cardiovascular risks of nortriptyline. Neither do they cause the initial gastrointestinal upset, headache, or the jitteriness of the SSRIs. However, excess sedation, impaired motor and cognitive performance, falls, and accidents are sizable problems, more so with the long-acting agents clonazepam and alprazolam. They are the most rapidly effective treatment of anxiety but may interfere with psychotherapeutic efforts to learn psychological and behavioral symptom control techniques (Workgroup on Panic Disorder, 1998).

Lorazepam and oxazepam are more appealing for the older patient. Both have short half-lives and oxazepam shows significant renal clearance, making it worthwhile for patients with liver disease. However, they must be taken at least twice daily to combat an anxiety disorder, are difficult to eliminate after long-term administration, and resist substitution. Buspirone is a weak antianxiety agent not related to the benzodiazepines or antidepressants. It rarely causes adverse reactions, must be taken two to three times daily for at least 10 days to initiate relief, and will not help persons withdrawing from benzodiazepines. It is effective for generalized anxiety disorder but not for panic. Beta-blockers, calcium channel blockers, and antipsychotics are not recommended for older adults with an anxiety disorder. On balance, most older adults with an anxiety disorder who have not been exposed to a benzodiazepine will be better served by an antidepressant.

Antidepressant Augmentation

Although SSRIs are widely prescribed for depression, close to a third of first-episode patients will not respond and nearly two-thirds either will not achieve or will not sustain a full remission of symptoms (Amsterdam & Hornig-Rohan, 1996). More than 10% who fully recover will experience a subsequent episode despite adequate ongoing treatment (Fredman & Rosenbaum, 1998). Persons who tolerate but do not respond to an SSRI or are dissatisfied with their response may be candidates for a trial of nortriptyline. Combined therapy with two serotonergic antidepressants (e.g., sertraline in the morning plus trazodone at night), an antidepressant with valproic acid, or an antidepressant combined with estrogen or thyroid replacement therapy is increasing in frequency, but there are few studies to guide the generalist practitioner. Recent polls of psychopharmacologists suggest that the addition of bupropion or methylphenidate is the first choice when seeking to augment SSRI treatment. Less preferred additions to an SSRI include mirtazapine, olanzapine, and buspirone (Fava et al., 1998). There are few if any data to support the use of androgens or dehydroepiandrosterone as antidepressants or therapeutic adjuncts (Lebowitz et al., 1997).

Augmentation strategies are generally employed when the patient has achieved only partial remission after no less than 6 weeks at an adequate dose with a single antidepressant or remained severely symptomatic after trials of medications from differing classes. Many patients will be less irritable, more motivated, and more interested in family life before they are aware of an elevation in mood. Although they genuinely feel no less depressed since they started therapy, their family and the practitioner will notice the improvement. Genuine nonresponders will show no evidence of significant change in any symptom domain. They should be reevaluated for unrecognized personality disorder, alcohol or medication abuse (Blow et al., 1992), and intractable social stressors (Costa & McCrae, 1994). The practitioner may have missed subtle somatic delusions and other plausible but improbable beliefs that are indicative of psychotic depression and will require combined antidepressant plus antipsychotic therapy. More commonly, the drug has failed and should be tapered and an alternative medication begun rather than trying augmentation. With the exception of psychotic depression, patients who fail to respond to an adequate trial of two different antidepressants used singly should be referred to a psychopharmacologist or geriatric psychiatrist and may be candidates for electroconvulsive therapy (ECT).

Medication for Bipolar (Manic–Depressive) Disorder

The use of lithium for bipolar disorder or to augment the response of antidepressants is problematic in the elderly in part because of reduced renal function and structural brain changes. Lithium may also be toxic despite normal therapeutic levels in the older patient (Parfrey et al., 1983). The anticonvulsant valproic acid (Maletta, 1992) is increasingly considered first choice for augmentation of antidepressant therapy, treatment, and prevention of mania. A therapeutic level is available and although hepatic toxicity is a risk, it is infrequent. Valproic acid inhibits hepatic enzymes that metabolize a variety of medications used frequently by older adults. Patients taking beta-blockers, type 1C antiarrhythmics, benzodiazepines, or anticoagulants may be prescribed valproic acid but should be monitored more closely until the dose is stabilized. Because mania appearing late in life is most often associated with stroke or dementia, valproic acid is clearly preferable to lithium. See Chapter 4 for a more detailed discussion of mania and psychosis in late life.

Antipsychotics

When psychosis accompanies a depressive disorder, low-dose haloperidol (0.5 mg) or perphenazine (2 mg) should be added to nortriptyline, nefazodone, trazodone, or tranylcypromine. Thioridazine (10 mg) is less likely to provoke extrapyramidal side effects than is haloperidol, but due to sedative and hypotension propensities it should be added only when an SSRI, venlafaxine, or bupropion is already in place. Haloperidol, perphenazine, and thioridazine are all available as liquid concentrates that allow for precise dose titration and ease of administration. Monotherapy in the treatment of psychotic depression is not good practice (Coryell, 1998). However, when psychosis occurs as a complication of dementia or is a brief stress reaction within the context of personality disorder, risperidone (0.25 mg initially) may be preferable for frail seniors who may not tolerate the sedative or hypotensive effects of thioridazine. There is insufficient data on which to recommend risperidone and the other atypical antipsychotics (olanzapine, quetiapine) for psychotic depression. Indeed, the atypicals show a complex pattern or receptor blockade (dopaminergic plus serotonergic and cholinergic), which raises questions about their use with an antidepressant possessing significant serotonergic or anticholinergic properties.

Electroconvulsive Therapy

Age-related factors increase the value of ECT for geriatric major depression (Myers et al., 1984a). ECT may be particularly useful in cases of medication inefficacy or intolerance, psychotic depression (Coryell, 1998), imminent suicidal risk, or morbid nutritional status. Advanced age, concurrent antidepressants, and cardiovascular compromise increase the risk of adverse reactions, with cardiovascular complications being the most frequent events. The cognitive impairment associated with ECT includes temporary postictal confusion, transient anterograde or retrograde amnesia, and, less commonly, permanent amnestic syndrome in which events surrounding the treatment are forgotten (American Psychiatric Association Task Force on ECT, 1990). Treatments may be limited to twice weekly and applied unilaterally to the nondominant hemisphere to minimize confusion. However, bilateral treatment may be more effective (Sackeim et al., 1993). Single treatment maintenance ECT can be administered as an outpatient procedure in ambulatory surgery settings over intervals of several weeks to months (Hay & Hay, 1992) and may offer higher rates of sustained recovery.

REFERENCES

Alexopoulos, G. S., Meyers, B. S., Young, R. C., et al. (1997). Vascular depression hypothesis. *Archives of General Psychiatry, 54,* 915–922.
American Psychiatric Association. (1994). *Diagnostic and statistical manual of mental disorders* (4th ed.). Washington, DC: Author.

American Psychiatric Association Task Force on ECT. (1990). *The practice of ECT: Recommendations for treatment, training, and privileging.* Washington, DC: American Psychiatric Press.

Amsterdam, J. D., Hornig-Rohan, M. (1996). Treatment algorithms in treatment resistant depression. *Psychiatric Clinics of North America, 19,* 371–386.

Beck, A. T., Epstein, N., Brown, G., et al. (1988). An inventory for measuring clinical anxiety: psychometric properties. *Journal of Consultation and Clinical Psychology, 56,* 893–897.

Beck, A. T., Ward, C. H., Mendelson, M., et al. (1961). An inventory for measuring depression. *Archives of General Psychiatry, 4,* 53–56.

Beck, J. C. (Ed.). (1989). *Geriatrics review syllabus.* New York: American Geriatrics Society.

Blazer, D. G., Hughes, D. C., Fowler, N. (1989a). Anxiety as an outcome of depression in elderly and middle-aged adults. *International Journal of Geriatric Psychiatry, 4,* 273–278.

Blazer, D., Woodbury, M., Hughes, D. C., et al. (1989b). A statistical analysis of the classification of depression in a mixed community and clinical sample. *Journal of Affective Disorders, 16,* 11–20.

Blow, F. C., Cook, C. A. L., Booth, B. M., et al. (1992). Age-related psychiatric comorbidites and level of functioning in alcoholic veterans seeking outpatient treatment. *Hospital and Community Psychiatry, 43,* 990–995.

Chambless, D. L., Caputo, G. C., Bright, P., et al. (1984). Assessment of fear in agoraphobics: The body sensations questionnaire and the agoraphobic cognitions questionnaire. *Journal of Consulting and Clinical Psychology, 52,* 1090–1097.

Clark, D. C. (1992, December 10). Remarks presented at the "Too Young to Die" Conference on the National Suicide Survey conducted by Empire Blue Cross and Blue Shield and the Gallup Organization, New York.

Conwell, Y., Melanie, R., Caine, E. D. (1990). Completed suicide at age 50 and over. *Journal of the American Geriatrics Society, 38,* 640–644.

Coryell, W. (1998). The treatment of psychotic depression. *Journal of Clinical Psychiatry, 59*(Suppl. 1), 22–27; discussion, 28–29.

Costa, P. T., McCrue, R. R. (1994). Depression as an enduring disposition. In L. S. Schneider, C. F. F. Reynolds, B. D. Lebowitz, et al. (Eds.), *Diagnosis and treatment of depression in late life* (pp. 155–168). Washington, DC: American Psychiatric Press.

Coyne, J. C. (1976). Depression and the response of others. *Journal of Abnormal Psychology, 85,* 186–193.

Fava, M., Mischoulon, D., Rosenbaum, J. (1998). Augmentation strategies for failed SSRI treatment: A survey of the Massachusetts General Hospital Clinical Psychopharmacology Unit. *American Society of Clinical Psychopharmacology Progress Notes, 9,* 7.

Flint, A. J. (1994). Epidemiology and comorbidity of anxiety disorders in the elderly. *American Journal of Psychiatry, 151,* 640–649.

Frank, E. (1994). Long-term prevention of recurrence in elderly patients. In L. S. Schneider, C. F. F. Reynolds, B. D. Lebowitz, et al. (Eds.), *Diagnosis and treatment of depression in late life* (pp. 317–330). Washington, DC: American Psychiatric Press.

Fredman, S. J., Rosenbaum, J. R. (1998). Recurrent depression, resistant clinician? *Harvard Review of Psychiatry, 5,* 281–285.

Gallagher, D., Rose, J., Rivera, P., et al. (1989). Prevalence of depression in family caregivers. *Gerontologist, 29,* 449–456.

Georgotas, A., McCue, R. E., Cooper, T. B., et al. (1988). How effective and safe is continuation therapy in elderly depressed patients? *Archives of General Psychiatry, 45,* 929–932.

Greenberg, D., Kennedy, G. J. (1991). Till death do us part: Marital therapy in a geriatric ambulatory practice. *Gerontologist, 31,* 118.

Gurland, B. J., Wilder, D. E., Berkman, C. (1988). Depression and disability in the elderly: Reciprocal relations and changes with age. *International Journal of Geriatric Psychiatry, 3,* 163–179.

Hamilton, M. (1959). The assessment of anxiety states by rating. *British Medical Journal, 32,* 50–55.

Hay, D., Hay, L. (1992). The role of ECT in the treatment of depression. In C. D. McCann & N. S. Endler (Eds.), *Depression: New directions in theory, research, and practice* (pp. 255–272). Toronto: Wall & Emerson.

Hemmelgarn, B., Suissa, S., Huang, A., et al. (1997). Benzodiazepine use and the risk of motor vehicle crash in the elderly. *Journal of the American Medical Association, 278,* 27–31.

Karasu, T. B., Docherty, J. P., Gelenberg, A., et al. (1993). Practice guidelines for major depressive disorder in adults. *American Journal of Psychiatry, 150*(Suppl. 4).

Katon, W., Vitialno, P., Anderson, K., et al. (1987). Panic disorder: Residual symptoms after the acute attacks abate. *Comprehensive Psychiatry, 28,* 151–187.

Katz, I. R. (1996). On the inseparability of mental and physical health in aged persons. *American Journal of Geriatric Psychiatry, 4,* 1–16.

Katz, I. R., Curil, S., Nemetz, A. (1988). Functional psychiatric disorders in the elderly. In L. W. Lazarus (Ed.), *Essentials of geriatric psychiatry* (pp. 113–137). New York: Springer.

Kelman, H. R., Thomas, C. (1990). Transitions between community and nursing home residence in an urban elderly population. *Journal of Community Health, 15,* 105–122.

Kennedy, G. J., Kelman, H. R., Thomas, C. (1991). Persistence and remission of depressive symptoms in late life. *American Journal of Psychiatry, 148,* 174–178.

Kennedy, G. J., Kelman, H., Thomas, C., et al. (1989). Hierarchy of characteristics associated with depressive symptoms in an urban elderly sample. *American Journal of Psychiatry, 146,* 220–225.

Kermis, M. D. (1986). The epidemiology of mental disorders in the elderly: A response to the Senate/AARP report. *Gerontologist, 26,* 482–487.

Klein, D. F. (1981). Anxiety reconceptualized. In D. F. Klein & J. G. Rabkin (Eds.), *Anxiety: New research and changing concepts* (pp. 235–263). New York: Raven Press.

Kohn, R., Westlake, R. J., Rasmussen, M. D., et al. (1997). Clinical features of obsessive–compulsive disorder in elderly patients. *American Journal of Geriatric Psychiatry, 5,* 211–215.

Krishnan, K. R., Hays, J. C., Blazer, D. G. (1997). MRI-defined vascular depression. *American Journal of Psychiatry, 154*, 497–501.

Kushner, M. G., Sher, K. J., Beitman, B. D. (1990). The relation between alcohol problems and the anxiety disorders. *American Journal of Psychiatry, 147*, 685–689.

Lebowitz, B. D., Pearson, J. L., Schneider, L. S., et al. (1997). Diagnosis and treatment of depression in late life: Consensus statement update. *Journal of the American Medical Association, 278*, 1186–1190.

Mackensie, T. B., Popkin, M. K. (1987). Suicide in the medical patient. *International Journal of Psychiatry in Medicine, 17*, 3–22.

Maletta, G. J. (1992). Treatment of behavioral symptomatology of Alzheimer's disease, with emphasis on aggression: Current clinical approaches. *International Psychogeriatrics, 4*, 117–130.

Menza, M. A., Robertson-Hoffman, D. E., Bonapace, A. S. (1993). Parkinson's disease and anxiety: Comorbidity and depression. *Biological Psychiatry, 34*, 465–470.

Myers, J. K., Weissman, M. M., Tischler, G. L., et al. (1984). Six month prevalence of psychiatric disorders in the community. *Archives of General Psychiatry, 41*, 959–967.

National Institutes of Health Consensus Development Panel. (1992). Diagnosis and treatment of depression in late life. *Journal of the American Medical Association, 268*, 1018–1024.

Parmalee, P. A., Katz, I. R., Lawton, M. P. (1993). Anxiety and its association with depression among institutionalized elderly. *American Journal of Geriatric Psychiatry, 1*, 46–58.

Parfrey, P. S., Ikeman, R., Anglin, D., et al. (1983). Severe lithium intoxication treated by forced diuresis. *Canadian Medical Association Journal, 129*, 979–980.

Parikh, R. M., Lipsey, J. R., Robinson, R. G., et al. (1987). Two-year longitudinal study of post-stroke mood disorders: dynamic changes in correlates of depression at one and two years. *Stroke, 18*, 579–584.

Perel, J. M. (1994). Geropharmacokinetics of therapeutics, toxic effects and compliance. In L. S. Schneider, C. F. F. Reynolds, B. D. Lebowitz, et al. (Eds.), *Diagnosis and treatment of depression in late life* (pp. 245–258). Washington, DC: American Psychiatric Press.

Radloff, L. S. (1977). The CES-D Scale: A self-report depression scale for research in the general population. *Journal of Applied Psychological Measurement, 1*, 385–401.

Rapp, S. R., Parisi, S. A., Walsh, D. A. (1988). Psychologic dysfunction and physical health among elderly medical inpatients. *Journal of Consulting and Clinical Psychology, 56*, 851–855.

Reynolds, C. F., Frank, E., Perel, J. M., et al. (1992a). Combined pharmacotherapy and psychotherapy in the acute continuation treatment of elderly patients with recurrent major depression: A preliminary report. *American Journal of Psychiatry, 149*, 1687–1692.

Reynolds, C. F., Hoch, C. C., Buysse, D. J., et al. (1992b). EEG sleep in spousal bereavement and bereavement-related depression of late life. *Biological Psychiatry, 31*, 69–82.

Rovner, B. W., Broadhead, J., Spencer, M., et al. (1989). Depression and Alzheimer's disease. *American Journal of Psychiatry, 146,* 350–353.

Rovner, B. W., German, P. S., Broadhead, J., et al. (1990). The prevalence and management of dementia and other psychiatric disorders in nursing homes. *International Psychogeriatrics, 2,* 13–24.

Sackeim, H. A., Prudic, J., Devanand, D. P., et al. (1993). Effects of stimulus intensity and electrode placement on the efficacy and cognitive effects of electroconvulsive therapy. *New England Journal of Medicine, 328,* 839–846.

Salzman, C. (1994). Pharmacologic treatment of depression in elderly patients. In L. S. Schneider, C. F. F. Reynolds, B. D. Lebowitz, et al. (Eds.), *Diagnosis and treatment of depression in late life* (pp. 181–244). Washington, DC: American Psychiatric Press.

Schultz, S. K., Castillo, C. S., Kosier, J. T., et al. (1997). Generalized anxiety in depression: Assessment over 2 years after stroke. *American Journal of Geriatric Psychiatry, 5,* 229–237.

Sheikh, J. I., King, R. I., Taylor, C. B. (1991). Comparative phenomenology of early-onset versus late-onset panic attacks: A pilot survey. *American Journal of Psychiatry, 148,* 1231–1233.

Sheikh, J. I., Yesavage, J. A. (1986). Geriatric Depression Scale: Recent evidence and development of a shorter version. *Clinical Gerontology, 5,* 165–172.

Smith, S. L., Sherrill, K. A., Colenda, C. C. (1995). Assessing and treating anxiety in elderly persons. *Psychiatric Services, 46,* 36–42.

Strain, J. J., Lyons, J. S., Hammer, J. S., et al. (1991). Cost offset from a psychiatric consultation–liaison intervention with elderly hip fracture patients. *American Journal of Psychiatry, 148,* 1004–1049.

Telch, M. J., Lucas, R. A. (1993). Combined pharmacologic and psychological treatment of panic disorder: Current status and future directions. In B. E. Wolfe & J. D. Maser (Eds.), *Treatment of panic disorder: A consensus development conference* (pp. 177–197). Washington, DC: American Psychiatric Press.

Teri, L., Curtis, J., Gallagher-Thompson D., et al. (1994). Cognitive-behavioral therapy with depressed older adults. In L. S. Schneider, C. F. F. Reynolds, B. D. Lebowitz, et al. (Eds.), *Diagnosis and treatment of depression in late life* (pp. 279–292). Washington, DC: American Psychiatric Press.

Testa, M. A., Anderson, R. B., Nackley, J. F., et al. (1993). Quality of life and antihypertensive therapy in men. *New England Journal of Medicine, 328,* 901–913.

Wallace, A. E., Kofoed, L. L., West, A. N. (1995). Double-blind, placebo-controlled trial of methyphenidate in older, depressed, medically ill patients. *American Journal of Psychiatry, 152,* 929–931.

Weissman, M. R., Klerman, G. L., Markowitz, J. S., et al. (1989). Suicidal ideation and suicide attempts in panic disorder and attacks. *New England Journal of Medicine, 321,* 1209–1214.

Wells, K. B., Burnam, M. A., Rogers, W., et al. (1992). The course of depression in adult outpatients. *Archives of General Psychiatry, 49,* 788–794.

Wells, K. B., Stewart, A., Hays, R. D., et al. (1989). The functioning and well-being of depressed patients: Results from the Medical Outcomes Study. *Journal of the American Medical Association, 262,* 914–919.

Williams, J. B. W. (1988). A structured interview guide for the Hamilton Depression Rating Scale. *Archives of General Psychiatry, 45,* 742–747.

Winograd, C. H. (1992). Geriatric assessment: Concepts, components, and settings. In J. E. Morely (Ed.), *Geriatric care* (pp. 179–188). St. Louis: GW Manning.

Wooley, M. A., Avins, A. L., Mirand, J., et al. (1997). Case-finding instruments for depression. Two questions are as good as many. *Journal of General Internal Medicine, 12,* 439–445.

Workgroup on Panic Disorder. (1998). Practice guideline for the treatment of patients with panic disorder. *American Journal of Psychiatry, 155*(Suppl.), 1–34.

Yost, E., Beutler, L., Corbishley, M. A., et al. (1986). *Group cognitive therapy: A treatment approach for depressed older adults.* New York: Pergamon.

Zisook, S., Shuchter, S. R., Sledge, P. (1994). Diagnostic and treatment considerations in depression associated with late-life bereavement. In L. S. Schneider, C. F. F. Reynolds, B. D. Lebowitz, et al. (Eds.), *Diagnosis and treatment of depression in late life* (pp. 419–430). Washington, DC: American Psychiatric Press.

Zung, W. W. (1986). Prevalence of clinically significant anxiety in a family practice setting. *American Journal of Psychiatry, 143,* 1471–1472.

Zung, W. W. (1990). The role of rating scales in the identification and management of the depressed patient in the primary care setting. *Journal of Clinical Psychiatry, 51*(Suppl.), 72–76.

3

The Dementias

There are 4 million Americans afflicted with dementia at a cost near $100 billion a year in fees to physicians, hospitals, nursing homes, and home care agencies. The indirect or hidden expense to the family members providing care is estimated to be an additional $100 billion. With the number of persons with dementia projected to double over the next 40 years (Ernst & Hay, 1994), even modest benefits to the individual will have a substantial cost offset if achieved in the population at large. Advances in the treatment of cognitive impairment and the genetic detection of individuals at risk before onset of the disease promise a genuine breakthrough. An awareness of the multiple causes of dementia-related disability will lead to realistic goals and beneficial treatment.

DEMENTIA DEFINED

All dementias share three elements. First, progressive decline differentiates dementia from developmental disorders that emerge in childhood but remain stable throughout adult life. Second, impairment of cognition is compound rather than circumscribed. Persons with dementia have learning and memory problems plus at least one of the following: impairments in the ability to communicate, to reason, to plan and to manipulate objects in space, to be oriented and alert, and to modulate emotion. This distinguishes dementia from the pure disorders of memory and the nonprogressive disorders of communication seen in the aphasias and stroke. Third, dementia in the early and middle stages does not impair consciousness, which separates it from delirium. Finally, dementia is a general complex of symptoms, which may also be part of an etiologically specific disorder as in neurosyphilis. In summary, dementia is a syndrome of progressive and global decline in cognitive capacities, severe enough to substantially interfere with the individual's well-being and social function.

EPIDEMIOLOGY

Because dementia is an age-related disorder, as the proportion of older adults increases both the incidence and prevalence of dementia will increase. Alzheimer's disease alone affects 8–15% of persons 65 or older. If we define severe dementia as that which requires either institutional care or full-time home care, then 4.6% of persons 65 and older are severely demented. Another 10% are moderately demented living semi-independently (Katzman, 1986). But among individuals 85 and older, more than 15% are severely demented with the prevalence approaching 50% among those with a demented first-degree relative (Mohs et al., 1987). The prevalence of dementia increases exponentially, doubling every 5 years at least to age 85. The wide variation in prevalence by gender, nationality, and ethnicity is poorly understood. The higher prevalence among women reflects their survival advantage over men rather than a higher incidence of the illness (Henderson, 1989). And despite improved survival rates associated with cardiovascular disease, an increase in vascular-related dementia may be expected (Kennedy et al., 1987), even if present cases are overdiagnosed (Small et al., 1997). Educationally disadvantaged minorities may also be disproportionately affected by the increasing prevalence of dementia (Lilienfeld & Perl, 1994).

GENETIC AND OTHER RISK FACTORS

Classification by age is important because early-onset Alzheimer's disease is more often familial rather than sporadic (Tanzi et al., 1987). Early-onset (before 65) familial Alzheimer's disease has been linked to mutations on chromosomes 1 (presinilin 2), 14 (presinilin 1), and 21 with some forms of late onset linked to chromosome 12. If a person inherits one of the presinilin-producing genes, they will develop Alzheimer's disease at an early age. The apolipoprotein allele E-4 (APOE-4), located on chromosome 19, is associated with the more common late-onset Alzheimer's disease but is not associated with markedly elevated risk as with the presinilins (National Institute on Aging, 1998). The autosomal dominant inheritance pattern of Alzheimer's disease associated with chromosome 21 is similar to that observed with Huntington's disease. Huntington's disease is inherited as a Mendelian dominant gene with dementia occurring in 50% of affected individuals. In Huntington's it is possible to specify the genetic presence or absence risk in absolute terms and to predict both age of onset and severity (Nance, 1998).

However, the determination of true risk is complicated for both the familial and sporadic cases of Alzheimer's disease. The age of onset varies, susceptible persons may not survive to the age of onset, and other mediating factors associated with advanced age may modify risk. As a result the consensus is against genetic screening for Alzheimer's disease (Small et al., 1997). Indeed families that proceed with testing frequently overinterpret the meaning of both positive and negative results despite caveats from the clinical team. Tests of spinal fluid for AD7C-NTP (de la Monte et al., 1997), τ and amyloid precursor protein, and others are promising but lack the sensitivity and specificity for routine use especially in early stages of the illness (National Institute on Aging/Alzheimer's Association Working Group, 1996). Although advanced age and family history are established risk factors, head trauma and lower educational attainment have also been linked to Alzheimer's disease.

At the present time, risk reduction for Alzheimer's disease seems distant. However, our ability to reduce cardiovascular risk factors and traumatic brain injury, which complicate if not cause dementia, is already at hand. The diversity in dementia presentation, associated conditions, and clinical course highlights the importance of measures to prevent the onset and progression of cardiovascular disease and diabetes. Weight control, exercise, lowering of cholesterol, treatment of diabetes and hypertension, elimination of tobacco use, and minimizing alcohol intake represent good preventive health at any age, more so for individuals with vascular dementia (Cummings, 2000). And there is a growing body of evidence that late-life depression accompanied by cognitive impairment often heralds the onset of dementia even when the impairment remits with antidepressant therapy (Alexopoulos et al., 1993; Jost & Grossberg, 1996).

DIAGNOSTIC CRITERIA AND PROCEDURES

Although a histological examination of brain tissues sets the criteria for "definite" Alzheimer's disease, the diagnosis of "probable" Alzheimer's dementia can be accurately made in 90% of cases by history from the patient and family and clinical examination (Small et al., 1997). "Possible" cases may have atypical features but no identifiable alternative diagnosis. Routine diagnostic laboratory procedures include complete blood count; blood chemistries; liver function studies; serological test for syphilis; thyroid-stimulating hormone, vitamin B_{12}, and folate levels; and cardiogram. Chest X ray, HIV test, and test of Lyme disease may also be included, based on physical exam and history. For patients with syncope or suspected seizures, an electroencephalogram may be ordered. A review of the ingestion of prescribed and over-the-counter medications, alcohol, and tobacco products is also part of the diagnostic process.

Although some clinicians feel imaging is routine, others identify more specific indications (Small et al., 1997). Because the incidence of irreversible dementia is age related, the detection rate for reversible causes with imaging studies may decrease with advanced age. Computerized tomography of the brain without contrast should be performed when focal neurological signs are present, when change in mental status is sudden, or when trauma or mass effects are suspected. Magnetic resonance imaging may be indicated when vascular dementia is suspected or when the course of illness is stairstep rather than the smooth decline of Alzheimer's disease. However, the white matter changes seen on T2-weighted images are not necessarily indicative of dementia (Small et al., 1997). The use of magnetic resonance imaging (MRI) to confirm the clinical diagnosis of vascular dementia also has therapeutic and prognostic significance for patient and family. Similarly functional imaging studies with positron emission tomography (PET) or single photon emission computerized tomography (CT) may detect the temporal–parietal metabolic deficits of Alzheimer's disease or the diffuse irregular deficits of vascular dementia prior to objective signs of memory impairment on cognitive screening (Cutler et al., 1985). Serial imaging studies are recommended at 6-month intervals if the diagnosis remains suspect. However, imaging studies and laboratory tests are no substitute for the history and mental status examination.

DIFFERENTIAL DIAGNOSIS

The nosology of dementia is confusing because of its historical origins and successful efforts to disaggregate types of the illness from the syndrome. The diagnosis is challenging particularly in the early stage because there are no definitive biological markers, the onset is often insidious, and other reversible causes of cognitive impairment either resemble or accompany dementia. The clinical history from patient and family, physical examination with emphasis on neurological findings, mental status examination with emphasis on cognitive assessment, and laboratory procedures are carried out to detect reversible or partially reversible disease. Table 3.1 lists characteristics that distinguish the various cognitive disorders as well as the specific dementias.

Delirium is perhaps the most common cognitive disorder. The hallmarks are waxing and waning symptoms, impaired attention, visual hallucinations, and demonstrable physiological disturbance.

TABLE 3.1. Differential Diagnosis of Cognitive Impairment in Adults

Condition	Distinguishing features
Dementia	Progressive decline, global cognitive impairment; memory deficits, recent and remote; aphasia, apraxia, agnosia, executive dysfunction; patients tend to minimize deficits
Developmental disorder	Childhood onset without progressive decline; history of diminished educational and work attainment; attention unimpaired
Delirium	Sudden onset with deficits in attention, fluctuating course; impairment reversible but recovery may be slowed by advanced age
Major depressive disorder with cognitive impairment	Memory and concentration complaints prominent; aphasia absent, apathy or irritability present; cooperation with testing difficult, risk of subsequent dementia elevated
Age associated, mild cognitive impairment	Age > 50, memory complaints prominent; performance below one standard deviation from the mean on tests normed with young adults, information retrieval slowed; learning, orientation, communication intact; functional independence preserved
Alzheimer's disease	Insidious onset with smooth, inexorable decline, cortical atrophy, apolipoprotein Eε4 allele and cardiovascular disease elevates risk, more rapid decline in middle stage; mood disturbance early, psychosis and behavioral disturbance later in the course
Vascular dementia	Sudden onset, fluctuating course with temporary improvements or prolonged plateau; multiple infarcts, diffuse white matter lesions, diabetes, cardiovascular disease present; focal neurological exam
Huntington's disease	Autosomal dominant but incomplete penetrance; atrophic caudate nuclei: premorbid DNA testing quantifies risk, age of onset, severity
Parkinson's disease	Characteristic tremor with unilateral onset, bradykinesia, bradyphrenia, cognition may be spared
Acute cognitive impairment due to stroke, traumatic brain injury	Focal neurological exam; circumscribed rather than global cognitive deficits may improve significantly over 6 months
Frontal lobe degeneration, Pick's disease	Personality, sociability, executive function prominently impaired; disinhibition, impaired judgment and social indifference significant; aphasia, apraxia, amnesia, loss of calculation less notable
Lewy body dementia	Sudden onset, fluctuating level of awareness, psychosis (visual and auditory hallucinations more often than delusions) prominent, Parkinsonian signs and falls; adverse response to typical antipsychotic
Creutzfeldt–Jakob disease	Rapid progression, death in 6–12 months, characteristic EEG, myoclonic jerks
Alcohol-related dementia	Massive, prolonged abuse, may remit with abstinence
Normal pressure hydrocephalus	Gait disturbance ("magnetic gait"), incontinence, ventricular enlargement disproportionate to cortical atrophy
AIDS dementia	HIV positive, may present with behavioral disturbance, Parkinsonian features

Symptoms should remit once the disturbance is reversed, but recovery may be delayed in older persons threatening a premature diagnosis of dementia. However, persons with dementia are more susceptible to delirium. Delirium can also be chronic and difficult to distinguish from dementia.

Cognitive impairment due to depressive disorders is distinguished by the patient's prominent complaints of difficulty with memory and concentration. Apathy, irritability, and reluctance to complete cognitive testing are apparent but without aphasia. The term "pseudodementia" was introduced by Madden et al. (1952) to describe cases in which the diagnosis of dementia was changed after a remission of cognitive deficits. Pseudodementia originally implied a misdiagnosis. However, present use of pseudodementia to describe the reversible cognitive impairment seen in late-life depression leads to confusion and should be abandoned (Reifler, 1986).

Age-associated memory impairment (AAMI), or benign senescent forgetfulness, is characterized by subjective memory complaints in persons age 50 or older whose performance falls by one standard deviation below the mean on formal memory tests normed for younger adults. Although lower memory scores are predictive of dementia, only 1–3% of these individuals will progress to global cognitive impairment (Richards et al., 1999). In contrast, 5–15% of persons with mild cognitive impairment (MCI) will develop dementia in the coming year. MCI is characterized by memory performance between one and one-half standard deviation below the mean score of tests of memory. As with AAMI, persons with MCI have memory complaints but do not meet diagnostic criteria for dementia. They exhibit slowed information retrieval, but orientation, communication, and functional independence are all intact. They also benefit from self-taught memory aids (Peterson et al., 1999). Trials are underway to determine if cholinesterase inhibitors, vitamin E, and anti-inflammatory agents prevent the progression of AAMI and MCI. A positive outcome, particularly with MCI, would have enormous public health implications and would propel screening and early intervention into widespread practice.

Alzheimer's disease is the most frequently encountered dementia. The onset is insidious; the decline is smooth but more rapid in the middle stage in which behavioral disturbances start to emerge. Individuals with Alzheimer's disease often minimize their deficits unlike persons with MCI or depression. Alzheimer's and Pick's disease represent cortical dementias in which there is primary neuronal degeneration (Huber & Paulson, 1985). Huntington's and Parkinson's disease represent the subcortical dementias. Dementia associated with Lewy bodies overlaps with both Parkinson's and Alzheimer's disease in presentation and distribution of pathology.

The secondary neuronal degeneration of the vascular dementias (multi-infarct, Binswanger's) is due to angiopathic disorders, most commonly ischemic heart disease and arrhythmias, hypertension, and diabetes. Hemiparesis, gait disorder, and other signs of past stroke also suggest vascular dementia (Hachinski, 1983). However, the pathology of vascular dementia is frequently of a mixed type (cortical and subcortical) with diverse presentations in which the loss of brain volume, ventricular dilatation, bradykinesia, and the cognitive deficits are difficult to distinguish from Alzheimer's disease.

Although perceptual distortions are common in dementia, when visual or auditory hallucinations are prominent, signs of Parkinson's disease are evident, the onset is abrupt, and the course is characterized by lucid moments alternating with confusion, Lewy body disease may be diagnosed (McKeith et al., 1996). Paranoid delusions, falls, and depression are also characteristic of diffuse Lewy body dementia. Opinions vary, but the proportion of dementia represented by Lewy body disease may approach 34%, making it more common than vascular dementia. More important, patients with diffuse Lewy body disease experience marked disruptions in dopaminergic systems, accounting for their exquisite sensitivity to antipsychotic medications (Luis et al., 1999).

Alzheimer's, vascular, and Lewy body disease make up the vast majority of dementia diagnoses. Figure 3.1 offers a simplified algorithm that will capture 95% of the dementias encountered by the average practitioner. The key elements are (1) character of onset and decline, (2) evidence of ischemic brain injury, and (3) prominent hallucinations and Parkinsonian features. Smooth decline following insidious onset is probably Alzheimer's disease. When the onset is abrupt, the course fluctuates, and there is significant evidence of ischemic brain injury, the dementia is likely to be vascular. When the onset is abrupt, the course is fluctuating, hallucinations are prominent, and Parkinsonian signs are evident, the diagnosis is Lewy body disease.

The rare dementias would be easy to overlook were it not for their distinctive features. Marked deficits in visual perception and praxis may suggest corticonuclear degeneration. Early deterioration in personality, loss of social inhibitions, and frontal lobe atrophy may indicate Pick's dementia (Heston et al., 1987). Physical signs such as the tremor and bradykinesia of Parkinson's disease, the choreoathetoid movements of Huntington's disease, the myoclonic twitching of Creutzfeldt–Jakob disease, or the pseudobulbar palsy of vascular dementia may not present before intellectual deterioration is observed.

Cognitive deficits are progressing and involve more than memory impairment.

Insidious onset with smooth
decline and motor function
minimally impaired?

YES NO →   Abrupt onset or fluctuating course,
    ↓   little if any psychosis?

ALZHEIMER'S
DEMENTIA   ↓
                                History of stroke or significant
                                ischemic brain injury on CT
                                scan or MRI?

                                YES NO →   Marked fluctuation in cognitive
                                    ↓   impairment, hallucinations
                                                      prominent, signs of Parkinson's
                                                      syndrome evident, falls?

                                VASCULAR DEMENTIA   YES
                                                       ↓
                                                      LEWY BODY DISEASE

FIGURE 3.1. Simplified algorithm for differential diagnosis in 95% of cases.

Changes in affect, typically depression but also hypomania and irritability, preceding signs of dementia, suggest a non-Alzheimer's diagnosis (Mahendra, 1985). Huntington's disease is typical of the subcortical dementias in that various cortical functions including communication, praxis, and visual perception are generally spared. However, memory impairment, apathy, and psychomotor retardation are marked and progressive. Emotional disturbances and personality change are regular features of Huntington's disease and frequently the first signs of the illness (Folstein & Folstein, 1983). Normal pressure hydrocephalus is characterized by incontinence, abnormal ("magnetic") gait, and ventricular atrophy out of proportion to cortical loss. The cognitive impairment of stroke or acute traumatic brain injury may predispose the person to dementia but may also improve over the 6 months following the accident. Like the dementia associated with the toxicity and nutritional deprivation of massive alcohol abuse, chronic injury in boxing and other contact sports and accidents is potentially preventable.

Dementia may also be secondary to infectious systemic disease such as syphilis or acquired immune deficiency syndrome (Koenig et al., 1986). Transmissible disorders of the prion type (Creuztfeldt–Jakob disease) may also cause dementia through exposure to infected foodstuffs or transplanted tissues or tissue extracts (Harrington et al., 1986). Thus dementia may be classified as infectious or transmissible.

Ultimately, Katzman (1986) advocated the more productive clinical nosology in which dementia is seen as reversible, irreversible, or partially reversible. Although few dementias are reversible, most have elements that will partially remit with interventions described later. Reifler and Larson's (1988) concept of excess or reversible disability in dementia is characterized by a rule of halves. One-half of persons with dementia have a concurrent physical or mental illness that contributes to their functional impairments. Half that number will experience at least temporary benefits from treatment of the comorbid condition. And in half that group the benefits will last a year or more.

COGNITIVE ASSESSMENT

To maintain a vulnerable patient's sense of self-determination, the clinical assessment should begin with family members present, progress to an individual interview for mental status examination and discussion of preliminary findings, and end with patient and family collaborating in the treatment plan. Cognitive screening should be conducted without family present to avoid distractions and any potential embarrassment over failed items. It is useful to discuss findings and recommendations in the individual interview and then gain the patient's permission to share the information with family. This model of individual autonomy in the context of family care orientation is designed to lessen defensiveness and forge alliances throughout the family system. A premium is placed on openness and full disclosure, which is essential in the management of future deterioration. However, certain individuals will be too anxious or suspicious to be examined alone or to accept a discussion of findings and recommendations in their presence. In such cases, tact and ingenuity are required to obtain consent for disclosure to the family. Because the patient is asked to actively demonstrate errors, considerable care is required to place the person at ease and to accurately administer the exam.

The use of a cognitive screening instrument allows the clinician to demonstrate the presence and, with longitudinal administrations, the course of deficits objectively. A number of related factors may influence cognitive performance yet not be indicative of dementia. These include inefficient learning strategies, slowed processing capacity, reduced attention, sensory deficits, and age-associated memory impairment (Grober et al., 1988). Age, education, and other demographic factors also alter performance (Folstein et al., 1985).

The Mini-Mental Status Examination (MMSE) is the most widely used screening exam for impaired cognition in the United States and has been translated to a number of languages and normed for age and education. However, the meaning of an impaired MMSE score is not always clear. Molloy and Standish (1997) have standardized the administration procedures for the MMSE to reduce test time and uncertainty about scoring (see Table 3.2). Their techniques also reduce test anxiety. A perfect score is 30 with mild to moderate impairment falling between 18 and 24. For persons with less than nine grades of education, a score of 17 or less is evidence of at least mild impairment. Whether mild, moderate, or severe, an impaired MMSE score is a more

TABLE 3.2. Standardized Mini-Mental State Examination

Preparations

Ensure that the patient is willing and that vision and hearing aids are in place if needed. Ask, *"Would it be all right to ask you some questions about your memory?"* Ask each question a maximum of three times. If the patient does not respond, score the item as 0. If the answer is incorrect, score 0. Do not hint, prompt, or ask the question again once an answer has been given. If the patient answers, *"What did you say?"* do not explain or engage in conversation—merely repeat the same directions up to a maximum of three times. If the patient interrupts or wanders from the task, redirect the person by saying, *"I will explain in a few minutes when we are finished. Now if we could just proceed please . . . we are almost finished."*

Begin by saying, *"I am going to ask you some questions and give you some problems to solve."*

	Max. score
1. (Allow no more than 10 seconds for each reply.)	
a. *"What year is this?"* (Accept exact answer only.)	1
b. *"What season is this?"* (In the last week of the old season or first of the new accept either.)	1
c. *"What month of the year is this?"* (On the first day of the new month or last day of the previous, accept either month.)	1
d. *"What is today's date?"* (The day before or after is acceptable, e.g., on the 7th accept the 6th or 8th.)	1
e. *"What day of the week is this?"* (Exact day only)	1
2. (Allow no more than 10 seconds for each reply.)	
a. *"What county/borough are we in?"*	1
b. *"What province/state/country are we in?"*	1
c. *"What city/town are we in?"*	1
d. If in the clinic: *"What is the name of this hospital/building?"* (Exact name of hospital/institution/building only)	1
If in the patient's home: *"What is the street address of this house?"* (Street name and house number or equivalent in rural areas)	1
e. If in the clinic: *"What floor of the building are we on?"* (Exact answer only)	1
If in the home: *"What room are we in?"* (Exact only)	1
3. *"I am going to name three objects. After I have said all three, I want you to repeat them. Remember what they are because I am going to ask you to name then again in a few minutes."* (Say the objects slowly at 1-second intervals.) *"BALL (1 second), CAR (1 second), MAN. Please repeat the three items for me."* (Score 1 point for each reply on the first attempt. Allow 20 seconds for the reply, if the patient cannot repeat all three on the first attempt, repeat until they are learned but no more than five times.)	3

(continued on next page)

TABLE 3.2. *(continued)*

4. *"Now please subtract 7 from 100 and keep subtracting 7 from what's left until I tell you to*   5
   stop." (May repeat three times if the patient pauses—allow one minute for answer.
   Once the patient starts do not interrupt until 5 subtractions have been completed.
   If the patient stops, repeat, "Keep subtracting 7 from what's left" for a maximum of
   3 times. See scoring examples below.)

5. *"Now what were the three objects that I asked you to remember?"* (Score 1 point each   3
   regardless of the order; allow 10 seconds.)

6. Show the patient a wristwatch and ask, *"What is this called?"* (Accept "wristwatch"   1
   or "watch" but not "clock" or "time.")

7. Show a pencil and ask, *"What is this called?"* (Do not accept "pen.")   1

8. *"I'd like you to repeat a phrase for me: say, 'No ifs, ands, or buts.' "* (Exact reply only)   1

9. *"Read the words on the page and then do what is says."* (Hand the patient the sheet with   1
   CLOSE YOUR EYES on it. Instructions may be repeated three times but patient must
   close eyes for correct score.)

10. Ask if the patient is right- or left-handed. The paper held in front of the patient   3
    should be taken with the nondominant hand. *"Take this paper in your right/left hand,*
    fold it in half and place it on the floor."
    Takes paper with nondominant hand = 1
    Folds it in half = 1
    Places it on the floor = 1

11. Give the patient a pencil and paper and say, *"Write any complete sentence on this piece*   1
    of paper." (Allow no more than 30 seconds. Sentence should make sense. Ignore
    spelling.)

12. Place intersecting pentagons design, pencil and paper in front of the patient. Say,   1
    "Please copy this design." (Allow multiple attempts up to 1 minute. To be correct the
    patient's copy must show a four-sided drawing within two five-sided figures. Ignore
    rotation and distortions.)

Scoring serial 7's

93, 86, 79, 72, 65	5 points
93, 88, 81, 74, 67	4 points
92, 85, 78, 71, 64	4 points
93, 87, 80, 73, 64	3 points

Note. Adapted by permission of the author, Dr. D. W. Molloy, McMaster University. Also see Molloy et al.
(1991).

sizable predictor of mortality than physical disability, number of conditions, or age (Kelman et al., 1994).

Of the widely used screens for cognitive impairment, the Clock
Drawing Test is the briefest, requiring less than 5 minutes to complete.
The patient is asked to draw a clock face with all the numbers and
hands and then to state the time as drawn. The number 12 must appear
on top (3 points), there must be 12 numbers present (1 point), there
must be two distinguishable hands (1 point), and the time must be
identified correctly (1 point) for full credit. A score less than 4 is considered impaired (Stahelin et al., 1997). The Orientation–Concentration
Test of Blessed et al. (1968) and the MMSE require 10 to 15 minutes.

The MMSE is more heavily weighted to cognitive capacities other than memory. Memory testing is the Blessed's strong point. The more comprehensive Mattis Dementia Rating Scale (1976) requires a minimum of 20 minutes. Other tests include Trail Making A and B, which measures executive function and the Boston Aphasia screen for communication deficits. Solomon's (1998) "7-Minute Neurocognitive Screening Battery" incorporates brief tests of orientation, aphasia (animal names), clock drawing, and the free and cued recall memory measure.

The Free and Cued Selective Reminding text may be useful to distinguish age-associated memory impairment from dementia. The Free and Cued Selective Reminding test reduces the age-related decrements in learning and processing to elicit genuine deficits in recall, which are characteristic of dementia. The measures may also be less sensitive to educational attainment (Grober et al., 1998). For intellectually gifted persons and those with higher educational attainment, and when decline is subtle, a lengthier examination or referral to a neuropsychologist is warranted. For annual screening of seniors in primary care without signs or symptoms of dementia, the MMSE combined with the Clock Drawing Test provides adequate sensitivity and specificity (Stahelin et al., 1997). The average decline in MMSE scores among Alzheimer's patients is 2 to 4 points per year. Serial assessments at 6-month intervals are helpful when the diagnosis remains suspect. However, like imaging studies, none of the cognitive screening or neuropsychological batteries can be considered diagnostic.

ASSESSMENT OF FUNCTIONAL IMPAIRMENT

An assessment of impairment in activities of daily living is critical (Kasper, 1990). Whereas the examination of cognition occurs between patient and practitioner, functional impairment is more reliably assessed with collateral informants, most often family. An assessment of activities of daily living covers the maintenance of physical hygiene and grooming but also the more instrumental tasks such as management of finances, property, and household chores. Patients may appear in immaculate condition as a result of attentive caregivers, yet not be able to shop, cook, bathe, dress, or pay bills without total assistance. The Functional Activities Questionnaire (Pfeffer et al., 1982), the Revised Memory and Behavior Problems checklist, (Teri et al., 1992b) are two instruments advocated by Small et al. (1997) which, when administered to a collateral informant, demonstrate decline in multiple domains of independent function and can objectively support the diagnosis. The Global Deterioration Scale and Functional Assessment Staging

(Auer & Reisberg, 1997) is another widely used measure of dementia-related dependency. It also has value for informing the patient and family of the progression of the illness and the need to document preferences for late-stage and end-of-life care.

GENERAL TREATMENT CONSIDERATIONS

The comprehensive approach to dementia care seeks to push the majority of dementia-related disability to the end of the patient's naturally occurring lifespan (Mayeux & Sano, 1999). There are five elements to the comprehensive approach. First is accurate diagnosis of the specific dementia and other conditions that contribute to the disability. Patients and families need to know what to expect, particularly when vascular dementia or Lewy body disease will make the course of illness and behavioral disturbances difficult to predict. Second is caregiver education, counseling and support. In any chronic deteriorating condition, family is the best medicine. Third is the pharmacological palliation of cognitive impairment, which is rapidly advancing. Fourth are interventions, both pharmacological and behavioral, to lessen behavioral disturbances. Fifth is attention to end-of-life and institutional care issues. Evidence cited later argues that preserving the person's independence even if the condition cannot be cured has become a realistic goal.

It is foremost in the treatment of dementia to avoid nihilism. Although the number and effectiveness of medications to reverse cognitive impairment remains limited (Patel, 1995), there are a variety of approaches both pharmacological and otherwise to counter the disability of behavioral disturbances (Teri et al., 1992a). Primary care physicians provide the majority of mental health services, including dementia care. However, when mental symptoms are disruptive and when family dynamics are strained, the assistance of clinicians with expertise in dementia is generally required. Assisting the demented individual to adjust to the loss of independence and to overcome periods of grief and suspiciousness is particularly meaningful (Miller, 1989). Also important are the opportunities to reassure family members that they may not be haunted by all the horrors they have heard about the disease (Rabins, 1984).

It is helpful to have a conceptual framework in which to recognize the clinical course and stages of dementia. Cohen et al. (1984) identify phases in the patient, which are similar to reactions to catastrophic events. In Cohen's framework the demented individual initially undergoes a process of recognition that something ill defined is wrong.

This is variably followed by denial of deficits and lost capacities and by anger over being confronted or reminded of impairment. Guilt and shame in the affected person or family occur as the implications of the diagnosis become apparent. Once emotional reactions subside, a more concrete phase follows in which there are active attempts to cope and to prepare. In some cases this is followed by a maturation in which patients and families affirm aspects of their lives that remain valuable and enduring. In the end, there is a separation from self in which awareness is extinguished. Problems arise when patient and family are out of phase. Not every individual progresses through this hypothetical framework, however, the value of recognizing these phases for the clinician lies in the realization that what seems an irrational reaction is part of the process of adaptation.

Staging of dementia is also important in that the cognitive enhancer medications (see next section) are FDA approved only for mild to moderate Alzheimer's disease. Nonetheless, many practitioners, patients, or their families are comfortable with "off label" use in cases of mild cognitive impairment, vascular and Lewy body dementias, and late-stage Alzheimer's disease. MMSE scores above 20, memory loss and disorientation, repetitiousness, loss of interests, and change in personality characterize mild Alzheimer's dementia. Although depression may appear early, delusions, agitation, sleep disturbance, and wandering are more characteristic of moderate dementia (Devanand et al., 1997). Persons with moderately advanced dementia have MMSE scores ranging between 10 and 19. They require supervision to complete activities of daily living such as dressing and to be safe from dangerous wandering. Severe dementia is evidenced by marked aphasia, loss of capacity to recognize family, incontinence, and dependency in all ADLs. Stated simply, mildly impaired persons are forgetful and sometimes disoriented but can care for most of their personal needs. Moderately impaired persons require supervision for care and safety. Severely impaired persons are totally dependent and are losing the capacity to recognize family.

MEDICATIONS TO PALLIATE
COGNITIVE IMPAIRMENT

Medications to palliate the cognitive impairment of dementia are listed in Table 3.3. However, the list will be outdated within months of publication. Breitner (1999) foresees new medications emerging in the next two decades, which will nearly eliminate the morbidity of Alzheimer's disease. Yet until those agents have been administered to a generation at

TABLE 3.3. Agents Used to Palliate the Cognitive Impairment of Dementia

Generic name	Trade name	Initial dose	Final dose	Arrhythmic potential	Hypotensive potential	Sedative potential	Precautions	Advantages
Anticholinesterases								
Donepezil	*Aricept*	5 mg daily	10 mg daily	Bradycardia	Low	Low	Transient, initial GI upset; abrupt withdrawal leads to abrupt decline	Once-a-day dosing, safety
Rivastigmine	*Exelon*	1.5 mg b.i.d.	6 mg b.i.d.	Low	Low	Low	Transient, initial GI upset; titrated up at 2-week intervals; abrupt withdrawal leads to abrupt decline; b.i.d. dosing	Wider dose range
Galantamine	*Reminyl*	3 mg b.i.d.	12 mg b.i.d.	Low	Low	Low	Transient, initial GI upset; titrated up at 2-week intervals; abrupt withdrawal leads to abrupt decline; b.i.d. dosing	Nicotinic receptor modulation
Antioxidants								
Selegiline	*Eldepryl*	5 mg daily	5 mg b.i.d.	Low	Moderate	Low	Potentially life-threatening diet and drug interactions are rare at recommended doses	Available as a transdermal patch
Alpha-tocopherol	*Vitamin E* (Hoffmann-LaRoche)	30 IU daily	1,000 IU b.i.d.	NA	NA	NA	Liver toxicity, coagulopathy	Low toxicity, OTC
Others								
Extract of *Ginkgo biloba*	*Ginkgold Tebonin forte*	60 daily	60 q.i.d.	Low	Low	Low	q.i.d. dosing; an "herbal" not subject to FDA quality controls; few data available at maximum dose	Low toxicity, OTC
Conjugated estrogens	*Premarin*	0.625 daily	1.25 daily	NA	NA	NA	Assess risk of thromboembolic complications, breast and uterine cancer, menstruation; 21-day treatment if uterus intact	Proven health benefits even if cognition not improved
Transdermal estradiol	*Estraderm*	0.05 every 21 or 28 days	0.1 every 21 or 28 days					

Note. GI, gastrointestinal; NA, not applicable; q.i.d., four times a day. Other abbreviations as in Tables 2.3 and 2.4.

risk, the pharmacological alternative will continue to be drugs that may palliate but cannot prevent the disability of dementia. Given the recent arrival of cholinesterase inhibitors, the extent to which practitioners use them, singly or in combination, varies widely. The presence of vascular disease, history of stroke, and subcortical opacities should not be exclusion factors for treatment (Cummings, 2000). For patients with suspected vascular dementia, the use of 325 mg aspirin daily in addition to cessation of smoking and reduction of serum lipids should be recommended (Nyenhuis & Gorelick, 1998). Yet it should be remembered that in frail older adults and those already medicated for a variety of conditions, adding medications means multiplying side effects. Nonetheless, the new agents herald a rational polypharmacy for dementia similar to that which has proved so beneficial in the treatment of childhood leukemia and adult hypertension (Drachman & Leber, 1997).

Cholinesterase inhibitors improve cholinergic neurotransmission. In mild to moderately impaired persons they may improve cognition, delay decline, lessen the disability in ADL (Rogers et al., 1996), improve psychological and behavioral disturbances including psychosis (Kaufer et al., 1996; Becker et al., 1998), and forestall nursing home admission (Knopman et al., 1996). Livingston and Katona (2000) performed a Numbers Needed to Treat (NNT) analysis based on randomized placebo controlled trials of cholinesterase inhibitors published between 1994 and 1998. NNT analyses calculate the number of patients receiving active treatment that are needed to demonstrate a beneficial effect compared to placebo. For example, 29 patients with atrial fibrillation would need to be treated with warfarin to prevent stoke in one patient. In patients at high risk for repeated myocardial infarction, 40 would need to be treated with propranolol to demonstrate the prevention of one reinfraction. In contrast with 10 mg of donepezil, 6 (95% confidence interval of 4–12) Alzheimer patients need to be treated to reverse cognitive decline by one year in one person. With 12 mg rivastigmine, 5 (95% confidence interval of 4–7) patients need to be treated. With either medication even fewer patients are required to demonstrate lack of deterioration over 6 months compared to placebo.

On average, these agents restore the person to a level of impairment seen 6 months previously and may alter the slope of decline. When withdrawn, the cognitive impairment falls to that of patients treated with placebo. Although the effect is palliative, the less impaired time and delay in nursing home admission that cholinergic enhancers provide may be precious, particularly for the minority of patients whose improvement is marked. The side effects of cholinergic enhancement are nausea, diarrhea, sweating, bradycardia, and insomnia. They are most often transient, occurring at initiation of treatment.

To lessen adverse reactions, the cholinesterase inhibitors should be taken after breakfast.

Tacrine was the first cholinesterase inhibitor to be FDA approved for Alzheimer's disease, but it is no longer marketed because of superior safety and ease of administration offered by other agents. Donepezil is similar to tacrine but possesses a more prolonged action, greater specificity for brain tissue, and much less risk of liver toxicity. The starting dose is 5 mg once daily after breakfast. Increasing to 10 mg after 1 month will provide greater chance of improving cognition but is more likely to provoke gastrointestinal distress. Phasing in the increase on an every-other-day schedule may enhance tolerability. On average donepezil will add 1 to 2 points of cognitive capacity on the MMSE. Roughly one patient in four will experience improvement readily noticeable to family and practitioner. Among those in whom benefits are not readily apparent, at least half will experience a flattening of decline over the next 6 to 9 months remaining above their baseline measures of impairment. Benefits may take 3 months to become evident and after 40 weeks of treatment, most responders will have reverted to the level of disability noted at the point where donepezil was started. However, patients in the earliest stage of dementia, when cognitive decline is relatively slow, are most likely to benefit. Middle-stage patients in whom the slope of decline is more acute will exhibit more transient improvement. Although donepezil is FDA approved for mild to moderate Alzheimer's disease, many practitioners find it has an alerting effect in late-stage patients as well. Some residents in nursing facilities will also benefit (Cummmings et al., 1999). Cholinesterase inhibitors should not be withdrawn upon admission to a nursing home. However once the patient is bed bound, free of behavioral disturbances, and no longer recognizes family or caregivers, the benefits of the drug are questionable.

Rivastigmine (Exelon) is a cholinesterase inhibitor administered once or twice daily. The dose ranges from 3 to 6 mg b.i.d. and should be gradually titrated up over 1 month to 6 weeks to avoid nausea (Vellas et al., 1998). Patients able to tolerate the gastrointestinal difficulties of higher doses may benefit more. Rivastigmine also inhibits butryl cholinesterase that may be more active in the latter stages of dementia (Rösler et al., 1999). Galantamine (Reminyl) is a cholinesterase inhibitor with nicotinic receptor modulating activities. It is taken twice daily at doses ranging from 6 to 12 mg. Its benefit and side effect profiles are similar to other cholinesterase inhibitors, and at the time of this writing it is under FDA review (Krall et al., 1999).

It is not clear whether persons with a marginal response to one cholinesterase inhibitor will exhibit more noticeable changes with another. However, those who are intolerant of one agent deserve a trial of another. Although the cholinesterase inhibitors should not be prescribed together, they may be combined with vitamins C (500 mg) and E (400 IU b.i.d). Because the common dementias may overlap diagnostically, every patient with the diagnosis of dementia should be offered a trial of a cholinergic enhancer (Cummings, 2000). Most patients will add vitamin E but should be discouraged from adding extract of *Ginkgo biloba* due to minimal benefit, cost, and possible coagulopathy. Otherwise the risk of drug interactions and physical side effects is low. However, some patients will react negatively to the return of insight. Nonetheless, the rarity of reported negative reactions does not substantially detract from the value of the cholinesterase inhibitors and vitamin E.

Extract of *Ginkgo biloba* (EGb) has few side effects and is widely used by patients in Europe and the United States. Its mechanism of action is presumed to be that of an antioxidant or anticoagulant. At 60 mg b.i.d., it demonstrated minimal but statistically significant effects on cognition and functional disability among patients with either vascular or Alzheimer's dementia treated from 26 to 52 weeks (LeBars et al., 1997). However, as a botanical it is not subject to FDA regulations regarding quality control, and the expense of the name brands (Tebonin forte, Ginkgold) used in published studies approaches that of prescription medications (Itil et al., 1996).

The research literature also describes other agents that boost the cholinergic signal. Xanomeline is a selective (M_1) postsynaptic muscarinic agonist, which boosts the cholinergic signal without inhibiting acetylcholinesterase. Postsynaptic cholinergic neurons in the cortex are relatively spared in Alzheimer's disease, adding to the appeal of the agent. It is administered at 75 mg t.i.d. Because it may alter the release of the amyloid precursor protein, it has been investigated for the possibility of altering the course of illness (Levy, 1998).

Selegiline, a selective monoamine oxidase B inhibitor, and vitamin E (alpha-tocopherol) reduce the rate of functional decline and delay nursing home placement in moderately impaired persons with dementia. However, cognitive performance is not enhanced and the combination of the two agents is no more beneficial than either alone (Sano et al., 1997). Selegiline at low doses of 5–10 mg daily was safe despite the potential hypertensive reaction to sympathomimetics and tyramine-rich foods. Vitamin E was also safe, but at the doses used in the study (1,000 IU t.i.d.) may be associated with liver toxicity and coagulopathy.

Preliminary data also suggest that estrogen may reduce the risk of dementia among older women (Paganini-Hill & Henderson, 1994) and enhance verbal memory (Kampen & Sherwin, 1994). Conjugated estrogens (0.625–1.25 daily) or transdermal estradiol (0.05–0.1 mg) are prescribed for 21 days for women with an intact uterus and 28 days for those who have had a hysterectomy. A large-scale placebo-controlled double-blind test of the estrogen hypothesis is under way in the Women's Health Initiative. Provided the older woman is free of risk factors for estrogen-related complications (see Chapter 9), the general health benefits of estrogen replacement warrant its use without regard to putative benefits for cognition.

Treatments for Alzheimer's disease have focused on cholinergic decline, oxidative stress, and, more recently, inflammation. Additional support for the neuroinflammatory hypothesis comes from more than 20 epidemiological studies. Patients taking anti-inflammatory drugs, or suffering from conditions for which such drugs are routinely used, have a substantially reduced risk of developing dementia (McGeer et al., 1996; Rogers et al., 1993). For example, Alzheimer's disease is less common in arthritis patients who frequently use anti-inflammatory agents. In the Baltimore Longitudinal Study of Aging, persons taking nonsteroidal anti-inflammatory drugs but not acetaminophen exhibited a lesser prevalence of the disease.

A number of studies are under way to test the anti-inflammatory treatment hypothesis. These include randomized trials of an anticholinesterase combined with a cyclooxygenase (COX) inhibitor. The demonstration that brain tissue expresses both isomers of COX—COX-1 and COX-2—has increased enthusiasm for studies of nonsteroidal anti-inflammatory drugs (NSAIDs), which inhibit the activity of one or both of these enzymes. Microglial cells which are part of the immune–inflammatory response surround amyloid plaques. Neuronal expression of COX-2 is upregulated in Alzheimer brains, and COX-2 activity increases the susceptibility of neurons to amyloid toxicity. Newly developed selective COX-2 inhibitors, which have similar anti-inflammatory activity but substantially reduced gastrointestinal, renal, and liver toxicity compared to nonselective NSAIDs, thus represent attractive candidates for clinical trials (Aisen, 1999). Although the National Institute on Aging (1998) cautions against the use of nonsteroidal anti-inflammatory agents to prevent cognitive decline, interest in the inflammatory hypothesis is intense.

ENVIRONMENTAL MODIFICATIONS

The physical environment should be modified to be safe and predictable. A regular schedule of ADLs, including rising, meals, medications, and exercise, prevents confusion and lessens the burden on memory. Unfamiliar people, places, and events require accommodation for which the patient is ill equipped. Travel, even to visit close family and friends, should be planned carefully. The withdrawal of activities requiring higher levels of autonomous function (e.g., use of firearms, opportunities to cook or smoke unsupervised, and automobile driving) requires compassion and at times imagination. In some states, a diagnostic report to the department of motor vehicles is required which gives both patient and practitioner added impetus to address the issue. Similarly, gas heat may be changed to electric and matches may be locked away. A lock on the door or placing the doorknob in an unfamiliar area, such as near the top of the door rather than at waist level, can help a patient remember not to wander away from home. Hussian and Brown (1987) described an effective approach to limiting unsafe wandering among institutionalized patients through the use of a visually averting grid pattern. Large signs with clear, simple instructions may be helpful. Caregivers should emphasize contrasting colors and experiment to determine optimal illumination.

MANAGEMENT OF BEHAVIORAL AND PSYCHOLOGICAL SIGNS AND SYMPTOMS

Some family caregivers prefer a less than candid stance with their impaired relative. But, as mentioned earlier during discussion of cognitive screening, honesty and straightforward communication about restrictions are the basis of preserving the dignity and respect that every person, demented or otherwise, deserves. This is not to say that erroneous beliefs need always to be challenged with reality. Provided that the affected individual shows no intent to act on the belief (e.g., to return to the workplace) little is gained from further weakening an already shaky sense of self. Better to reinforce the pride in functioning that underlies the expressed intent by simply reflecting, "Yes, your work is important."

Problem behaviors are often an expression of the caregiving context and the caregiver's capacities as well as the patient's disease. The causes are usually multiple. Intervention to make the disturbed behavior less disruptive is a more realistic goal than is outright elimination. A wait-and-see attitude may be reasonable when transient depression occurs, but agitation and psychosis are more likely to be persistent and disruptive (Devanand, 1997). Teri et al. (1997) found that combined behavioral and psychoeducational approaches significantly improved depressive symptoms in the majority of dementia patients and their caregivers.

Characterization of the three-point sequence, or ABC's, of problematic behavior is central to the task of management (Teri et al., 1997). First, the caregiver is asked

A. To identify the "Antecedents" or triggering events such as changes in daily routine of the environment, interpersonal conflict, emotional or physical stressors. The antecedents can then be removed or minimized as a preventive measure.
B. To describe the "Behavior" in detail, how often it occurs, when and where it is most likely to happen, how long it lasts. Caregivers may need to step back and observe or take note to provide sufficient detail and to set the baseline for objective measurement of improvement. This observation period also refines recognition of antecedents and how the problem behavior fits into other aspects of the patient's life.
C. To identify the "Consequences" of the behavior, how the caregiver or others react to reinforce or deter the activity, and what happens when the activity ceases.

With the ABC's in hand, a treatment plan can be enacted. Preventive measures are best but must be practical. Caregivers should identify a small, achievable goal, which everyone can agree on and around which problems, solutions, and alternatives may be identified. They should build on success by monitoring the value of the plan, providing positive feedback, and incorporating new interventions as the opportunity arises. The strategy may need to be changed. The caregiver will need to be flexible but consistent throughout.

The key to behavioral intervention is improved communication and patient perception. Adequate time must be allowed to communicate. Visual cues and verbal suggestions should be coupled. Caregivers should maintain good nonverbal behavior by staying at eye level with the patient. They should avoid provocative stances or gestures, speak softly and slowly, use "sound bite"-sized statements or instructions, check that the patient understands and is ready, eliminate visual distractions and reduce ambient noise, and attend to one thing at a time. They must make sure that glasses and hearing aids and spares are available; they should expect them to be misplaced.

SPECIFIC PROBLEM BEHAVIORS AND SYMPTOMS

Agitation

Agitation is a common, persistent problem and the etiology varies. Delirium may be the most frequent acute cause. Particularly when the change in behavior is abrupt, acute illness should be suspected. However, environmental stressors such as sleep deprivation and unfamiliar or chaotic surroundings can induce confusion indistinguishable from toxic delirium. Patients may be "talked down" and reoriented, but attempts to flee or remove intravenous lines or life supports will require medication, most often haloperidol.

Depression, psychosis, anxiety, boredom, and pain also contribute to agitation (Greenwald et al., 1989). Frontal-lobe degeneration impairs the person's judgment and capacity to sequence steps to gain attention or comfort. Patients whose needs cannot be accurately expressed due to aphasia may also become agitated. Their inability to comprehend spoken cues may compromise staff efforts to reassure them. Recognizing the impediments to communication will lessen the caregiver's frustration and justify the time and patience required to reduce if not prevent agitation. Age-related impairments in hearing and vision add to the problem.

Verbally Disruptive Behaviors

Verbally disruptive behaviors include screaming, abusive language, moaning, and repetitive verbalizations. These behaviors disturb others and may signal the person's unmet needs. Screaming is one of the most distressing forms of agitation (Cohen-Mansfield et al., 1990). In theory, screaming may result from cortical disinhibition, or be reinforced (conditioned) by attention. However, it more often results from physical discomfort, sensory deprivation, or social isolation (Cohen-Mansfield & Werner, 1997). Frequently the patient is unable to explain or identify an unmet need. The caregiver must infer possible causes, which include pain, fecal or urinary urgency, constipation, anxiety, depression, psychosis, sensory isolation, boredom, and lack of exercise. Often the behavior can be reduced in frequency and volume without resorting to sedation. Exposure to videotapes generated by family and music appropriate to the person's background and culture reduce the problem. However, individual social interaction is more effective. Examples include simple conversation, range-of-motion exercises, and sensory stimulation with photos, fabrics, fragrances, and occupational therapy games (Cohen-Mansfield & Werner, 1997). Frequent, brief checks for toileting, snacks, and physical stimulation once incorporated into the staff's routine are not burdensome.

Family and staff generally prefer a little unpleasant vocalization to a patient made inaccessible with psychotropics. With psychotropic medications the risk:benefit:burden ratio of treatment is a critical concern. However, risk to the patient and risk to others must be parceled out. The concept of negotiated autonomy helps to avoid futile power struggles over patient rights. Negotiated autonomy means that once the patient is dependent on others, the autonomy of those others becomes a shared concern. Behavior that is disagreeable to others with whom the patient resides or on whom the patient depends is a justified focus of intervention. Thus accommodation rather than autonomy is the issue.

Sundowning

Increased confusion at evening time can usually be managed by recognizing that the change in the environmental routine triggers the problem. Patients who become troubled at change of shift in the nursing home or hospital may be responding to the increase in stimulation. Others may be bothered by the reduction in stimulation as the day winds down and daylight fades. In either situation, providing the optimum of stimulation is preferable to medication. Food, brief personal contact, music, or improvement in hearing or vision impairments are only some of the alterations in the care routine that reduce sundowning. When suspiciousness or agitation becomes disruptive and is not lessened by modulating the environmental stimuli, medication may be necessary.

Delusions, Hallucinations, Paranoia, Suspiciousness

It is important to distinguish persistent false beliefs or perceptions from transitory illusions that result from impairments in vision, hearing and cortical deficits (Wragg & Jeste, 1989). Briefly mistaking one family member for another can be upsetting but rarely leads to disturbed behavior. On the other hand, global suspiciousness, unwarranted accusations, and fears of abandonment, which interfere with care, may be psychotic. If the psychosis does not interfere with care or distress the person, then medication may not be needed. Similarly, if antecedents can be identified, they may be manipulated to reduce the problem to manageable proportions. Change in routine and caregiving personnel should be minimized. Better lighting to reduce shadows and correct sensory deficits and a modulated level of activity and attention may also be effective. The suspicious person may be set at ease by reassurance and redirection to a less threatening theme or activity. Distraction, physical activity, and gentle touch (the elbow is neutral territory) may also restore trust. Attention provided when suspicions are silenced will lay a foundation for trust and reassurance at more problematic times. Arguing or coercive reality orientation will only increase suspiciousness and distress.

However, when patients act on their delusions through seclusiveness, threats, accusations, or assault, antipsychotic medication will be necessary. Similarly, refusal to attend a day-care center, admit a home health aide, or allow health maintenance procedures may be the result of paranoia rather than a reasoned preference. Paranoia can also take the form of delusional jealousy with accusations of infidelity, which can be heartbreaking for the spouse. Even suspicious patients usually retain enough regard for an empathic physician that they will consent to medication to restore sleep, alleviate stress, or help control their temper. The patient can be informed that family or nursing staff will place liquid medication in their juice or cereal each morning if they agree. Consent need not be renewed with each dose.

Depressive Symptoms

Transient depressive symptoms are not uncommon in dementia, but persistent depressed mood and suicidal behaviors are less frequent. As a result, behavioral interventions should be the first line of intervention when depressive symptoms emerge but do not suggest a major depressive disorder. These interventions are also important adjuncts to antidepressant medications. Depressed expressions may be evoked when the patient is reminded of sad events, when frustration overwhelms, and when the person feels neglected or alone. To lessen depressive expressions, caregivers should focus on pleasant memories, avoid or minimize frustrating, unpleasant circumstances, and increase pleasurable activities and social interaction. Clearly this requires added time and attention from staff and may need to be maintained to be preventive.

Sleep Disturbance

Sleep disturbance is common in dementia and disrupts both the patient and the caregiver's rest. A brief assessment of sleep pattern, time spent in bed, and daytime activities will identify the need for changing the sleep schedule, adding exercise, or prescribing medication. If physical discomfort awakens the patient, an analgesic at bedtime may help. Holding fluids after 6 P.M. may reduce the frequency of nighttime urination. Although the behavioral approach is the mainstay of treatment, it is the caregiver's behavior that must be modified if the demented person's sleep is to improve. As a result, the burdens and benefits of treatment need to be estimated for both the patient and caregiver. Sedation will solve the problem but predisposes the patient to falling. Hypersomnia is less often a problem than insomnia. For patients who sleep too much, coffee or tea may be useful. Other patients who are apathetic or nap too frequently may benefit from low-dose methylphenidate (5–15 mg after breakfast or lunch).

Indiscreet or Unwelcome Sexual Behavior

Demented persons seeking sexual gratification should not be labeled pathological even though they may disturb caregivers and facility staff. "Sexual acting out" may be the result of lack of privacy or an appropriate partner. However, when sexual advances are unwelcome or when self-stimulation is not managed discreetly, more may be required than directing the patient to a private area. The problem should be discussed directly with the patient at the time of the behavior and disapproval indicated for the circumstances surrounding the act, not the impulse. A matter-of-fact approach with family members and staff also helps alleviate their reluctance to discuss the issue. Modeling openness and a willingness to help the patient regain control is preferable to a punitive attitude. Pathological sexuality in dementia is more often seen with frontal-lobe disease and represents a disinhibition rather than willfulness. Staff and family will be less morally outraged once the neurological basis of the behavior is explained. Therapy with medroxyprogesterone or conjugated estrogens has been used to lessen sexual aggression in demented males. Psychotropic medications used for this purpose should be reserved for incidents of assaultiveness or masturbatory self-mutilation.

Difficulties Accepting Personal Care

Efforts to assist with feeding, bathing, and transfer from bed to chair or toilet are sometimes met with assaultive behavior particularly when the caregiver is not familiar with the patient. Assaultiveness results from protective reflexes and disinhibition directly related to the dementia. Apraxia, aphasia, and agnosia, common in Alzheimer's disease but made worse by age-related impairment in vision and hearing, reduce the patient's ability to complete or comprehend simple tasks or to recognize the caregiver.

It is helpful to educate staff that the objectionable behavior is the result of neurological deficits and protective responses rather than malice. With time, staff become accustomed to the patient's needs and, through trial, effort, and intuition, develop an effective routine for care. Placing mittens on the patient's hands at bath time can prevent scratching. Two persons may be required for bathing to prevent assault. The time saved by team approach to "problem bathers" more than compensates for the added personnel. Physical or chemical restraints for the purpose of bathing often result in more rather than less expenditures in staff time and effort. Nonetheless, for some patients, low doses of lorazepam (0.25 mg) are necessary to prevent combativeness without overly sedating the patient. Late in dementia, patients become so impaired that they are unable to allow others to feed them or to swallow without risking aspiration. Difficulty with feeding may signal terminal decline. Artificial nutrition and hydration through a gastrostomy tube is not recommended (Gillick, 2000).

Willful Behavior and Personality Disorders

Despite accusations that objectionable behavior is "done on purpose," most often staff and family will be mistaken in attributing willfulness to the demented person's behavior (Mittelman et al., 1995). However, individuals with the dramatic–impulsive cluster of personality disorders (histrionic, borderline, narcissistic, antisocial) may also become demented. Differentiating their impulsiveness, extreme emotionality, or manipulations from the impaired judgment and emotional lability of dementia is difficult. Also, lack of empathic regard for caregivers further limits their capacity to appreciate the consequences of their actions. Problematic interpersonal relations across adult life are the key indicator that psychotropic medications may not be beneficial. Limit setting and confrontation are more effective. Because the behavior is part of an enduring pattern, staff should adjust their expectations accordingly. The patient's outbursts of anger, efforts to manipulate or intimidate, and attention-seeking behavior may be unavoidable, but staff have the choice of how to respond. Acknowledging that their reaction to objectionable behavior is understandable will alleviate shame and guilt and allow a more reasoned approach to restoring the patient's equilibrium and the staff's sense of competence.

Falls

Gait disturbance due to apraxia, quadriceps weakness, rigidity, sedatives, and poor vision predispose the dementia patient to falls, soft tissue injury, and fractures. Physical therapy and change in medications may reduce the risk but not eliminate it. Falls can be eliminated with restraints but the quality of life is degraded. This dilemma should be shared with staff and family to reach a balance between safety and freedom. The substituted judgment of family in an informed or negotiated model of consent is most helpful (Moody, 1988). Faced with the progressive decline of a loved relative, the family may choose near-term freedom from restraints rather than long-term freedom from injury.

Wandering, Pacing

The patient who walks about the backyard or enclosed garden of a nursing home presents no problem. However, when someone with dementia wanders away from supervision or becomes lost, safety becomes the issue. In the acute-care setting, where wandering poses a genuine risk, placing the patient under close observation may be necessary. A family member may volunteer to provide supervised walking. Alternatively, physical therapy or other forms of low-risk exercise may be substituted. Exercise for the demented person is an underutilized modality to remedy behavioral disturbance. Caregivers should seek to determine whether there is a temporal or event related pattern to the wandering. Do reminders of leaving (hat, coat) need to be removed? Pictures of family prominently displayed in the patient's room may assist when helping the patient to return. If the patient is searching for someone or something familiar, the pictures and personal possessions may satisfy. It should be kept in mind that pacing or wandering may signal unmet needs or discomfort. Staff may need to experiment with toileting, snacks, or analgesics to find the right solution.

Catastrophic Reactions

Persons with dementia can be transiently overwhelmed, displaying anxious confusion, suspiciousness, or tearful self-reproach. This catastrophic response follows overstimulation and a sense of failure or threat. An overbearing attitude, rapid questions, excessive commands, and too much noise or activity can provoke the response. Criticism, whether real or implied, and intrusive efforts to correct or reorient the person may also contribute. Patient fatigue or conflict with certain individuals may also be to blame. To counter a catastrophic reaction it is helpful to change the subject or defer the task to a less distressing time. A soothing tone with empathic comments spoken slowly and eye contact may abort the response. At times it will be necessary to create a distraction or remove the patient from the source of conflict or to supply a pleasurable alternative. However, staff must not let the situation get out of hand before resorting to medication.

Unsafe Driving

An empathic confrontation may be sufficient when cognitive impairment is mild and the patient is insightful about the prognosis and risks. Asking the patient to pass a driver's test with the licensing authority may resolve the problem. However, when the demented person refuses to acknowledge the risks, the family should be advised to disable the vehicle or confiscate the keys.

MEDICATIONS TO LESSEN BEHAVIORAL AND PSYCHOLOGICAL DISTURBANCES

"Start low, go slow" is the catch phrase of prescribing for older adults. However, the most common error when using medication to control behavioral disturbance is failure to follow through and to monitor the effects. Mechanical restraints should only be used as an emergency procedure while awaiting for the effects of medication to take hold. Physical restraint heightens anxiety and results in a struggle to break free with undesirable physiological consequences (Evans & Strumpf, 1993). Readers are referred to Chapters 2, 4, and 5 for greater detail and prescribing guidelines for individual agents.

Sedatives

A short-acting benzodiazepine (lorazepam 0.5 mg orally or intramuscularly) can help the patient through procedures such as CT scan or MRI. Intravenous injection of haloperidol is reserved for episodes of life-threatening agitation in the context of fracture, stroke, or myocardial infarction. For sleep disturbance, low doses of the sedating antidepressant trazodone (25 mg) may be effective, but hypotension will ensue as the dose is increased (Houlihan et al., 1994). The sedating antipsychotic thioridazine again in low doses (10 mg) may also be beneficial. The short-acting benzodiazepines will induce sleep but may also impair cognition.

Antipsychotics

Haloperidol (0.5 mg), thioridazine (10 mg), and risperidone (0.5 mg) are available in liquid forms which allows the dose to be given in food or beverage, thereby assisting patients who have difficulty swallowing or accepting medications from caregivers. The benefits of haloperidol are its relatively low sedative and hypotensive effects. Haloperidol, because of its lack of cardiovascular effects and availability of an injectible form, is preferable for short-term use in acute-care settings where delirium complicates dementia. The drawback with haloperidol is the rigidity that results from extrapyramidal effects at higher doses. The advantages of thioridazine are its sedative property and freedom from extrapyramidal effects. It is, however, hypotensive as the dose is increased. Although considerably more expensive than typical antipsychotics, the atypical antipsychotics are preferable for longer-term treatment. Risperidone, a mildly sedative atypical antipsychotic, is neither Parkinsonian nor hypotensive at low doses (.25–2 mg daily). Katz et al. (1999) found it considerably superior to placebo for the treatment of suspiciousness and aggressive behavior in dementia. However, at 2 mg, extrapyramidal signs began to appear. Olanzapine (2.5–10 mg) is less likely to induce extrapyramidal effects, is more sedative than risperidone, may cause somnolence, increased blood glucose and body weight, and gait disorder, but is rarely hypotensive. It reduces agitation, aggression, and other manifestations of psychosis (Street, 1999). Quetiapine (Seroquel) is more sedative than olanzapine but no more likely to cause extrapyramidal effects. It is also relatively free of interactions with other drugs. At a mean dose of 100 mg (25 mg initially then up to 50 mg b.i.d.) it reduces behavioral disturbances, most notably hostility among older adults with psychosis due to dementia or other disorders (McManus et al., 1999). In summary, although the newer antipsychotic medications are modestly effective in dementia, their side effect profile makes them clearly superior to typical antipsychotics.

Antidepressants

Depressive symptoms are more common than depressive disorders in dementia, but the safety and variety of antidepressants have lowered the threshold with which an antidepressant may be offered. However, a lack of efficacy studies among dementia patients means the prescriber will make the choice of agents based on side effects and target symptoms. For the agitated or sleep-deprived depressed patient, trazodone is an effective antidepressant but is hypotensive and very sedative (25 mg initial dose). Nefazodone (50 mg b.i.d.) is virtually free of amnestic and arrhythmic effects and is less sedative than trazodone. Sertraline (25 mg to begin) is not sedative and improves the signs of depression among nursing home residents in the late stages of dementia (Magai et al., 2000). As with the longer-acting citalorpam, it is also less likely than some other SSRIs to alter the metabolism of other medications. Paroxetine (10–20 mg daily) is a more calming SSRI. Like sertraline it is free of cardiovascular and amnestic risk but may cause nausea and jitteriness in a minority of persons. For the frail patient in whom no risk of side effects can be tolerated, bupropion (75 mg b.i.d.) which is selectively noradrenergic, is reasonable. In similar instances methylphenidate (5–15 mg after breakfast and lunch) may be prescribed and has the advantage of rapid onset of therapeutic response for the apathetic or somnolent patient. Venlafaxine (25 mg b.i.d.) has the advantage of lacking sedative and hypotensive properties but may impair appetite. Mirtazapine (7.5 mg) will improve sleep and appetite.

Antianxiety Agents

Antidepressants are frequently effective in combating anxiety. Nefazodone, paroxetine, and venlafaxine are appealing in this regard and will be less sedating than the benzodiazepines and therefore less likely to impair awareness. However, frail patients who cannot tolerate any degree of sedation may be administered buspirone (10–30 mg b.i.d.), which is free of amnestic effects.

Antiaggression Agents

Although antipsychotics have been the main treatment of aggression, valproate (125 mg b.i.d. to start) has gained increasing recognition as an antiaggression agent as well as a mood stabilizer. It is relatively safe and is not amnestic, arrhythmogenic, or hypotensive, but it should be monitored with therapeutic levels (Maletta, 1992). Carbamazepine has also shown promise (Tariot, 1999), but both agents may alter anticoagulant levels. Antiadrenergic (beta-blockers) have also been advocated for this purpose but are more likely to compromise cardiovascular function. Gabapentin and lamotragine are newer antiepileptic agents with reports of antimanic properties; however, their use in older patients with dementia is not well documented (Semenchuk & Labiner, 1997).

CAREGIVER BURDEN AND DYSFUNCTIONAL FAMILY DYNAMICS

The majority of dementia care is provided by female family members who vary widely in their capacity to adapt to the burden of caring for a relative (Butler, 1996) (see treatment of caregiver burden in Chapters 7 and 8 and the mediation of family conflict in Chapter 14). The family is a crucial focus of intervention. Rehabilitation of the patient should always include consultation with the family, and failure of the family to appear should alert the clinician to future problems. Dysfunctional family dynamics may become evident during a crisis but should be anticipated in the early phase of the evaluation. Sibling rivalries among the children and unresolved marital discord complicate the family effort to provide care. Parent–child conflicts may reappear and be beyond resolution once the parent's cognition wanes. Dominant forces of influence in the family shift as one relative or another assumes the burden of care. Most families are remarkably creative in providing care. Others seem enmeshed, trapped in maintaining conflict rather than resolving it (Boss et al., 1990). The clinician's task is to confront these problems with skill and perseverance (Light & Lebowitz, 1989).

Clinical depression is a problem for 20 to 60% of the family members who become primary caregivers (Cohen & Eisdorfer, 1988; Gallagher et al., 1989). The focus of care in these instances shifts to the family member and includes psychotherapy and/or antidepressant medication. In rare instances elder abuse, most often in the form of neglect, will require more coercive intervention and will necessitate direct involvement with community agencies. Certain patient behaviors are particularly distressing to loved ones, and these include incontinence, nighttime wandering, and assaultiveness (Coleridge & George, 1986). Perhaps cruelest of all is the patient's loss of capacity to recognize the loved caregiver (Gwyther, 1990). Even early in the disease family members may be mistaken for strangers. It is helpful to explain that perceptual disorders may in part account for this form of disorientation (Rabins, 1984). Also factual, readable materials help families educate themselves about the illness and caring for their relative. Excellent guides for the family include Mace and Rabin's (1999) *36 Hour Day* now available in seven languages, Cohen and Eisdorfer's (1986) *Loss of Self*, Gwyther's (1988) *Care of Alzheimer's Patients: A Manual for Nursing Home Staff*, and Jarvik and Small's (1988) *Parentcare: A Commonsense Guide for Adult Children*. The Alzheimer's Association has extensive but concise material freely available to families in local offices and web sites.

PRACTITIONER AS *DE FACTO* GUARDIAN
AND OTHER MEDICAL–LEGAL ISSUES

Patients without family or involved friends present a special problem to the practitioner, one that can best be handled by a generalist who has cared for the individual over an extended period. In such cases the practitioner may function as a *de facto* guardian, becoming the primary advocate for medical procedures or nursing care. This places a unique responsibility on the practitioner to operate in the best medical interest of a patient whose capacity to participate in decision making is ever diminishing. It is this disease-imposed loss of autonomy due to impaired cognition that differentiates the *de facto* medical conservator from the paternalistic physician.

Physicians, nurses, psychologists, and social workers are increasingly being called on to provide affidavits and expert testimony regarding older individuals' capacity to manage assets and property and to make essential life decisions. Detailed instructions for evaluations of capacity as well as warnings of the pitfalls appear in Chapter 14. A credible evaluation should include a diagnostic assessment that emphasizes the evaluation of functional capacity and is substantiated by validated measures of cognitive impairment and functional deterioration (Baker et al., 1986). Ideally, the evaluation should include a visit to the allegedly incapacitated person's home where the evaluator can directly observe his or her capacity to manage personal documents, mail, medications, financial transactions, and telephone communications. A history of functional decline from collateral informants and a review of medical assessments to ensure that reversible causes of mental impairment have not been neglected are mandatory. The report should delineate life skills that are preserved as well as those that are deficient. For example, an individual may take pride in keeping house and preparing meals but not be able to balance the checkbook or make change in the market. A court-ordered financial guardian and assistance with shopping is required but a housekeeper is not. Here again the practitioner can play the role of *de facto* guardian by championing the patient's skills without neglecting the functional deficits.

MANAGEMENT OF FINANCIAL RESOURCES

In the early stage of the disease, when incapacity is minimal and easily contained, the physician should anticipate future need for supportive services and urge family and patient to accept referral before the need becomes acute. Arrangements for home health aides, day treatment, respite care, and residence in nursing facilities can be patched together with a good deal of continuity. However, providing these arrangements exceeds the capacity of any one individual and is best coordinated by a social worker or other professional functioning as a case manager. Legal advice for the management of financial assets is another important area of consideration for the family. Nursing home placement will devastate even substantial estates, and prolonged care at home is also expensive (Overman & Stoudemire, 1988). Durable power of attorney assigned to a family member while the patient is still capable of exercising the necessary judgment will ensure adequate access to resources once the person is no longer able to manage financial decisions (see Chapter 14 for a more complete presentation).

PREPARATIONS FOR END-OF-LIFE CARE

Cost considerations aside, patients and families need assistance throughout the treatment process to confront end-of-life care issues. The appointment of a durable power of attorney for health care decisions (health care proxy) is the first step. A backup proxy may also be appointed. Some ethicists prefer the appointment of a health care proxy to the use of advanced directives in that the proxy is empowered to act across an array of contingencies, which may be difficult to anticipate. However, the use of "feeding tubes" (gastrostomy or nasogastric tube), "breathing machines" (respirators), or "artificial kidney" (hemodialysis) for reasons beyond treatment of acute illness will be rejected by most older patients if time and compassion are provided for the discussion. Cardiac resuscitation should also be carefully discussed before it is indicated. Quality of mentation after resuscitation in the community or hospital will be severely compromised in persons with dementia. Resuscitation in the operating room is the exception when recovery to baseline is to be expected. Late in the stage of dementia, when the patient has lost awareness of caregivers and surroundings, the use of antibiotics or hospitalization for acute illness may be rejected as well by some caregivers. These are not easy decisions, but they are more easily approached when the practitioner anticipates the need and is experienced in the discussion (see Chapter 14 for a more complete presentation).

SUMMARY

A comprehensive approach to dementia care based on evidence from the scientific literature promises to reduce the disability of dementia substantially in the near future. It contains several elements: accurate diagnosis of the specific dementia and amelioration of comorbid conditions; patient and family education with special attention given to the misleading fluctuations seen in vascular and Lewy body dementias; caregiver counseling and support; pharmacological palliation of impaired cognition; interventions to lessen the excess disability of behavioral disturbances; discussion of end-of-life decisions, and institutional care. However, the use of medications and modifications in staff's or family's approach to the patient will still require ingenuity and perseverance. Consultation from a specialist can prove invaluable, but most of the management will continue to be the responsibility of the family, primary care practitioners, or nursing home staff. Skillful treatment based on accurate diagnosis will improve the demented individuals' and their family's well-being despite the degenerative nature of the illness. Even modest benefits to the individual when spread over the large numbers of older Americans who will become demented means a sizable reduction in projected costs of dementia care.

REFERENCES

Aisen, P. S. (1999, August 19). *Current status of anti-inflammatory drug studies in Alzheimer's disease*. Paper presented at the Ninth Congress of the International Psychogeriatric Association, Vancouver, British Columbia, Canada.

Alexopoulos, G. S., Meyers, B. S., Young, R. C., et al. (1993). The course of geriatric depression with "reversible dementia": A controlled study. *American Journal of Psychiatry, 150,* 1693–1699.

Auer, S., Reisberg, B. (1997). The GDS/FAST system. *International Psychogeriatrics, 9,* 167–171.

Baker, F. M., Perr, I. N., Yesavage, J. A. (1986). *An overview of legal issues in geriatric psychiatry.* Washington, DC: American Psychiatric Association.

Becker, R. E., Colliver, J. A., Markwell, S. J., et al. (1998). Effects of metrifonate on cognitive decline in Alzheimer's disease: A double-blind, placebo-controlled, 6-month study. *Alzheimer Disease and Related Disorders, 12,* 54–67.

Blessed, G., Tomlinson, B. E., Roth, M. (1968). The association between quantitative measures of dementia and senile change in the cerebral gray matter of elderly subjects. *British Journal of Psychiatry, 114,* 797–811.

Boss, P., Caron, W., Horbal, J., et al. (1990). Predictors of depression in caregivers of dementia patients: Boundary ambiguity and mastery. *Family Process, 29,* 245–254.

Breitner, J. C. S. (1999). The end of Alzheimer's disease? *International Journal of Geriatric Psychiatry, 14,* 577–586.

Butler, R. N. (1996). Sounding board: On behalf of older women. *New England Journal of Medicine, 334,* 794–796.

Cohen, D., Eisdorfer, C. (1986). *The loss of self.* New York: Norton.

Cohen, D., Eisdorfer, C. (1988). Depression in family members caring for a relative with Alzheimer's disease. *Journal of the American Geriatrics Society, 36,* 885–889.

Cohen, D., Kennedy, G., Eisdorfer, C. (1984). Phases of change in the patient with Alzheimer's dementia: A conceptual dimension for defining health care management. *Journal of the American Geriatrics Society, 32,* 11–15.

Cohen-Mansfield, J., Werner, P. (1997). Management of verbally disruptive behaviors in nursing home residents. *Journal of Gerontology: Medical Sciences, 52,* M369–M377.

Cohen-Mansfield, J., Werner, P., Marx, M. S. (1990). Screaming in nursing home residents. *Journal of the American Geriatrics Society, 38,* 785–792.

Coleridge, P. T., George, L. K. (1986). Predictors of institutionalization among caregivers of patients with Alzheimer's disease. *Journal of the American Geriatrics Society, 34,* 493–498.

Cummings, J. L. (2000). Cholinesterase inhibitors: A new class of psychotropic compounds. *American Journal of Psychiatry, 157,* 4–15.

Cummings, J. L., Katz, I. R., Tariot, P., et al. (1999, April 17–24). *Donepezil in the treatment of Alzheimer's disease in a nursing home population.* Paper presented at the 51st annual meeting of the American Academy of Neurology, Toronto, Ontario, Canada.

Cutler, N. R., Haxby, J. V., Duara, R., et al. (1985). Brain metabolism as measured with PET: Serial assessment in a patient with familial Alzheimer's disease. *Neurology, 35*(1), 184.

de la Monte, S. M., Ghanbari, K., Frey, W. H., et al. (1997). Characterization of the AD7C-NTP cDNA expression in Alzheimer's disease and measurement of a 41-kD protein in cerebrospinal fluid. *Journal of Clinical Investigation, 100,* 3093–3104.

Devanand, D. P. (1997). Use of the Columbia University Scale to Assess Psychopathology in Alzheimer's disease. *International Psychogeriatrics, 9,* 137–142.

Devanand, D. P., Jacobs, D. M., Tang, M.-X., et al. (1997). The course of psychopathology in mild to moderate Alzheimer's disease. *Archives of General Psychiatry, 66,* 205–210.

Drachman, D. A., Leber, P. (1997). Treatment of Alzheimer's disease: Searching for a breakthrough, settling for less. *New England Journal of Medicine, 336,* 1245–1247.

Ernst, R. L., Hay, J. W. (1994). The U.S. economic and social costs of Alzheimer's disease revisited. *American Journal of Public Health, 84,* 1261–1264.

Evans, L. K., Strumpf, N. E. (1993). Frailty and physical restraints. In Y. Perry, J. Morley, R. Coe (Eds.), *Aging and musculoskeletal disorders* (pp. 324–333). New York: Springer.

Folstein, M., Anthony, J. C., Parhad, I., et al. (1985). The meaning of cognitive impairment in the elderly. *Journal of the American Geriatrics Society, 33,* 228–235.

Folstein, S. E., Folstein, M. F. (1983). Psychiatric features of Huntington's disease. *Psychiatric Developments, 2,* 193–206.

Gallagher, D., Rose, J., Rivera, P., et al. (1989). Prevalence of depression in family caregivers. *Gerontologist, 29,* 449–456.

Gillick, M. R. (2000). Rethinking the role of tube feeding in patients with advanced dementia. *New England Journal of Medicine, 342,* 206–210.

Greenwald, B. S., Kramer-Ginsberg, E., Marin, D. B., et al. (1989). Dementia with coexistent major depression. *American Journal of Psychiatry, 146,* 1472–1478.

Grober, E., Bushke, H., Crystal, H., et al. (1988). Screening for dementia by memory testing. *Neurology, 38,* 900–903.

Grober, E., Lipton, R. B., Katz, M., et al. (1998). Demographic influence on free and cued selective reminding performance in the elderly. *Journal of Clinical and Experimental Neuropsychology, 20,* 221–226.

Gwyther, L. P. (1988). *Care of Alzheimer's patients: A manual for nursing home staff.*

Washington, DC: American Health Care Association and the Alzheimer's and Related Disorders Association.

Gwyther, L. P. (1990). Letting go: Separation–individuation in a wife of an Alzheimer's patient. *Gerontologist, 30,* 698–702.

Hachiniski, V. (1983). Multi-infarct dementias. *Neurologic Clinics, 1*(1), 27–36.

Harrington, M. G., Merril, C. R., Asher, D. M., et al. (1986). Abnormal proteins in the cerebrospinal fluid of patients with Creutzfeldt–Jakob disease. *New England Journal of Medicine, 315,* 279–283.

Henderson, A. S. (1989). Psychiatric epidemiology and the elderly. *International Journal of Geriatric Psychiatry, 4,* 249–253.

Heston, L. L., White, J. A., Mastri, A. R. (1987). Pick's disease: Clinical genetics and natural history. *Archives of General Psychiatry, 44,* 409–411.

Houlihan, D. J., Mulsant, B. H., Sweet, R. A., et al. (1994). A naturalistic study of trazodone in the treatment of behavioral complications of dementia. *American Journal of Geriatric Psychiatry, 2,* 78–85.

Huber, S. J., Paulson, G. W. (1985). The concept of subcortical dementia. *American Journal of Psychiatry, 142,* 1313–1317.

Hussian, R. A., Brown, D. C. (1987). Use of two-dimensional grid patterns to limit hazardous ambulation in demented patients. *Journal of Gerontology, 42,* 558–560.

Itil, T. M., Erlap, E., Tsambis, E., et al. (1996). Central nervous system effects of Ginkgo biloba, a plant extract. *American Journal of Therapeutics, 3,* 63–73.

Jarvik, L., Small, G. (1988). *Parentcare: A commonsense guide for adult children.* New York: Crown.

Jost, B. C., Grossberg, G. T. (1996). Evolution of psychiatric symptoms in Alzheimer's disease: A natural history study. *Journal of the American Geriatrics Society, 44,* 1078–1081.

Kampen, D. L., Sherwin, B. B. (1994). Estrogen use and verbal memory in healthy postmenopausal women. *Obstetrics and Gynecology, 3,* 979–983.

Kasper, J. D. (1990). Cognitive impairment among functionally limited elderly people in the community: Future considerations for long-term care policy. *Milbank Quarterly, 68,* 81–109.

Katz, I. R., Jeste, D. V., Mintzer, J. E., et al. (1999). Comparison of risperidone and placebo for psychosis and behavioral disturbances associated with dementia: A randomized, double-blind trial. *Journal of Clinical Psychiatry, 60,* 107–115.

Katzman, R. (1986). Alzheimer's disease. *New England Journal of Medicine, 314,* 964–973.

Kaufer, D. I., Cummings, J. L., Christine, D. (1996). Effect of tacrine on behavioral symptoms in Alzheimer's disease: An open label study. *Journal of Geriatric Psychiatry and Neurology, 9,* 1–6.

Kelman, H. R., Thomas, C., Kennedy, G. J., et al. (1994). Cognitive impairment and mortality among older community residents. *Journal of the American Public Health Association, 84,* 1255–1260.

Kennedy, G., Hofer, M., Cohen, D., et al. (1987). Significance of depression and cognitive impairment in patients undergoing programmed electrical stimulation of cardiac arrhythmias. *Psychosomatic Medicine, 49,* 410–421.

Knopman, D., Schneider, L. S., Davis, K., et al. (1996). Long term tacrine (Cognex) treatment effects on nursing home placement and mortality: The Tacrine Study Group. *Neurology, 47,* 166–177.

Koenig, S., Gendelman, H. E., Orenstein, J. M., et al. (1986). Detection of AIDS virus in macrophages in brain tissues from AIDS patients with encephalopathy. *Science, 233,* 1089–1093.

Krall, W. J., Srmek, J. J., Cutler, N. K. (1999). Cholinesterase inhibitors: A therapeutic strategy for Alzheimer's disease. *Annals of Pharmacotherapy, 33,* 441–450.

LeBars, P. L., Katz, M. M., Berman, N., et al. (1997). A placebo-controlled double-blind randomized trial of an extract of Ginkgo biloba for dementia. *Journal of the American Medical Association, 278,* 1327–1332.

Levy, M. L. (1998). Cholinergic therapy for Alzheimer's disease. *Annals of Long Term Care, 6,* 92–96.

Light, E., Lebowitz, B. D. (Eds.). (1989). *Alzheimer's disease treatment and family stress: Directions for research.* Rockville, MD: National Institute of Mental Health.

Lilienfeld, D. E., Perl, D. P. (1994). Projected neurodegenerative disease mortality among minorities in the United States, 1990–2040. *Neuroepidemiology, 13*(4),179–186.

Livingston, G., Katona, C. (2000). How useful are cholinesterase inhibitors in the treatment of Alzheimer's disease?: A number needed to treat analysis. *International Journal of Geriatric Psychiatry, 15,* 203–207.

Luis, C. A., Barker, W. W., Gajaraj, K., et al. (1999). Sensitivity and specificity of three clinical criteria for dementia with Lewy bodies in an autopsy-verified sample. *International Journal of Geriatric Psychiatry, 14,* 526–533.

Mace, N. I., Rabins, P. V. (1999). *The 36-hour day.* Baltimore: Johns Hopkins University Press.

Madden, J. J., Luhan, J. A., Kaplan, L. A., et al. (1952). Non-dementing psychoses in older persons. *Journal of the American Medical Association, 150,* 1567–1570.

Magai, C., Cohen, C., Kennedy, G. J., et al. (2000). A controlled clinical trial of sertraline in the treatment of depression in nursing home residents. *American Journal of Geriatric Psychiatry, 8,* 66–75.

Mahendra, B. (1985). Depression and dementia: The multi-faceted relationship. *Psychological Medicine, 15,* 227–236.

Maletta, G. J. (1992). Treatment of behavioral symptomatology of Alzheimer's disease, with emphasis on aggression: Current clinical approaches. *International Psychogeriatrics, 4,* 117–130.

Mattis, S. (1976). Mental status examination for organic mental syndrome in the elderly patient. In L. Bellak & T. B. Karasu (Eds.), *Geriatric psychiatry: A handbook for psychiatrists and primary care physicians* (pp. 79–121). New York: Grune & Stratton.

Mayeux, R., Sano, M. (1999). Treatment of Alzheimer's disease. *New England Journal of Medicine, 341,* 1670–1679.

McGeer, P. L., Schulzer, M., McGeer, E. G. (1996). Arthritis and anti-inflammatory agents as possible protective factors for Alzheimer's disease: A review of 17 epidemiologic studies. *Neurology, 47,* 425–432.

McKeith, L. G., Galasko, D., Kosaka, K., et al. (1996). Consensus guidelines for the clinical and pathologic diagnosis of dementia with Lewy bodies (DLB): Report of the consortium on DLB international workshop. *Neurology, 47,* 1113–1124.

McManus, D. Q., Arvantis, L. A., Kowalcyk, B. B. (1999). Quetiapine, a novel antipsychotic: Experience in elderly patients with psychotic disorders. Seroquel Trial 48 Study Group. *Journal of Clinical Psychiatry, 60*(5), 2992–2998.

Miller, M. D. (1989). Opportunities for psychotherapy in the management of dementia. *Journal of Geriatric Psychiatry and Neurology, 2,* 11–17.

Mittelman, M. S., Ferris, S. H., Shulman, E., et al. (1995). The effects of a multicomponent program on spouse-caregivers of Alzheimer's disease patients: Results of a treatment/control study. In L. L. Heston (Ed.), *Progress in Alzheimer's disease and similar conditions* (pp. 259–270). Washington, DC: American Psychiatric Association Press.

Mohs, R. C., Breitner, J. C. S., Silverman, J. M., et al. (1987). Alzheimer's disease: Morbid risk among first-degree relatives approximates 50% by 90 years of age. *Archives of General Psychiatry, 44,* 405–408.

Molloy, D. W., Alemayehu, E., Roberts, R. (1991). A standardized Mini-Mental State Examination (SMMSE): Its reliability compared to the traditional Mini-Mental State Examination (MMSE). *American Journal of Psychiatry, 148,* 102–105.

Molloy, D. W., Standish T. I. M. (1997). A guide to the standardized Mini-Mental State Examination. *International Psychogeriatrics, 9,* 87–94.

Moody, H. R. (1988). From informed consent to negotiated consent. *Gerontologist, 28,* 64–70.

Nance, M. A. (1998). Huntington disease: Clinical, genetic and social aspects. *Journal of Geriatric Psychiatry and Neurology, 11,* 61–70.

National Institute on Aging. (1998). *Progress report on Alzheimer's disease* (NIH Publication No. 993616). Bethesda, MD: Author.

National Institute on Aging/Alzheimer's Association Working Group. (1996). Apolipoprotein E genotyping in Alzheimer's disease. *Lancet, 347,* 1091–1095.

Nyenhuis, D. L., Gorelick, P. B. (1998). Vascular dementia: A contemporary review of epidemiology, diagnosis, prevention, and treatment. *Journal of the American Geriatrics Society, 46,* 1437–1448.

Overman, W., Stoudemire, A. (1988). Guidelines for legal and financial counseling of Alzheimer's disease patients and their families. *American Journal of Psychiatry, 145,* 1495–1500.

Paganini-Hill, A., Henderson, V. W. (1994). Estrogen replacement and risk of Alzheimer's disease in women. *American Journal of Epidemiology, 140,* 256–261.

Patel, S. V. (1995). Pharmacotherapy of cognitive impairment in Alzheimer's disease: A review. *Journal of Geriatric Psychiatry and Neurology, 8,* 81–95.

Peterson, R., Smith, G., Waring, S., et al. (1999). Mild cognitive impairment: Clinical characterization and outcome. *Archives of Neurology, 56,* 303–308.

Pfeffer, R. I., Kurosaki, T. T., Harrah, C. H. Jr., et al. (1982). Measurement of functional activities in older adults in the community. *Journal of Gerontology, 37,* 323–329.

Rabins, P. V. (1984). Management of dementia in the family context. *Psychosomatics, 25,* 369–375.

Reifler, B. V. (1986). Mixed cognitive-affective disturbances in the elderly: A new classification. *Journal of Clinical Psychiatry, 47,* 354–356.

Reifler, B. V., Larson, E. (1988). Excess disability in demented elderly outpatients: The rule of halves. *Journal of the American Geriatrics Society, 36,* 82–83.

Richards, M., Touchon, J., Ledesert, B., et al. (1999). Cognitive decline in aging: Are AAMI and AACD distinct entities? *International Journal of Geriatric Psychiatry, 14,* 534–540.

Rogers, S. L., Friedhof, L. T., Apter, J. T., et al. (1996). The efficacy and safety of donepezil in patients with Alzheimer's disease: Results of a U.S. multicenter, randomized, double-blind, placebo controlled trial. *Dementia, 7,* 293–303.

Rogers, J., Kirby, L. C., Hempleman, S. R., et al. (1993). Clinical trial of indomethacin in Alzheimer's disease. *Neurology, 43,* 1609–1611.

Rösler, M., Anand, R., Cicin-Sain, A., et al. (1999). Efficacy and safety of rivastigmine in patients with Alzheimer's disease: International randomized controlled trial. *British Medical Journal, 318,* 633–638.

Sano, M., Ernesto, C., Thomas, R. G., et al. (1997). A controlled trial of selegiline, alpha-tocopherol, or both as treatment or Alzheimer's disease. *New England Journal of Medicine, 336,* 1216–1222.

Semenchuk, M. R., Labiner, D. M. (1997). Gabapentin and lamotrigine: Prescribing guidelines for psychiatry. *Journal of Practical Psychiatry and Behavioral Health, 3,* 334–342.

Small, G. W., Rabins, P. V., Barry, P. P., et al. (1997). Diagnosis and treatment of Alzheimer disease and related disorders. *Journal of the American Medical Association, 278,* 1363–1371.

Solomon, P. R., Hirschoff, A., Kelly, B., et al. (1998). A 7-minute neurocognitive screening battery highly sensitive to Alzheimer's disease. *Archives of Neurology, 55,* 349–355.

Stahelin, H. B., Monsch, A. U., Spiegel, R. (1997). Early diagnosis of dementia via a two-step screening and diagnostic procedure. *International Psychogeriatrics, 9,* 123–130.

Street, J. S. (1999, August 15–20). *The role of atypical antipsychotic agents in Alzheimer's disease.* Abstract presented at the Ninth Congress of the International Psychogeriatric Association, Vancouver, British Columbia, Canada.

Tanzi, R. E., Gusella, J. F., Watkins, P. C., et al. (1987). Amyloid beta protein gene: cDNA, mRNA distribution, and genetic linkage near the Alzheimer locus. *Science, 235,* 880–884.

Tariot, P. N. (1999). Treatment of agitation in dementia. *Journal of Clinical Psychiatry, 60*(Suppl. 8), 11–20.

Teri, L. (1997). Assessment and treatment of neuropsychiatric signs and symptoms in cognitively impaired older adults: Guidelines for practitioners. *Seminars in Clinical Neuropsychiatry, 2,* 152–158.

Teri, L., Logsdon, R., Uomoto, J., et al. (1997). Behavioral treatment of depression in dementia: A controlled trial. *Journals of Gerontology, 32B*, P159–P166.

Teri, L., Rabins, P., Whitehouse, P., et al. (1992a). Management of behavior disturbance in Alzheimer disease: Current knowledge and future directions. *Alzheimer Disease and Associated Disorders, 6*, 77–88.

Teri, L., Truax, P., Logsdon, R., et al. (1992b). Assessment of behavioral problems in dementia: The revised memory and behavioral problems checklist. *Psychology and Aging, 7*, 622–631.

Vellas, B., Inglis, F., Potkin, S., et al. (1998). Interim results from an international clinical trial with rivastigmine evaluating a 2-week titration rate in mild to severe Alzheimer's disease patients. *International Journal of Geriatric Psychopharmacology, 1*, 140–144.

Wragg, R. E., Jeste, V. D. (1989). Overview of depression and psychosis in Alzheimer's disease. *American Journal of Psychiatry, 146*, 577–587.

4

Psychosis and Mania

Treatment options for psychotic disorders and mania have improved considerably in the last decade, offering a more optimistic prognosis. The observation that deterioration following psychosis is not inevitable has brought about new enthusiasm for both treatment and research. But the similarities between late-onset schizophrenia, delusional disorder, mania, and the psychoses of depression, dementia, and stroke can make the diagnosis difficult among older adults. Compounding the diagnostic problem is the overlap between the psychotic disorders and psychotic episodes seen in individuals with personality disorders who are transiently overwhelmed by stressful events. Although a psychiatric consultant is often required, primary care personnel should know how to evaluate and treat the common manifestations of psychosis. They should be able to distinguish disabling disorders from benign, transient states and the shared expressions of cultural or religious groups which may exceed the provider's experience. With skill and perseverance, the practitioner will be able to help the patient preserve relationships and secure needed care even though insight and judgment may not be fully restored. Table 4.1 lists diagnostic criteria for the psychoses and mania. Table 4.2 summarizes differential diagnosis and treatment.

ACHIEVING AND SUSTAINING THE ALLIANCE

The practitioner's priority is an alliance with the patient, family, or third party who identified the problem. Denial and lack of insight do not preclude a working relationship. Delusional persons are accustomed to disbelief. The practitioner's willingness to understand the pa-

TABLE 4.1. Diagnostic Criteria for Psychotic Disorders and Manic Episodes

Schizophrenia

A. Symptoms
- Positive symptoms (delusions, hallucinations)
- Disorganized speech (derailment, incoherence)
- Disorganized or catatonic behavior
- Negative symptoms (flat affect, impoverished speech and interests)

B. Social and occupational dysfunction
C. 6-month duration including prodrome

Paranoid Type

A. Preoccupation with delusions or auditory hallucinations
B. Absence of
- Disorganized speech
- Catatonic or disorganized behavior
- Disturbance in affect

Schizophreniform disorder

A. Criteria for schizophrenia (but with recovery)
B. Duration at least 1 but not more than 6 months

Schizoaffective disorder

A. Symptoms of schizophrenia
B. Hallucinations or delusions present for 2 weeks without mood disturbance
C. Meets criteria for mood disorder for substantial period
D. Type: Bipolar or depressive

Delusional disorder

A. False beliefs not of a shared cultural or religious origin
B. Capacity for self-care preserved
C. Impairment in social activities and personal relations
D. Other symptoms of psychosis absent

Brief psychotic disorder

A. Symptoms of schizophrenia (but with recovery)
B. Duration at least 1 day but less than 1 month

Shared psychotic disorder (folie à deux)

A. One person's delusion infects a close associate
B. The delusions are shared and similar

Psychotic disorder due to general medical condition

A. Prominent delusions or hallucinations
B. Medical disorder is the direct physiological cause
C. Is not a manifestation of delirium

(*continued on next page*)

TABLE 4.1. (*continued*)

Substance-induced psychotic disorder

A. Prominent delusions or hallucinations
B. Substance (most often prescribed or over-the-counter medication) is the direct physiological cause
C. Is not a manifestation of delirium

Manic episode

A. Mood is persistently and abnormally elevated, irritable, or expansive for at least 1 week. Either psychosis or severe social impairment is present.
B. Three of the following are present during the episode (four if irritability only)
   • Grandiose or inflated self-regard
   • Decreased need for sleep
   • Loquacious, pressured speech
   • Flight of ideas, racing thoughts
   • Distractible
   • Agitation, increased goal-directed activity
   • Increased pursuit of pleasures with high self-destructive potential
C. Symptoms are not substance induced or due to delirium

Hypomanic episode

A. Mood is persistently and abnormally elevated, irritable, or expansive for at least 4 days duration
B. Same number and kind of symptoms as for manic episode
C. Symptoms represent an unequivocal, uncharacteristic and socially disruptive change in behavior
D. Resulting impairment is not markedly disruptive nor associated with psychosis

Note. Adapted from American Psychiatric Association (1994). Copyright 1994 by the American Psychiatric Association. Adapted by permission.

tient's perspective may offer welcome relief to persons who have been subjected to ridicule. At the same time, pathologically suspicious patients are wary of intimacy often despite painful loneliness. They need trust, and trust cannot be established merely by good intentions or professional status. Demonstrated reliability, availability, and respect for the person's individuality are more likely to serve than exaggerated empathy. Tact and tolerance will allow sufficient trust to sustain the diagnosis and treatment process. Accepting the delusions or hallucinations as real will only provoke suspicion. The practitioner need not agree with the delusions or verbally acknowledge the presence of hallucinations. Better to accept the psychotic perceptions as evidence of a need for assistance. Directive, confrontational efforts to correct the false beliefs of delusions or to categorically deny the reality of hallucinations will only provoke resentment.

The patient's agenda rarely includes correction of false beliefs or perceptions. However, it is possible to identify distressing issues with the patient and third party, form a consensus, and share plans to reduce the problem. For example, with the delusional person who is convinced that the landlord is piping poison gas into the apartment via the radiator, it may be sufficient to reply, "I may not be able to fight the landlord for you but I can see how stressful the situation is for you. Let me give you something to reduce the effects of the stress so you can manage your [insomnia, nerves, depression] better." Similarly, the husband whose jealous delusions lead to threats against his wife may agree to medication to avoid loss of control and separation. Focusing on the physical effects of the distress may also allow for diagnostic studies needed to identify reversible contributors to the disturbance including impaired vision or hearing, polypharmacy, endocrine or metabolic disorder, undetected central nervous system disease, or neoplasm. Once patient and practitioner agree on a therapeutic target, interventions and contributing factors may be explored.

Changes in the patient's circumstances may bring a long-standing but previously hidden problem to the practitioner's attention. Invested, caring family or neighbors may have sheltered the person throughout life, compensating for the interpersonal deficits which become apparent only when the social network fails due to death, disability, or illness. Alternatively, the patient may have managed independently until needs for personal assistance or invasive medical procedures unsettle a fragile sense of security. The practitioner's foresight and efforts to restore equilibrium are basic to success with all the psychotic disorders.

Gaining permission from the patient to share the results of diagnostic procedures and treatment recommendations with other concerned parties sets the groundwork for future collaboration. Providing a clear expectation that "we work as a team" avoids the perceived threat of betrayed confidence. Teamwork is also critical to clinical efficiency. Particularly when disturbances in judgment or impulse control are expected, initial networking with team members will seem time well spent when crises arise. Family and other involved parties need information and guidance to realistically cope with the patient's difficulties. They should be made aware that complete insight is an unrealistic goal but greater social compatibility and independence are not. Delusions that do not interfere with care or personal well-being and do not overtly distress others around the patient may be left alone. Some family members or associates of the patient will take the accusations as a personal affront or feel compelled to convince the patient of their falsity. This is particularly difficult with late-onset psychosis which is typically insidious, not terribly bizarre, and does not cause obvious disability. It is difficult indeed to be forgiving when one's best efforts

TABLE 4.2. Differential Diagnosis and Treatment of Psychosis and Mania in Late Life

Diagnosis	Distinguishing features	Psychosocial interventions	Biomedical interventions
Delirium	Sudden onset, variable attention span, signs of systemic illness, visual or tactile hallucinations	Reality orientation, reassurance	Reversal of systemic illness, p.r.n. use of low-dose typical antipsychotic
Dementia	Insidious onset, attention span unimpaired, distorted beliefs and perceptions usually reactive but may be persistent, presence of aphasia, apraxia	Validation therapy rather than reality orientation, behavioral interventions and environmental alterations by staff or family	Address vision or hearing deficits, low-dose atypical antipsychotic
Stroke	Sudden onset, right hemisphere signs, apraxia	Reassurance, reality orientation	Supportive care, p.r.n. use of low-dose typical antipsychotic
Seizure disorder	Sudden onset of behavioral change, most often associated with stroke or dementia	Reassurance, education	Rule out space-occupying lesion or toxic etiology; antiepileptic drug
Personality (paranoid, narcissistic, schizotypal) disorder	Paranoid accusations, usual lifelong history of interpersonal difficulties may be compensated for by family or associates, recent stress event	Empathic focus on consequences of behavior, patient needs, and respons-ibilities rather than apportionment of blame or justification of feelings; psychotherapy during periods of stress	Episodic rather than continued use of atypical antipsychotic or antidepressant during periods of stress
Early-onset schizophrenia	Onset in early adulthood, negative symptoms, residual signs of illness and disability	Supportive, directive care with case management, vocational and psychosocial rehabilitation, family counseling	Atypical antipsychotic, antidepressant, or mood stabilizer if indicated
Late-onset schizophrenia	Most often delusional, decline in self-care	Supportive, directive care, with case management, family counseling	Low-dose atypical antipsychotic, antidepressant, or mood stabilizer if indicated
Delusional disorder	Adequate occupational attainment, intellect and self-care intact, absence of hallucinations	Empathic, supportive rather than reality orientation, family counseling	Low-dose atypical antipsychotic, antidepressant, or mood stabilizer if indicated
Early-onset mania (bipolar mood disorder, manic type)	Mood disorder characterized by recovery and relapse, satisfactory interpersonal and occupational attainment, grandiose, irritability, poor judgment	Psychotherapy and education for patient and family focused on maintaining medication, social relations, problem solving	Mood stabilizer or lithium may require typical antipsychotic or electroconvulsive therapy

(continued)

TABLE 4.2. (*continued*)

Diagnosis	Distinguishing features	Psychosocial interventions	Biomedical interventions
Late-onset mania	Most often associated with stroke, dementia, hyperthyroidism, or induced by medication; may be exacerbation of unrecognized early-onset bipolar disorder	Psychotherapy and education for patient and family focused on maintaining medication, social relations, problem solving	Definitive treatment of underlying condition (hyperthyroidism, hypertension), mood stabilizer (avoid lithium), may require typical antipsychotic, electroconvulsive therapy
Psychotic depression	Prominent mood disturbance, somatic or paranoid delusions	Psychotherapy and education to maintain medication and interpersonal relationships	Combined antidepressant with antipsychotic, electroconvulsive therapy
Drug-induced psychosis in Parkinson's disease	Hallucinations, delusions emerging after treatment with levodopa	Caregiver counseling	Reduce levodopa to lowest effective dose, low-dose clozapine with white cell monitoring, or quetiapine or olanzapine
Adjustment or stress reaction with psychosis	Sudden onset, clear precipitant	Supportive psychotherapy, reassurance	Short-term course of atypical antipsychotic
Benign hallucinosis	Illusory perceptual distortion usually with impaired vision or hearing, not associated with social impairment	Reassurance, family support, avoid stigma of psychotic or dementing disorder	Do not medicate unless associated depression or anxiety disorder is present
Cultural or religious beliefs outside the practitioner's experience	Shared, common part of identifiable social group rather than an individual eccentricity	Avoid stigmatizing patient as mentally ill	Do not medicate unless associated depression or anxiety disorder is present

Note. Typical antipsychotics include haloperidol, fluphenazine, thioridazine; atypical antipsychotics include risperidone, olanzapine, quetiapine, and clozapine.

result in ungrounded insults of malicious intent. Yet families are remarkably resourceful and resilient. Family therapy, the cornerstone of psychotherapeutic work in the psychoses, should be directed at understanding strengths and how to shore up the caring relationship. It may be impossible to resolve long-standing conflicts. But mediation can nonetheless restore a working equilibrium.

THE SCHIZOPHRENIAS

Although the burden of dementia is substantial, the premature mortality and total years lost in personal productivity and autonomy make schizophrenia the most devastating mental illness of adult life. The prevalence is 1% in both the developed and developing nations. Close to 2 million people are treated for the illness every year with upward of 100,000 in hospitals every day. Sixty percent of affected individuals will receive disability benefits within the first year of onset. Ten percent will suicide within that first year. The majority of those who survive will neither marry nor have children (Andreasen, 1999). For patients young or old, the critical elements of successful treatment are a comprehensive, individualized approach including medication, family support, and education and aggressive case management outreach known as assertive community management for persons at high risk for hospitalization. Although 90% of persons with schizophrenia receive antipsychotic medication, only 50% receive the recommended array of psychosocial and rehabilitative services. Failure to add an antidepressant for depressive episodes and to provide for psychosocial treatments (family intervention, therapeutic day programs) are the most frequent inadequacies. States vary in the availability of therapeutic programs. Yet the failure to treat depression, which is no less common in persons with schizophrenia than in anyone else, should be more easily remedied (Lehman et al., 1998).

Until recently, schizophrenia was seen as an illness starting in the young adult years. Social and intellectual deterioration were inevitable. By late life the prevalence of schizophrenia in the community was thought to be less than 1% as a result of premature mortality and premature dementia resulting in nursing home admission. More recent data suggest that schizophrenic psychoses are more prevalent in late life but do not inevitably lead to dementia (Jeste et al., 1997; Rabins et al., 1997). A number of clinical scientists now argue that schizophrenia has a distinct late-onset form occurring between ages 45 and 65 (Castle et al., 1997). Although most cases of schizophrenia in males occur in the second and third decades of life, the illness demonstrates a bimodal age of onset among women with a significant second peak occurring in the menopausal years (Jeste et al., 1997; Häfner, 1997). The loss of initiative and blunted emotionality persist; delusions and hallucinations diminish with age. The result is a more varied course including return of capacity for independent living in a significant minority of persons in middle age (Cohen, 1995). Nonetheless, older persons with schizophrenia experience a quality of life similar to that of dementia patients and generate increased health care costs compared to their younger peers (Cuffel et al., 1997).

Late-onset schizophrenia resembles early-onset disease in several ways. The positive symptoms are more prominent in women and impairments in visual and auditory processing are common, as is a family history of psychosis and a personal history of adjustment problems in childhood. Sensory impairments, particularly hearing difficulties which were thought to contribute to the onset of paranoia, may be the result of difficulty acquiring and accommodating to glasses and hearing aids as a result of the illness. The overall pattern of cognitive impairment is similar in early- and late-onset disease as are findings of nonspecific white matter and ventricular abnormalities on brain MRI. The course is persistent, and mortality is increased. Late-onset disease is more frequent in women, shows less severe negative symptoms, and is mostly delusional and paranoid in character. Also, impairments in learning, abstraction, and cognitive flexibility are not as severe. Most important, favorable responses are obtained at lower doses of antipsychotics, although full remission of symptoms is rare.

In summary, schizophrenia in old age is more prevalent than previously thought. Incident cases may appear after age 45, and the cost of care may have been underestimated. Most older patients remain symptomatic but are not demented and generally reside in community settings rather than nursing homes. Symptoms may be reduced with lower doses of antipsychotics than would be required in early life. However, the prevalence of tardive dyskinesia approaches 50% within 24 months of typical antipsychotic treatment representing a fivefold increase over that which is seen in younger persons. Hence, the atypical antipsychotics at low doses are clearly preferred.

DELUSIONAL DISORDER

In delusional (paranoid) disorder, false beliefs and inferences seriously impair social judgment and cannot be interpreted as originating from religious or cultural group norms. Pathological suspiciousness, jealousy, exaggerated self-regard, and erotic obsession are the most frequent manifestations. Most aspects of personality and cognitive performance remain intact. However, failure to pay bills, failure to attend to physical illness or disability, and accusations against others for which there is next to no basis in fact bring these people to the attention of social service agencies. Antipsychotic medication will in most instances substantially restore the person's capacity to manage, but only one in four will abandon the delusions and gain clear insight into their difficulties (Rabins, Pearlson, 1994).

MANIA

Late-onset mania is often misdiagnosed and as a result is likely to be more common than previously reported (Tariot et al., 1993). The presentation is more complex and less typical of classical bipolar (manic–depressive) illness. Diagnostic certainty is often clouded by the presence of cognitive impairment, suggesting dementia. Late-onset mania is more often secondary or closely associated in etiology to other medical disorders, most commonly stroke, dementia, or hyperthyroidism but also medications including antidepressants, steroids, estrogens, and other agents with known central nervous system properties (Young et al., 1997). A search for treatable components that contribute acutely to the person's disability should be pursued. Risk factors for cerebrovascular disease, including excessive use of alcohol, tobacco, suboptimal control of hypertension, diabetes, and other cardiovascular risk factors, should be explored.

The work-up will also identify indicators, such as structural brain changes or dementia, that assist in longer-term prognosis. The prognosis is generally less favorable than for earlier-onset mania. A careful history from family or friends may uncover repeated hypomanic episodes which did not seriously impair the individual but in retrospect are clear indicators of early-onset disease. The difficulties in recognizing the diagnosis, contributing conditions, age-related vulnerability to medication side effects, and frequency with which structural brain changes are associated all make treatment more difficult. Structural brain changes most frequently include subcortical hyperintensities seen on MRI (McDonald et al., 1991).

Late-onset mania is more frequently seen among men than women. The manic episode often presents with confusion, disorientation, distractibility, and irritability rather than elevated, positive mood. Conversely, the clinical interview may be characterized by irrelevant content delivered with an argumentative, intense yet fluent quality. Patently unrealistic plans concerning finances or travel, exaggerated self-regard, and contentious claims to certainty in the face of evidence to the contrary are also seen. The statements may be plausible rather than bizarre but are too improbable to be real. The unsuspecting examiner is often puzzled by the difficulty of the interchange until the diagnosis of mania is considered.

The presence of psychosis, sleep disturbance, and aggressiveness, particularly in the nursing home, may suggest dementia or depressive disorder rather than mania. Because mania in late life is genuinely less frequent than depression or dementia and less frequently recognized, these patients are most often treated with antipsychotics, antidepressants, or benzodiazepines which provide only partial relief. The mood stabilizers (antiepileptics) are preferred but their superiority has not been definitively established for late-onset bipolar illness or the mania that emerges following stroke or dementia.

The Lithium Problem

Although seniors who have experienced good results with lithium should not be switched to an alternative, a number of concerns argue against lithium for the initiation of treatment. Advanced age, absence of family history of bipolar disorder, and mania secondary to another medical condition, particularly stroke or dementia, all predict poor response to lithium. Because lithium is cleared by the kidneys, the age-related decline in renal function means older adults are at increased risk of toxicity. Structural brain changes which may not be clinically apparent are associated with higher risk of lithium intolerance. Finally, interactions with psychotropics and other medications which are less dangerous and less common in younger patients complicate the use of lithium in older adults. Clearly, the appearance of toxicity warrants a change to other agents. Other indicators which should be checked at least annually in patients treated with lithium include fasting blood sugar, thyroid function, creatinine clearance, blood urea nitrogen, and electrolytes. Worsening diabetes, thyroid status, congestive heart failure or arrhythmia, and psoriasis are among the more frequent nonemergency reasons for change to alternative treatment (McDonald & Nemeroff, 1996).

Signs of lithium toxicity include gastrointestinal complaints, ataxia, slurred speech, delirium, or coma and may occur even when the plasma level is below the conventional therapeutic range of 1.0 mEq/liter in the elderly. However, mild tremor and nystagmus frequently accompany lithium treatment and should not be considered signs of toxicity. Toxicity will predictably result when dehydration due to fever, vomiting, diarrhea, or sweating reduces the extracellular volume of distribution because lithium is reabsorbed in preference to sodium. Renal failure, diuretics, reduced intake of salt or fluids, and concomitant use of nonsteroidal anti-inflammatory agents—excepting aspirin and sulindac—increase the risk of toxicity (Rahgeb, 1990). Long-lasting cerebellar dysfunction is the most common neurological sequelae of lithium toxicity, although dementia, parkinsonism, peripheral neuropathies, and brainstem symptoms have also been reported (Verdoux & Bourgeois 1990). Cautious rehydration will counter suspected lithium toxicity, which may be prolonged before the patient's mental status clears. In acute renal failure, dialysis or forced saline diuresis will be required (Parfrey et al., 1983).

Pharmacological Treatment of Mania

Although antipsychotics are frequently prescribed for mania, there is a growing consensus that anticonvulsants, called mood stabilizers in this context, are preferable both for acute treatment and for the prevention of recurrence in late-life mania and bipolar disorder (Keck et al., 1992) (see Table 4.3). The anticonvulsant valproic acid is increasingly considered first choice for augmentation of antidepressant therapy, treatment, and prevention of mania. A therapeutic level is available and although hepatic toxicity is a risk, it is infrequent. Valproic acid inhibits hepatic enzymes that metabolize a variety of medications in frequent use by older adults. Patients taking beta-blockers, type 1C antiarrhythmics, benzodiazepines, or anticoagulants may be prescribed valproic acid but should be monitored more closely until the dose is stabilized. Although valproic acid is preferred, there will be a delay in its antimanic effects. Persons whose manic excitement is extreme or dangerous will require an antipsychotic. Although weight gain and hyperglycemia are drawbacks, controlled trials suggest that olanzapine will be helpful either singly or in combination with a mood stabilizer for acute mania (Tohen et al., 1999; Sharma & Pistor, 1999). It is also FDA approved for that purpose.

Gabapentin and lamotrigine are recently introduced medications approved for the treatment of epilepsy. There is considerable enthusiasm but limited data on their use as mood stabilizers in late-life mania, depression, or psychosis (Semenchuk & Labiner, 1997). Their low rate of drug interactions, protein binding, freedom from the need to monitor therapeutic levels or liver toxicity, and unique clearance make them particularly attractive (Knoll et al., 1998; Ghaemi et al., 1998; Sussman, 1998).

ANTIPSYCHOTICS AND THE AVOIDANCE OF MOVEMENT DISORDERS

Practitioners will encounter older persons with histories of psychosis throughout adult life and decades of typical antipsychotic administration (see Table 4.4), most frequently haloperidol, perphenezine, and thioridazine. There are two limitations of typical antipsychotics: (1) They are not uniformly effective and, (2) they reliably induce movement disorders as the dose and duration of administration are increased. Movement disorders emerge spontaneously with advanced age but are rarely disabling unless they evolve into Parkinson's disease or represent drug-induced pseudo-parkinsonism (Jeste et al., 1999). Although the typical antipsychotics are the most frequent cause of pseudo-parkinsonism, the SSRIs and on occasion the TCAs have also been implicated.

The drug-induced movement disorders are a direct result of dopa-

TABLE 4.3. Agents Used to Stabilize Mood, or to Combat Mania or Aggression in Late Life

Generic name	Trade name	Initial dose (mg)	Final dose (mg)	Sedative potential	Precautions	Advantages
Benzodiazepines						
Clonazepam	*Klonopin*	0.5 b.i.d.	5 b.i.d.	Moderate	Prolonged T½, falls, controlled substance, may exacerbate aggression or confusion in dementia	Rapid onset, fewer drug interactions, sedation
Lithium compounds						
Lithium carbonate	*Eskalith*	300 daily	300 t.i.d.	Low	Renal clearance is sole route of elimination, toxicity may appear below therapeutic range; tremor is a benign universal side effect; nausea, vomiting are signs of toxicity; risk of hypothryoidism	Patient preference, otherwise none; therapeutic level 0.6–1.2 mEq/liter
Controlled release	*Eskalith CR*	450 daily	450 b.i.d.			
Anticonvulsants						
Sodium valproate	*Depakote*	250 b.i.d.	1,000 b.i.d.	Moderate	Delayed onset of action, drug interactions, GI upset, tremor, weight gain, edema, thrombocytopenia; CBC and chemistries at baseline, then every 6 months; inhibits hepatic enzymes and increases other drug levels	Better tolerated than carbamazepine; therapeutic level 50–100 µg/ml
Carbamazepine	*Tegretol Epitol*	100 b.i.d.	500 b.i.d.	Moderate	Delayed onset of action, drug interactions, dizziness, unsteady gait; CBC and chemistries at baseline, then every 6 months; enhances cytochrome P450 activity and decreases other drug levels	Therapeutic level 4–12 µg/ml
Gabapentin	*Neurontin*	200 h.s.	900 t.i.d.	Moderate	Wholly dependent on renal clearance for elimination, therapeutic range not established, little experience in the elderly	Not protein bound, liver toxicity and drug interactions unlikely
Lamotrigine	*Lamictal*	25 h.s.	200 daily	Moderate	Prolonged half-life, appearance of rash calls for immediate cessation, therapeutic range not established, little used in the elderly	Does not alter P450 activity, drug interactions unlikely

Note. Abbreviations as in earlier tables.

95

TABLE 4.4. Selected Antipsychotics for Older Adults

Generic name	Trade name	Initial dose (mg)	Final dose (mg)	Movement disorders potential[a]	Hypotensive potential	Sedative potential	Precautions	Advantages
Sedative antipsychotics								
Thioridazine	*Mellaril*	10	100	Low	Dose-related	Moderate to high	Hypotensive and amnestic as dose increases, quinidine-like effects	Available as liquid, no EPS, sedative
Nonsedative antipsychotics								
Perphenazine	*Trilafon*	2	16	High	Low	Low	EPS, TD likely as dose increases, increases TCA level	Available as liquid and i.m. injection
Haloperidol	*Haldol*	0.5	20	High	Low	Low	EPS, TD likely as dose increases	Available as liquid, i.m. and i.v. injection
Fluphenazine	*Prolixin*	0.5	20	High	Low	Low	EPS, TD likely as dose increases	Available as liquid and i.m. injection
Extended-release antipsychotics								
Haloperidol decanoate	*Haldol decanoate*	12.5 i.m. every 14–28 days	200 i.m. every 28 days	Moderate	Low	Low	i.m. injection every 28 days, 90 days to steady state	Less EPS than oral, compliance
Fluphenazine enanthate	*Prolixin enanthate*	12.5 i.m. every 7–14 days	50 i.m. every 14–21 days	Moderate	Low	Low	i.m. injection every 14–21 days, 1:1 equivalence to oral dose, 20 days to steady state	Less EPS than oral, compliance
Atypical antipsychotics								
Risperidone	*Risperdal*	0.25	6	Low for TD, moderate for EPS	Moderate, dose-related	Moderate	EPS likely at doses above 2 mg; high potency; cost	Available in liquid form; depot form in development
Olanzapine	*Zyprexa*	2.5	15	Low	Moderate	Moderate	Anticholinergic as dose increases, high cost, hypoglycemia, weight gain	May produce less EPS, TD; FDA approved for acute mania
Quetiapine	*Seroquel*	25	750	Low	Moderate	More than moderate	Slit lamp exam for cataracts	Sedative, no anticholinergic effects, less EPS, TD
Clozapine	*Clozaril*	6.25	50	Low	Moderate	Moderate	Monitor WBC weekly, withdraw drug if less than 3,000, anticholinergic	Proven benefit for patients with idiopathic Parkinson's disease

Note. EPS, extrapyramidal (parkinsonian) symptoms; TD, tardive dyskinesia; i.m., intramuscular; i.v., intravenous.
[a]Acute dystonias are rare in the elderly but acute extrapyramidal (parkinsonian) symptoms and delayed tardive dyskinesias are frequent particularly with prolonged use of nonsedating antipsychotics.

mine receptor D_2 blockade and take on several forms. Acute painful dystonias are rare in the elderly. They emerge within hours of typical neuroleptic treatment, respond quite well to intramuscular diphenhydramine, and tend not to recur. Akithisia is a jittery, restless feeling which may be difficult to distinguish from anxiety but grows worse as the medication dose is increased. The onset of drug-induced parkinsonism (extrapyramidal side effects) with typical neuroleptics is dose related. It can be alleviated with anticholinergic medications, but these agents pose problems for older adults whose cholinergic tone is reduced by age or other medications with anticholinergic properties such as the TCAs.

Tardive dyskinesia follows longer-term treatment with typical neuroleptics. It may be irreversible even when the medication is stopped or an atypical is substituted. Compared to younger patients, older adults have a three- to fivefold increased risk of tardive dyskinesia (Woerner et al., 1998). Spasticity of the tongue and lips and writhing movements of the trunk may be observed and can be disfiguring if not disabling. Movement disorders can be minimized by limiting the choice of neuroleptics to the atypicals: olanzapine, risperdone, and quetiapine. The atypicals exhibit less dopamine D_2 receptor antagonism and more serotonin 5-HT2-receptor antagonism than do typical neuroleptics. The lesser D_2 blockade and different balance of dopaminergic to serotoninergic antagonism relative to typical antipsychotics results in less extrapyramidal symptoms (Cummings, 1999). Thioridazine is less likely to provoke extrapyramidal side effects and irreversible movement disorders but will lower blood pressure and impair balance as the dose is increased (Liu et al., 1998). Movement disorders are frequently seen but are usually not disabling with low doses of haloperidol and perphenazine. Thus if symptoms are well controlled and the movement disorder does not impair function or appearance, patient and practitioner may prefer not to change to the newer atypical antipsychotics, which are costly. If cost is a concern and treatment will be short term, the typical neuroleptics are acceptable.

However if treatment becomes long term, an atypical should be substituted by cross-tapering. The typical neuroleptic is reduced by 25% every 3 to 4 days until only 25% of the original dose remains. At that point the atypical is introduced at lowest dose. In 3 to 4 days the atypical is increased and the typical is eliminated. The practitioner further increases the atypical based on the recurrence of symptoms, most typically sleep disturbance. For example, to cross-taper from 2 mg haloperidol to risperidone, one would reduce the haloperidol by 0.5 mg every 3 to 4 days until the patient is taking 0.5 mg, at which point

25 mg risperidone is introduced. The haloperidol is eliminated 3 to 4 days later and the patient is observed. If sleep becomes disturbed or signs of the psychosis exacerbate, the risperidone is increased to 0.5 mg with further increases depending on the emergence or persistence of symptoms.

When psychosis occurs late in life as a delusional disorder or complication of dementia or as a brief reaction within the context of personality disorder, the more costly atypical antipsychotics risperidone, olanzapine, or quetiapine may be preferable for frail seniors who may not tolerate the sedative or hypotensive effects of thioridazine. Parsa and Bastani (1998) recommend quetiapine for the treatment of psychosis in Parkinson's disease to avoid worsening bradykinesia seen with typical antipsychotics and at doses of 2 mg or more with risperidone. Olanzapine may also be a good choice for the same reasons. Clozapine, the first atypical antipsychotic medication, does not induce movement disorders. At doses given to young persons with schizophrenia, it is anticholinergic and induces agranulocytosis in as many as 2% of patients. However, the Parkinson Study Group (1999) found that low doses (6.25–50 mg) given to older patients with levodopa-induced psychosis significantly reduced psychosis and tremor without impairing cognition. White blood cell (WBC) counts were monitored weekly and only 2 patients out of more than 60 were withdrawn for leukopenia (WBC = 2,900–3,000) which resolved after clozapine was stopped. Thus despite its side effect profile, clozapine, at low doses with WBC monitoring may be beneficial for a small but clearly defined set of older patients.

When psychosis arises out of delirium and requires treatment to manage dangerous behavior (agitation, pulling out i.v. lines), haloperidol remains the safest choice due to its relative freedom from cardiovascular side effects. There are insufficient data available to recommend the atypical antipsychotics for psychotic depression. The complex pattern of receptor blockade (dopaminergic, serotonergic, cholinergic) brought about by the atypicals raises questions about their use with antidepressants possessing significant serotonergic or anticholinergic properties (Muller-Siechender et al., 1998). Most reports indicate that a tricylic plus a typical antipsychotic are preferable (Coryell, 1998). However favorable reports combining an atypical with other agents to treat psychotic depression are emerging but not in exclusively geriatric samples (Rothchild et al., 1999). Recent controlled trials found both venlafaxine and fluvoxamine effective as a single drug therapy (Zanardi et al., 2000).

Haloperidol, perphenazine, thioridazine, and risperidone are all available as liquid concentrates, which allows for precise dose titration and ease of administration. Some patients will not reliably accept oral medication and prefer long-acting injectible antipsychotic medication from a visiting nurse or clinic staff. However, an injectible antipsychotic is no substitute for an ongoing trusting relationship. The prolonged half-life Haldol decanoate means that efforts to stabilize the patient's symptoms with an initial injection of 12.5 to 25 mg and subsequent monthly increases will take time. Long-acting injectible antipsychotics are more profitably used upon discharge from an inpatient admission in which symptoms have been controlled with oral medication. Haldol decanoate is given by deep intramuscular injection every 28 days at 50 times the daily oral dose which stabilized the psychosis. For a daily oral dose of 1 mg, the every-28-day Haldol decanoate injection would be 50 mg. The total dose should not exceed 200 mg every 28 days.

ELECTROCONVULSIVE THERAPY FOR MANIA OR PSYCHOSIS

It is important to recognize that electroconvulsive therapy has a long history in the treatment of mania and psychotic depression and may be indicated for the severely disturbed older psychotic patient when agitation or the threat of violence becomes extreme. Age-related factors increase the value of ECT for geriatric mental disorders (Myers et al., 1984). It may be particularly useful in cases of medication inefficacy or intolerance, psychotic depression, imminent suicidal risk, or morbid nutritional status (Coryell, 1998). Advanced age, concurrent antidepressants, and cardiovascular compromise increase the risk of adverse reactions, with cardiovascular complications being the most frequent events. The cognitive impairment associated with ECT includes temporary postictal confusion, transient anterograde or retrograde amnesia, and less commonly permanent amnestic syndrome in which events surrounding the treatment are forgotten. Treatments may be limited to twice weekly and applied unilaterally to the nondominant hemisphere to minimize confusion. However, bilateral treatment may be more effective (Sackeim et al., 1993). Single-treatment maintenance ECT can be administered as an outpatient procedure in ambulatory surgery settings over intervals of several weeks to months and may offer higher rates of sustained recovery.

SUMMARY

Psychosis impairs the patient's capacity to make health decisions and to maintain personal relations and social connections. Persons whose perceptions, beliefs, and decisional capacities are impaired by psychosis require the practitioner's insight and empathy to obtain the care they so clearly need. Their families need support and acknowledgment of the caregiving burden. A trustworthy, matter-of-fact approach targeted to immediate needs and concrete goals will alleviate distress and ultimately help the person not to act on hallucinations or delusions. Antipsychotics and mood stabilizers will be beneficial once an alliance has been formed. Forging a lasting, workable alliance with the patient, family, and other caregivers, despite denial and lack of insight, is one of the more satisfying aspects of clinical practice.

For consumer information and advocacy contact:

The National Alliance for the Mentally Ill (NAMI), 200 North Glebe Road, Suite 1015, Arlington, VA 22203; Phone: 703-524-7600, 800-950-NAMI; *www.nami.org*.

The National Depressive and Manic–Depressive Association (NDMDA), 730 North Franklin Street, Suite 501, Chicago, IL, 60610-7243; Phone: 312-642-0049, 800-82-NDMDA; fax: 312-642-7243.

Public Inquiries Branch, National Institute of Mental Health, Room 15C-05, 5600 Fishers Lane, Rockville, MD 20857.

REFERENCES

American Psychiatric Association. (1994). *Diagnostic and statistical manual of mental disorders* (4th ed.). Washington, DC: Author.

Andreasen, N. (1999). Understanding the causes of schizophrenia. *New England Journal of Medicine, 430,* 645–647.

Castle, D. J., Wessely, S. W., Howard, R., et al. (1997). Schizophrenia with onset at the extremes of adult life. *International Pyschogeriatrics, 8,* 712–717.

Cohen, C. I. (1995). Studies of the course and outcome of schizophrenia in later life. *Psychiatric Services, 46,* 877–889.

Coryell, W. (1998). The treatment of psychotic depression. *Journal of Clinical Psychiatry, 59*(Suppl. 1), 22–27; discussion, 28–29.

Cuffel, B. J., Jeste, D. V., Patterson, T. L., et al. (1997). Treatment costs and use of community mental health services for schizophrenia by age-cohorts. *American Journal of Psychiatry, 153,* 870–876.

Cummings, J. L. (1999). Managing psychosis in patients with Parkinson's disease. *New England Journal of Medicine, 340,* 801–803.

Ghaemi, S. N., Katzow, J. J., Desai, S. P., et al. (1998). Gabapentin treatment of mood disorders: A preliminary study. *Journal of Clinical Psychiatry 59,* 426–429.

Häfner, H. (1997). Special issue on late-onset schizophrenia and the delusional disorder in old age. *European Archives of Psychiatry and Clinical Neuroscience,* *247,* 173–218.

Jeste, D. V., Rockwell, E., Harris, M. J., et al. (1999). Conventional vs. newer antipsychotics in elderly patients. *American Journal of Geriatric Psychiatry, 7,* 70–76.

Jeste, D. V., Symonds, L. L., Harris, M. J., et al. (1997). Non-dementia non-praecox dementia praecox? Late onset schizophrenia. *American Journal of Geriatric Psychiatry, 5,* 302–317.

Keck, P. E., McElroy, S. L., Nemeroff, C. B. (1992). Anticonvulsants in the treatment of bipolar disorder. *Journal of Neuropsychiatry and Clinical Neurosciences, 4,* 395–405.

Knoll, J., Stegman, K., Suppes, T. (1998). Clinical experience using gabapentin adjunctively in patients with a history of mania or hypomania. *Journal of Affective Disorders, 49,* 229–233.

Lehman, A. F., Sreinwachs, D. M., and co-investigators of the PORT Project. (1998). Translating research into practice: The schizophrenia Patient Outcomes Research Team (PORT) treatment recommendations. *Schizophrenia Bulletin, 24,* 1–10.

Liu, Y. L., Stagni, G., Walden, J. G., et al. (1998). Thioridazine close-related effects on biomechanical force platform measures of sway in young and old men. *Journal of the American Geriatrics Society, 46,* 431–437.

McDonald, W. M., Krishnan, K. R. R., Doraiswamy, P. M., et al. (1991). The occurrence of subcortical hyperintensities in patients with mania. *Psychiatry Research, 40,* 211–220.

McDonald, W. M., Nemeroff, C. B. (1996). The diagnosis and treatment of mania in the elderly. *Bulletin of the Menninger Clinic, 60,* 174–196.

Muller-Siecheneder, F., Muller, M. J., Hillert, A., et al. (1998). Risperidone versus haloperidol and amitriptyline in the treatment of patients with a combined psychotic and depressive syndrome. *Journal of Clinical Psychopharmacology, 18,* 111–120.

Parfrey, P. S., Ikeman, R., Anglin, D., et al. (1983). Severe lithium intoxication treated by forced diuresis. *Canadian Medical Association Journal, 129,* 979–980.

Parkinson Study Group. (1999). Low-dose clozapine for the treatment of drug-induced psychosis in Parkinson's disease. *New England Journal of Medicine, 340,* 757–763.

Parsa, M. A., Bastani, B. (1998). Quetiapine (Seroquel) in the treatment of psychosis in patients with Parkinson's disease. *Journal of Neuropsychiatry and Clinical Neurosciences, 10,* 216–219.

Rabins, P. V., Black, B., German, P., et al. (1997). The prevalence of psychiatric disorders in elderly residents of public housing. *Journal of Gerontology: Medical Science, 51,* M319–M324.

Rabins, P. V., Pearlson, G. (1994). Part II: Paraphrenia, schizophrenia or ? In E. Chiu & D. Ames (Eds.), *Functional psychiatric disorders of the elderly* (pp. 316–325). Cambridge: Cambridge University Press.

Ragheb, M. (1990). The clinical significance of lithium-nonsteroidal anti-inflammatory drug interactions. *Journal of Clinical Psychopharmacology, 10,* 350–354.

Rothschild, A. J., Bates, K. S., Boehriinger, K. L., et al. (1999). Olanzapine response in psychotic depression. *Journal of Clinical Psychiatry, 60,* 116–118.

Semenchuk, M. R., Labiner, D. M. (1997). Gabapentin and lamotrigine: Prescribing guidelines for psychiatry. *Journal of Practicing Psychiatry and Behavioral Health, 3,* 334–342.

Sharma, V., Pistor, L. (1999). Treatment of bipolar mixed state with olanzapine. *Journal of Psychiatry and Neuroscience, 24,* 40–44.

Sussman, N. (1998). Background and rationale for use of anticonvulsants in psychiatry. *Cleveland Clinic Journal of Medicine, 65,* SI7–SI14.

Tariot, P. N., Podgorski, C. A., Blazina, L., et al. (1993). Mental disorders in the nursing home: Another perspective. *American Journal of Psychiatry, 15,* 1063–1069.

Tohen, M., Sanger, T. M., McElroy, S. L., et al. (1999). Olanzapine versus placebo in the treatment of acute mania. *American Journal of Psychiatry, 156,* 702–709.

Verdoux, H., Bourgeois, M. (1990). A case of lithium neurotoxicity with irreversible cerebellar syndrome. *Journal of Nervous and Mental Disease, 178,* 761–762.

Woerner, M. G., Alvir, J. M., Saltz, B. L., et al. (1998). Prospective study of tardive dyskinesia in the elderly: Rates and risk factors. *American Journal of Psychiatry, 155,* 1521–1528.

Young, R. C., Klerman, G. L. (1992). Mania in late life: Focus on age at onset. *American Journal of Psychiatry, 149,* 867–876.

Young, R. C., Moline, M., Kleyman, F. (1997). Estrogen replacement therapy and late life mania. *American Journal of Geriatric Psychiatry, 5,* 179–181.

Zanardi, R., Franchini, L., Serretti, A., et al. (2000). Venlafaxine versus fluvoxamine in the treatment of delusional depression: A pilot double-blind controlled study. *Journal of Clinical Psychiatry, 61,* 26–29.

5

Sleep Disturbances

$\mathbf{D}$isturbed, restless sleep is a common complaint among older adults. Excessive daytime drowsiness affects less than 2% of older persons, but as many as one-third complain of problems initiating or sustaining sleep (Foley et al., 1995). Insomnia is more frequent among women and persons who are widowed, separated, or divorced and among those of lower socioeconomic status. It tends to be relapsing and when persistent is an antecedent of the onset and recurrence of depression (Kupfer & Reynolds, 1997; Kennedy et al., 1991). Nearly 40% of hypnotic medications are prescribed to older adults despite the attendant risks of cognitive impairment, accidents, and dependency (Campbell et al., 1995). The interplay of age-related changes in sleep physiology, social factors, physical and mental illness, and medications make the diagnosis of sleep disturbance challenging. However, the very multiplicity of causes suggests an array of effective interventions both pharmacological and behavioral. Improved sleep hygiene is the ultimate goal.

ASSESSMENT

In addition to difficulty falling asleep and staying asleep, older patients often report that they do not feel rested or restored upon awakening. A few days of insomnia or restless sleep may be precipitated by acute illness or life events, but complaints of 3 weeks' duration suggest chronic sleep disturbance with a more complex cause. Duration of the symptoms is thus important both for diagnosis and for treatment. Obsessive worry about sleep and the use of alcohol or sedatives may be both a cause and a consequence of insomnia. A transient sleep problem can become persistent by self-defeating solutions such as spending too much time in bed or abandoning a regular schedule of sleep and waking. Primary insomnia is a diagnosis of exclusion in which mental disorders, physical illness, medications, or simple scheduling difficulties do not explain the associated impairment in social or cognitive function. Primary hypersomnia or excessive daytime drowsiness has similar exclusionary criteria but is associated with nocturnal myoclonus (periodic leg movements), restless leg syndrome, sleep apnea (respirator lapse), and snoring. Periodic leg movement disorder and restless leg syndrome are also associated with complaints of insomnia and nonrestorative sleep and appear to increase with age (Brown, 1997). In either case, symptoms causing substantial impairment for a month or more meet diagnostic criteria.

Whether the sleep disturbance is primary or secondary, an appreciation of the electrophysiology of normal sleep and changes related to age or mental illness sets the stage for effective assessment and realistic treatment. Table 5.1 displays electroencephalography of sleep which characterizes four domains, each with clinical significance. These include relaxed wakefulness, light or shallow sleep, dream or rapid eye movement (REM) sleep, and deep or restorative sleep. Relaxed wakefulness prepares the individual for sleep. A number of behaviors and exogenous stimuli can interfere with this preparatory domain. In Table 5.2, the characteristics of REM and non-REM sleep are compared showing the autonomic activity that accompanies dreaming. The behavioral disorders of REM sleep in which patients respond physically to dream content, experience the dream as a waking hallucination, or have recurrent nightmares are rare but may be seen in the dementias or following stroke. More common is respiratory or cardio-

TABLE 5.1. Electroencephalography of Sleep

Level of arousal	EEG rhythm and associated activity
Relaxed awake	Alpha (8–12 Hz) prevails posteriorly, beta (>12 Hz) anteriorly
Shallow sleep Stage 1	Theta (4–8 Hz), low amplitude, mixed frequency
Rapid eye movement	Loss of muscle tone, autonomic arousal (HR, RR, B/P), penile tumescence, spike and wave bursts (7 Hz) from pons, lateral geniculate, occipital cortex, duration increases
Stage 2	Sigma (12- to 16-Hz bursts) sleep spindles, K complexes (slow wave + spindles)
Deep sleep Stage 3 Stage 4	>50% sigma, <50% delta (1–2 Hz) <50% sigma, >50% delta

Note. Data from Spar and La Rue (1997).

TABLE 5.2. Characteristics of REM Sleep Compared to Non-REM Sleep

REM sleep	Non-REM sleep
Dream, light sleep	Restorative, deep sleep
Circadian component	Homeostatic component
Low point of temperature rhythm	Slow-wave sleep
Autonomic activation	Autonomic quiescence
Fluctuating heart rate, rate ratio, blood pressure, cardiac output	Lowered heart rate, rate ratio, blood pressure, cardiac output
Irregular breathing	Regular breathing
↓ Response to CO_2 inhalation	↑ Response to CO_2 inhalation
Frequent apnea	Rare apnea
Onset: Cholinergic	Onset: Serotonergic
Pontine tegmentum	Basal forebrain, midbrain raphe

Note. Data from Reynolds (1991).

vascular compromise associated with the physiological demands of dreaming which imperil the older person with poorly controlled heart or lung disease.

As shown in Table 5.3, REM sleep is relatively preserved in old age, a poetic justice given the observation that deep, restorative sleep declines late in life. It also shows a distinct circadian component occurring later in sleep and attuned to the nadir in body temperature. In contrast, shallow sleep increases with advanced age. Frequently awakenings (microarousals) throughout the night during shallow sleep and the advancement of the deep-sleep phase into the earlier hours are also part of the normal aging of sleep. These changes in part account for older adults becoming larks (early to bed, early to rise) whereas their grandchildren feel like owls, asleep in the morning, alert all night. However it is important to recall that the circadian nature of sleep is

TABLE 5.3. Sleep Characteristics of Normal Aging versus Psychiatric Disorders

Aging	Depression	Anxiety/panic	Dementia
Microarousals	↓ REM latency	Disturbed onset	↑ REM latency
↓ Slow-wave	↑ 1st REM period	Disturbed	↑ Episodes of apnea
Phase	↑ REM density	maintenance	↓ Phase activity
advancement	Slow-wave	Nocturnal panic	Arrhythmic, chaotic
REM	advancement	attack	Sleep decline parallels
advancement	Early awakening		cognitive decline
Day napping			
↑ Time in bed			
20% use hypnotics			

Note. Data from Reynolds (1991).

regulated by *zeitgebers,* environmental cues which entrain the sleep–wake cycle. As individuals age, they may reduce their level of physical activity and modify their previously set routine of bedtime and arising required for employment or child care. As a result, they become more vulnerable to sleep disturbance from all causes. Thus both physiological and social changes of late life make it difficult to reset nature's internal clock. The result can be reversal of the sleep–wake cycle, a disturbance of circadian rhythm due to phase delay, or phase advancement depending on whether the pattern of sleep onset, dreaming, and deep sleep occurs too early or too late.

More commonly practitioners encounter sleep disturbances resulting from and compounding the distress of physical and mental illness and their associated medications. Depression, anxiety disorders, and dementia all have a characteristic pattern of sleep disruption (see Table 5.4). Family caregivers of persons with dementia and disturbed sleep can anticipate interrupted sleep, which further degrades the quality of rest. Chronically lying in bed worrying about the day's mental residue can lead to a persistent insomnia. The bereaved elder who has lost a bed partner may have lost the comfort of sleep as well.

TABLE 5.4. Differential Diagnosis of Late-Life Sleep Disturbance

Primary insomnia	Difficulty initiating or maintaining restorative sleep, three times a week for 1 month, with daytime fatigue, irritability or impaired function, not due to scheduling or parasomnia; 6-month prevalence 12.0%, incidence 7.3%
Primary hypersomnia	Excessive daytime drowsiness usually associated with snoring, sleep apnea or leg movements; 6-month prevalence 1.6%, incidence 1.8%
Other etiologies	• Age-related "sleep decay," scheduling, habits, unrealistic expectations • Psychiatric disorders; depression, dementia, anxiety, psychosis • Parasomnias; somatic disorders exacerbated by sleep (angina, cognitive heart failure, esophageal reflux) • Dependency on sedative hypnotics, alcohol • Night time nicotine, caffeine • Night time antiadrenergic, antihistamine, antiparkinson medications • Periodic limb movement disorder; four or more movements at 20- to 40-second intervals, usually the legs • Restless-leg syndrome; painful or crawling sensation relieved only by movement

Note. Data from American Psychiatric Association (1994).

Kupfer and Reynolds (1997) suggest that the most common problem in assessing sleep disturbance at any age is failure to understand the complexity of the underlying causes. As noted elsewhere in this volume, with seniors it is more effective to sort out multiple etiologies than to seek to rule out all but the "major" contributor. Thus the approach must be systematic and long term in its goals. Even when the etiology seems obvious (e.g., major depressive disorder), a self-report sleep log kept for 2 weeks may indicate self-defeating or inefficient sleep habits. Ask the patient to record the exact times of bedtime, arising, and meals and the use of stimulant beverages, alcohol, tobacco, medications, and periods of exercise or physical activity. The quantity and quality of sleep should also be noted.

The patient may not be the sole source for a sleep history. If the patient has a bed partner or other sleep witness, ask about snoring, excessive daytime drowsiness, respiratory lapses (apnea), and episodes of confusion or assaultiveness that arise out of sleep. Respiratory and behavioral disturbances may best be diagnosed by referral for polysomnography, which will track heart rhythm and respiration, and the electroencephalogram. Sedation in the presence of sleep apnea or other breathing disturbance is dangerous in that respiratory drive may be compromised. Patients should also be referred to a sleep specialist once combined behavioral and pharmacology efforts have failed to counter insomnia (Reite et al., 1995).

TREATMENT

Education and behavioral interventions rather than medications are the mainstay of managing late-life sleep disturbance. Appraisal of the presenting problem, medical conditions, patient expectations, and incentives for and obstacles to change are critical to develop realistic goals. Modest improvement may be more realistic than a cure for chronic insomnia, particularly for older persons accustomed to sedative/hypnotics. First the practitioner should provide information about the physiological changes in sleep that occur with advanced age. Older adults need to continually "set and wind the internal clock" to maintain sleep hygiene. This entails stimulus and temporal control (Bootzin & Perlis, 1992). The sleep history or log will indicate habits that interfere with the stimulus to sleep. Exercise in the evening, a late meal, or liberal fluid intake at night will disrupt sleep, as will nicotine, stimulant beverages, and alcohol. Individuals who read, snack, or watch TV in bed should be counseled to reserve bedtime for sleep or intimacy only. If not sleepy, they should not retire. If not asleep within a quarter hour, they should leave the bedroom and read in dim light avoiding the alerting effects of TV or full illumination. Return to the bedroom only when sleepy. Stimulus control is simply classical conditioning in which time in bed becomes time asleep.

Both the stimuli and timing for rest and waking must be controlled for improved sleep efficiency. Ask the patient to follow a strict 7-day-a-week schedule for arising and bedtime which is to apply whether or not the previous night's sleep was satisfactory. Naps are eliminated or reduced to a single, short period in the afternoon. Time in bed is reduced to 7–8 hours to ensure that the sleep is efficient and continuous rather than fragmentary. The older person who tries to make up for lost sleep by spending extra time in bed further fragments the architecture of sleep with a greater number of microarousals and circadian disruption. In contrast, purposefully reducing sleep time through a restriction schedule induces a modest sleep deprivation, which in turn solidifies the night's sleep. Graded release of the restriction by adding a quarter-hour weekly is then used to maintain the sleep efficiency achieved during the period of deprivation (Kupfer & Reynolds, 1997).

Education, stimulus, and temporal control are helpful for most persons with sleep problems. However, other nonpharmacological interventions may be needed for persons who fail to sustain good sleep hygiene or who rely on sedative/hypnotics. Cognitive-behavioral therapies which combine elements of stimulus and temporal control but in a more structured format generally offer longer-term benefits (Morin et al., 1994). Progressive relaxation training (Bernstein & Borkovec, 1973) may be ineffective if not combined with a program of stimulus and scheduling control (Edinger et al., 1992). Bright light (2,000–4,000 lux) administered from 8 P.M. to midnight for as few as 2 nights may improve sleep in older person with primary sleep maintenance insomnia (Campbell et al., 1995).

Pharmacological interventions (see Table 5.5) will be necessary for a number of patients who are not satisfied with the results of behavioral approaches to insomnia and for those with periodic limb movements or restless-legs syndrome (Morin et al., 1994). As a first step, withdraw stimulant beverages and over-the-counter medications which interfere with either the quality of sleep or daytime performance. Over-the-counter medications which impair sleep include analgesics with caffeine (Anacin, Excedrin, Empirin), some cough and cold preparations, and decongestants with phenylpropanolamine or pseudoephedrine. Prescribed medications which may cause insomnia include atenolol, thyroid preparations, cortisone, theophylline, levodopa, and quinidine. Older patients should also be discouraged from

TABLE 5.5. Select Agents Used for Sleep Disturbance in Older Adults

Generic name	Trade name	Initial dose (mg)	Final dose (mg)	Amnestic potential	Hypotensive potential	Sedative potential	Precautions	Advantages
Short-lived benzodiazepines								
Lorazepam	Ativan	0.5	2	Moderate	Low	High	Falls, dependence, controlled substance	Short T½, no active metabolite
Oxazepam	Serax	15	30	Moderate	Low	High	Falls, dependence, controlled substance	Short T½, no active metabolite
Temazepam	Restoril	15	30	Moderate	Low	High	Falls, dependence, controlled substance	Short T½, no active metabolite
Benzodiazepine-"like" hypnotics								
Zolpidem	Ambien	5	10	Low	Low	High	May not sustain sleep or be sufficient in major disorders, dependence	Ultra short T½, no active metabolite, Level IV controlled substance
Zaleplon	Sonata	5	10	Low	Low	High	Very rapid onset, longer T½	Level IV controlled substance
Sedative antipsychotics								
Thioridazine	Mellaril	10	100	Dose related	Dose related	Moderate	Hypotensive and amnestic as dose increases, quinidine-like effects	Available as liquid, not a controlled substance
Sedative antidepressants								
Trazodone	Desyrel	25–50	300	Low	High	High	Hypotensive	No withdrawal, not a controlled substance
Nefazodone	Serzone	50	200	Low	Moderate	Moderate	Dry mouth	No withdrawal, not a controlled substance
Paroxetine	Paxil	10	40	Low	Low	Moderate	Nausea, tremor, drug interactions	No withdrawal, not a controlled substance
Mirtazapine	Remeron	7.5	15–30	Low	Low	Moderate	Prolonged T½, renal clearance, dry mouth, weight gain	No withdrawal, not a controlled substance
Hormonal agents								
Melatonin	Several	2	2	Low	Low	Low	Not FDA regulated, preparations may vary and include other ingredients	Over-the-counter, no withdrawal
Herbals, botanicals								
Matricaria recutita	German chamomile	As tea t.i.d. h.s.		None	None	Low	Not FDA regulated, allergic reactions	Over-the-counter, no withdrawal, very mild
Valeriana officinalis	Valerian	150 b.i.d.	300 h.s.	None	None	Low	Not FDA regulated, products may vary and include other ingredients, delayed onset	Over-the-counter, no withdrawal, very mild

using over-the-counter medications which are marketed as sleep aids. These include agents whose sole component is diphenhydramine (Nytol, Sleep-Eze, Sominex) and the diphenhydramine-containing "PM" analgesic preparations. Melatonin is also frequently used as a hypnotic but is not regulated by the Food and Drug Administration (FDA) and varies considerably in content from one brand to the next. However, in one single-blind placebo-controlled study, melatonin was associated with improved sleep efficiency in older adults (Garfinkel et al., 1995).

Once counterproductive medications have been eliminated use the following principles to direct the pharmacotherapy of sleep disorders. First, the lowest effective dose of an agent without active metabolites should be employed and used intermittently throughout the week, not every night. Renal or hepatic insufficiency may prolong the action of even short-lived agents. The goal is modest improvement in sleep rather than total eradication of the patient's complaints. Second, inform the patient from the outset that sleeping pills are a temporary solution and should be gradually tapered off after 3 to 4 weeks. Changes in behavior offer the best chance of long-term improvements in sleep but require the most effort. Rebound insomnia will require more gradual withdrawal. Finally, short-acting agents which are less likely to impair daytime performance are preferred (Kupfer & Reynolds, 1997)

Specific medications, doses, and precautions for late-life sleep disturbance are tabulated at chapter's end. However, several added perspectives are worth noting to guide the choice of a specific agent. The bulk of evidence supporting the treatment of insomnia comes from studies of benzodiazepines and zolpidem. They are remarkably safe and effective for transient, situational disturbances. Yet because of the inconvenience of triplicate prescriptions, difficulties withdrawing the patient from the medication, and fears of cognitive impairment and accidents, some practitioners prefer to prescribe a sedative antidepressant, amytriptyline, nortriptyline, or the antihistamine diphenhydramine. However, trazodone, nefazodone, or paroxetine are much better choices for chronic insomnia in seniors. These agents also have appeal as substitutes for benzodiazepines or other "sleepers" on which the patient has become dependent. The benzodiazepines are effective for periodic limb movement disorder and restless-leg syndrome, but in theory the sedative antidepressants may be as well. There is little if any literature on the use of sedative antidepressants when REM behavioral disturbance is diagnosed. I have cared for one older water colorist whose onset of vascular dementia was preceded by both vivid visual

TABLE 5.6. Treatment of Late-Life Sleep Disturbances

For insomnia

Behavioral approaches
    Education
    Strict 7-day schedule for sleep; stimulus and temporal control
    Restrict time in bed, reduce napping
    Environmental modification for comfort, warmth, and noise reduction
    Reduce nighttime fluids, alcohol, nicotine, caffeine, and stimulant tea
    Regular exercise, morning or late afternoon but not at night

Pharmacological approaches
    Indications
        Transient, situational disorders
        When behavioral interventions fail
        Adjunctive treatment of depression, anxiety, psychosis
    Additional considerations
        Tolerance and withdrawal problems with benzodiazepines
        Antipsychotic may be preferable for sleep disturbance of dementia but
        may impair motor function
        Sedative antidepressants and benzodiazepines may impair daytime
        function
        Drug interactions, aged metabolism, avoid antihistamines
        Sedatives may exacerbate sleep apnea

For periodic leg movement disorder, restless-leg syndrome

Hypnotics will override arousal but may not suppress movements

For REM sleep behavior disorder (refer for sleep laboratory evaluation)

Make-safe the bedroom; if sleep apnea is absent, use hypnotics or antipsychotics

For sleep apnea (refer for sleep laboratory evaluation)

Behavioral—weight loss, sleeping on side
Pharmacological—acetazolamide
Prosthetic—continuous positive airway pressure (CPAP)
Surgical—airway revision or tracheotomy

Note. Data from Kupfer and Reynolds (1997); Brown (1997).

hallucinations and REM behavior disturbance which had been kept a secret within the family until the patient injured herself. A low dose of thioridazine did not eliminate the hallucinations but did suppress the dangerous behavior of the REM disturbance. Nonetheless, the current use of antidepressants as sedatives is at best state-of-the-art rather than evidence based. For commentary on pharmacological treatment of sleep disturbance in dementia, see Chapter 3.

SUMMARY

Sleep complaints are pervasive among seniors and are typically complex in etiology. However, there is a mature literature useful to guide assessment and treatment. The elements of treatment as summarized in Table 5.6 include (1) education, (2) reversal of counterproductive habits and behaviors, (3) withdrawal or substitution of prescribed or over the counter medications which degrade sleep quality, (4) effective treatment of mental disorders which may underlie the patient's presenting complaint, and (5) the judicious use of sedative antidepressants or benzodiazepines. However, some older patients will resist all efforts to reduce or eliminate a favored hypnotic which they associate with restful sleep but the practitioner sees as potentially unsafe. Rather than threaten to terminate care, an informed consent approach may meet the prescriber's ethical need to address the risk without abandoning the patient. Risk of continued hypnotic use, a willingness to offer substitution therapy or seek an expert opinion, and the need to revisit the issue at reasonable intervals should be discussed in a nonpunitive interview with the patient (and family if agreed to) and documented in the record.

REFERENCES

American Psychiatric Association. (1994). *Diagnostic and statistical manual of mental disorders* (4th ed.). Washington, DC: Author.

Bernstein, D., Borkovec, T. D. (1973). *Progressive relaxation training.* Champaign, IL: Research Press.

Bootzin, R. R., Perlis, M. L. (1992). Nonpharmacologic treatments of insomnia. *Journal of Clinical Psychiatry, 53*(Supp.), 37–41.

Brown, L. K. (1997). Sleep and sleep disorders in the elderly. *Nursing Home Medicine, 5,* 346–353.

Campbell, S. S., Terman, M., Lewy, A. J., et al. (1995). Light treatment for sleep disorders: Consensus report. V. Age-related disturbances. *Journal of Biological Rhythms, 10,* 151–154.

Edinger, J. D., Hoelscher, T. J., Marsh, G. R., et al. (1992). A cognitive therapy for sleep-maintenance insomnia in older adults. *Psychology and Aging, 7,* 282–289.

Foley, D. J., Monjan, A. A., Brown, S. L., et al. (1995). Sleep complaints among elderly persons: An epidemiologic study of three communities. *Sleep, 18,* 425–432.

Garfinkel, D., Laudon, M., Nof, D., et al. (1995). Improvement of sleep quality in elderly people by controlled-release melatonin. *Lancet, 346,* 541–544.

Kennedy G. J., Kelman, H. R., Thomas, C. (1991). Persistence and remission of depressive symptoms in late life. *American Journal of Psychiatry, 148,* 174–178.

Kupfer, D. J., Reynolds, C. F., III. (1997). Management of insomnia. *New England Journal of Medicine, 336,* 341–346.

Morin, C. M., Culbert, J. P., Schwartz, S. M. (1994). Nonpharmacologic interventions for insomnia: A meta-analysis of efficacy. *American Journal of Psychiatry, 151,* 1172–1180.

Reite, M., Buysse, D., Reynolds, C., et al. (1995). The use of polysomnography in the evaluation of insomnia. *Sleep, 18,* 58–70.

Reynolds, C. F. (1991). Sleep disorders. In J. Sadavoy, L. Jarvik, & L. Lazarus (Eds.), *Comprehensive review of geriatric psychiatry* (pp. 249–261). Washington, DC: American Psychiatric Press.

Spar, J., La Rue, A. (1997). *Concise guide to geriatric psychiatry* (pp. 233–240). Washington, DC: American Psychiatric Association.

6

Personality, Somatoform, and Pain Disorders

An informed, realistic approach to patients with personality or somatoform disorders in old age will substantially improve their quality of life and the practitioner's level of satisfaction. (See Table 6.1 for DSM-IV diagnostic criteria of these disorders.) Many practitioners will develop an intuitive approach to the care of these unfortunate individuals. For those who seek assistance, the referral must be handled with patience and tact to avoid provoking fears of abandonment and rage over rejection. An explicit goal of sustaining the primary relationship and an emphasis on the practitioner's need for help are essential components of the recommendation for a mental health specialist to "join the team."

PERSONALITY DISORDERS

Personality disorders are persistent, maladaptive exaggerations of character manifested by difficulties in cognition, emotionality, personal relations, and impulse control. They may result in distorted perceptions and interpretations of life events; blunted or exaggerated feelings; problematic dealings with family, intimates, and caregivers; or a troublesome lack of restraint. The onset is no later than early adulthood, but the disorder may not be apparent until some event makes it impossible to ignore. When a personality trait becomes so inflexible and counterproductive that the individual's social function or personal comfort is substantially impaired, then a personality disorder may be diagnosed.

There is much confusion in both the clinical assessment and scientific study of personality disorders in late life. DSM-IV suggests that

TABLE 6.1. Personality, Somatoform, and Pain Disorders Simplified

DSM-IV Axis II or "minor" mental disorders

Personality disorders (personality traits exaggerated to the point of impairment)
Odd, eccentric (Cluster A)
Paranoid (suspicious, grandiose)
Schizotypal (schizophrenia like)
Schizoid (distant, aloof)
Dramatic, impulsive (Cluster B)
Antisocial (self destructive, predatory loners)
Histrionic (overly emotional, demonstrative)
Borderline (intense, volatile attachments)
Narcissistic (vain, insecure)
Anxious Cluster C
Avoidant (phobic)
Dependent (needy)
Obsessive–compulsive (intrusive preoccupations and rituals)
Not otherwise specified
Passive–aggressive (negativistic)
Personality change due to a medical disorder ("organic personality")

DSM-IV Axis I or "major" mental disorders

Somatoform disorders (physical disability due to psychological causes)
Hypochondriasis (angry search for illness)
Conversion (voluntary motor or sensory deficits solve conflicts)
Somatization (multiple systems)
Body dysmorphic (unrealistic disabling preoccupation with appearance)
Pain disorder (out of proportion to anatomic limitations)

Note. Adapted from American Psychiatric Association (1994). Copyright 1994 by the American Psychiatric Association. Adapted by permission.

personality disorder is infrequent among the elderly. Yet some authors find that personality disorder is no less frequent among the aged, particularly those with depressive disorders, than among younger persons (Bergman, 1971; Burns, 1988). An underestimate of the importance of personality disorder in late life has arisen in part as a result of the emphasis on symptom reduction rather than return to full function. From Francis Bacon to Hughlings Jackson, the split between science and practice remains evident when personality disorders are discussed (Gabbard, 1997).

Cluster Diagnoses

Personality disorders as listed in DSM-IV are divided into three clusters. The odd, eccentric disorders, listed as Cluster A, include paranoid, schizotypal (schizophrenia-like) and the schizoid (aloof). The patient's distorted perceptions and interpretations of events or other's motives and an intolerance of intimacy are the core problems which the provider, family, or care team encounter. Cluster B comprises the overly dramatic, impulsive disorders including antisocial, histrionic, borderline, and narcissistic types. These disorders are characterized by extreme, overwhelming emotions and unstable interpersonal relations which can cause the affected person to act on impulse with counter-productive or objectionable outcomes. Fears of abandonment and rage over narcissistic slights whether real or imagined are common.

In Cluster C, the avoidant, dependent, and obsessive–compulsive personality disorders, the common theme is anxiety. Anxiety reaches symptomatic levels when the individual is confronted with a situation most persons would neither avoid nor depend on others to resolve. When ritualized behaviors cannot be completed or when stereotyped, repetitive thoughts become excessively intrusive, the disorder is obses-sive–compulsive.

Personality disorder not otherwise specified (NOS) is reserved for individuals who meet the general criteria for dysfunction but not one of the entities described in the clusters and for those who fit categories not present in DSM-IV such as passive–aggressive (negativistic) per-sonality. Patients with a mix of problematic personality traits are more frequently encountered than those who fit a discrete category; hence, the utility of the cluster approach to diagnosis. Also, under stress a previously adaptive personality trait may become so exaggerated and dysfunctional that a personality disorder seems the appropriate diag-nosis (Oldham, 1994).

Epidemiology

The prevalence of personality disorders varies greatly depending on whether the sample is drawn from the clinic or the community. Esti-mates range from a low 0.8% in community residents (Robins et al., 1984) to 20% of older patients with a comorbid major mental illness (Fogel & Sadavoy, 1996). Among the young and middle-age commu-nity residents, the rates range from 0.5–2.5% for paranoid; 3% for schizotypal; 3% male, 1% female for antisocial; 2% for borderline; 2–3% for histrionic; 1% for narcissistic; 0.5–1.0% for avoidant; 1% for obsessive–compulsive among young and middle-age adults. Among mental health clinics, schizoid is the least and dependent the most fre-quently diagnosed personality disorder. Antisocial personality disor-der is more often diagnosed in men; borderline, histrionic, and dependent disorders are more frequently diagnosed in women. Per-sonality disorders may predispose an individual to anxiety or mood disorders and may complicate his or her course and treatment. Indeed, 10–20% of older persons with major depressive disorders have a personality disorder as well (Abrams et al., 1994). It is thought that the more dramatic personality disorders, particularly antisocial, become less a problem in late life as impulsiveness withers with age (Fogel & Sadavoy, 1966). Obsessive–compulsive and schizotypal personality disorders persist into late life (Molinari & Marmion, 1993).

There is evidence in younger persons that genetic components for affective lability, narcissism, and identity problems exist. Environmental effects may predominate elsewhere (Livesley et al., 1993). However, the influence of genetics in the context of environmental influences over the course of a long life is difficult to estimate. In keeping with everyday experience, personality traits seem to be stable over the life course even when major life events have intervened (McCrae & Costa, 1988). McCrae et al.'s (1999) study of personality traits among more than 7,000 persons found similar patterns of change and stability despite differences in nationality and culture. Neuroticism, extroversion, and openness declined while agreeableness and conscientiousness increased, suggesting a common maturational process that transcends culture and recent history.

Differential Diagnosis

The DSM-IV lists the personality disorders as Axis II or minor mental illnesses to distinguish them from the major or Axis I disorders such as depression, dementia, schizophrenia, and anxiety disorders among others. Certain personality disorders, most notably the paranoid, schizotypal, avoidant, and obsessive–compulsive, are paler reflections of the more disabling major mental illnesses. These major illnesses include respectively, delusional (paranoid) disorder, schizophrenia, social phobia, and obsessive–compulsive disorder. Paranoid, schizotypal, schizoid, and borderline disorders are also conceptually related to the major psychotic disorders. The schizoid, histrionic, narcissistic, antisocial, and dependent disorders have more of the attributes of a personality style or trait. This coupling of an attenuated mental illness with an exaggeration of personality is key to recognizing why these unfortunate older persons have such great difficulties with medical and nursing care, as well as marital, family, and community life (Gabbard, 1997).

Personality disorders are distinguished from a change in personality, which is more likely the result of major depression, delirium, dementia, or an overwhelming change in life circumstances. Stroke, traumatic brain injury, seizure disorders, neurodegenerative disorders, and endocrinopathies are examples of other conditions that may significantly change personality. It is the lifelong pattern of personal distress and social dysfunction with a more recent exacerbation that justifies the personality disorder diagnosis. By convention, a personality disorder diagnosis is not made during an episode of major mental illness, such as depression, and not appropriate when the major disorder preceded the apparent onset of the personality disorder. Transient exaggerations in previously adaptive traits represent adjustment reactions rather than personality disorders.

Individuals with personality disorders may develop concurrent illness such as generalized anxiety disorder or affective disorder, but here the long-standing personality trait coupled with social impairment by history should be obtained. Collateral informants are critical to a reliable diagnosis of personality disorder, particularly when distortions of perception and interpretation are in question.

Data on personality disorders among native-born and immigrant minority elders are limited in the extreme, and the diagnostician must be wary of suspecting a disorder at first blush when the culture or ethnic differences between patient and practitioner are marked. Conversely, discounting the possibility of a personality disorder simply because the literature or a collateral informant suggests the patient belongs to stereotypically stoic or demonstrative or suspicious cultural group should be guarded against. A collateral informant or family member who shares the patient's background can be invaluable source of information regarding norms which the patient's behavior may exceed.

Treatment

Although a personality disorder may be lifelong, the events that bring the disorder to clinical attention may be more episodic and thus modifiable. And when the event represents irrevocable change, such as a long-stay nursing home admission, adaptation need not be ideal to be viable. The goal is to help patients and their immediate community regain equilibrium rather than to reorganize character (Yesavage & Karasu, 1982). Patients with personality disorder are most likely to identify a symptom or interpersonal problem or crisis as the target for change rather than their characteristically difficult traits. Thus the shorter-term interpersonal, cognitive-behavioral, or problem-solving approaches are more likely to be acceptable (Woods, 1995). Interactions stylized to fit the patient's character can be adapted to each of the clusters and individualized for the specific disorder and presenting problem. Recognizing the diagnosis and formulating a treatment plan is useful for establishing an alliance with the patient and identifying interventions when the disorder becomes sufficiently disabling or when a frank anxiety or mood disorder occurs (Oldham, 1994).

In Cluster A, the paranoid, schizoid, or schizotypal person may become intolerably anxious or transiently psychotic when interpersonal barriers are breached. Demands for trust or intimacy occasioned by hospitalization, nursing home admission, medical or legal procedures, bereavement, retirement, or the onset of disability require an empathic but dispassionate stance (Sadavoy & Fogel, 1992). The practitioner should acknowledge the genuine difficulties with trust and intimacy but discreetly remind the patient of immediate needs when essential medical procedures or the benefits of social supportive services are rejected. A business-like approach which acknowledges the discomfort behind paranoid accusations can put the patient at ease and allow an increment of trust without joining in the paranoia. For schizoid, aloof persons, their need for respite from interpersonal demands should be respected. The patient's social withdrawal and lack of feeling or responses are explained to staff as self-protective rather than unappreciative or bigoted. A conservative rather than aggressive care plan will prove more acceptable to the schizoid person who initially refuses services when obviously ill.

For the overly dramatic, impulsive disorders of Cluster B (histrionic, narcissistic, borderline, or antisocial), the intensity of affect, particularly anger, need not be cause for excess alarm. These feelings are as ephemeral as they are intense. Staff should not overreact. The consultant should help the patient choose less problematic or intense expressions of feelings. The consultant demonstrates that strong feelings need not be catastrophic for the patient or the care team. Whatever the patient may feel, it is how one acts that most directly affects others. When impulsiveness leads to self-destructive behavior or objectionable acts, confrontation and limit setting are needed to regain control. Insight into how the behavior is ultimately self-defeating or unacceptable no matter how justified it may seem is a praiseworthy goal, but managing the behavior is the more immediate concern. Containing or minimizing objectionable behaviors may be a more reasonable target than outright elimination. The anxious–fearful patients of Cluster B may be particularity prone to depression (Scheidner et al., 1992).

Practitioners should be alert to the unconscious phenomenon of "object splitting" among patients with Cluster B disorder. Here the patient unrealistically perceives individual caregivers as either rescuers or persecutors. This transference is accompanied by an equally problematic countertransference in which the caregiver reacts with anger at being accused and rejected or with unrealistic responses to fantasies of rescue. The idealized care provider can easily become the despised target of the patient's rage once the person encounters the frustration of delayed gratification. Because splitting is automatic, it is difficult to prevent but not impossible to repair. Communication between all parties providing services to the person keeps the care team from taking sides in a futile contest of wills. When difficult treatment decisions arise, meeting with the team along with the patient and family can avoid fragmentation into adversarial camps. A behavioral contract specifying expectations and contingencies can be drawn up in the meeting. Family and staff agree to provide a consistent approach across disciplines and to work shifts to prevent the patient from playing one person off another in a manipulative attempt. The patient agrees to take responsibility for having needs met through open negotiation rather than objectionable or manipulative behavior. Contract breaches and renegotiating are to be expected and do not necessarily indicate a failed plan. Rather a consistent pattern of attention on the staff and family's part which will reduce rather than eliminate the problematic behavior is success for all parties. Stated bluntly, the patient may not be able to comply, but staff will feel much less angry, ambivalent, and inadequate if they are consistent. Scapegoating, staff demoralization, and therapeutic chaos can be prevented (Sadavoy & Dorian, 1983). Environmental modifications may also be necessary to contain impulsiveness or counter manipulations.

Medications

Psychotropic medications are indicated when a major depressive or anxiety disorder develops and when episodic psychosis or sleep disturbance occurs. However, without addressing the underlying dynamics and interpersonal and environmental problems, medications will offer the patient little relief (Fogel & Sadavoy, 1996). More often symptoms distressing the patient will not conform to simple diagnostic criteria. In either event, the pharmacological approach is symptomatic and often temporary (Soloff, 1998; Hori, 1998). The most troubling symptom is the one targeted for treatment. And treatment may be episodic rather than long term. Medication is offered to get the person through present difficulties rather than to prevent the inevitable emergence of difficulties in the future.

For either anxiety or depression, a course of antidepressant treatment is recommended. The antidepressant nortriptyline is mildly sedative and effective for depression, anxiety and irritability as well. Paroxetine is a mildly sedative SSRI but more likely to exhibit drug interactions than is sertraline and citalopram which are not sedative, anticholinergic, or hypotensive. These latter agents may be preferred for frail elders. Severe sleep disturbance may be combated with trazodone but hypotension may occur as the dose is increased. Nefazodone or mirtazapine due to sedative effects may be alternatives to trazodone.

Benzodiazepines should be avoided because of difficulties with dependency and cognitive impairment and lack of long-term efficacy (Hori, 1998). Buspirone may be a mildly effective and safe antianxiety agent. However, its latency of effect makes it less desirable for acute anxiety but reasonable when anxiety is chronic. Fluvoxamine is the antianxiety agent approved for obsessive–compulsive disorder and the logical choice when obsessive or compulsive personality traits get out of hand.

Short-term use of low-dose antipsychotics is helpful when suspiciousness, rage, or impulsiveness reaches psychotic proportions, particularly in the paranoid, borderline, and schizotypal disorders. Thioridazine is beneficial provided the person is not frail or hemodynamically compromised. For frail persons olanzapine, quetiapine, or risperidone cause fewer parkinsonian effects than haloperidol and are somewhat sedative. In an emergency, haloperidol remains the agent of choice due to ease of administration (rapidly absorbed oral liquid, as well as i.m. and i.v. preparations) and safety.

SOMATOFORM AND PAIN DISORDERS

When evidence of mental illness is expressed exclusively in the form of physical symptoms that do not conform to patterns of physical illness, a somatoform disorder may be present. Somatoform disorders are considered major (DSM IV-Axis I) mental illnesses and include hypochondriasis, conversion, somatization, body dysmorphic, and pain disorders. These illnesses are prevalent in 1% or less of older community residents but may be as common as one in every three older adults in general medical clinics (Fogel & Sadavoy, 1996). They are more often encountered by generalists than by mental health specialists. Although advanced age has long been associated with somatic preoccupation, a number of studies suggest otherwise (Barsky et al., 1991; Lyness et al., 1993, Costa & McCrae, 1987). Indeed, hypochondriasis in late life should be considered either a distinct disorder or a manifestation of depression rather than the result of unsuccessful aging (Kay & Bergman, 1966).

Differential Diagnosis and Nosology

There are four core characteristics of the somatoform disorders essential to both diagnosis and treatment. First, the patient's disability and need for medical care are genuine. Any suggestion that the condition is trivial will either reinforce the impairment or send the patient searching for unnecessary examinations. Second, the symptoms are not voluntary or consciously chosen to achieve an end, as in factitious disorder or malingering. Neither are symptoms the delusional components of a psychotic disorder. Third, the somatoform disorders differ from psychological factors affecting medical condition in that a physical cause or condition either cannot be diagnosed or makes a relatively modest contribution to the person's incapacity. Fourth, persons with somatoform disorders have adopted a "sick role," which offers the illusion of escape through the frustration of illness (Kellner, 1989). The patient flees criticism from which there is no acceptable alternative, or isolation due to socioeconomic disadvantages, or a deteriorating marriage. The individual demonstrates a withdrawal of interest in others which is refocused on the patient's body, leaving the appearance of being manipulative and self-centered. Guilt is transformed into anxiety about health. Hostility is atoned for through self-punishment via physical symptoms and loss of pleasure in simple physical function (Busse, 1976).

Because seniors with somatoform disorders will also have concurrent physical conditions, a sort-out rather than rule-out approach to treatment is more likely to preserve the person's independence and well-being. Symptoms of depression, particularly suicidal thought, should also be pursued (Duberstein, 1995). Polypharmacy and overutilization of analgesics or sedatives should be explored. A collateral informant is crucial to establishing the diagnosis without alienating the patient who will resent the exploration of psychological factors (Fogel & Sadavoy, 1996). And a long-standing clinical relationship is a tremendous advantage when the practitioner is faced with the need to assign an apparently new symptom to the established diagnosis of somatoform disorder or to explore other possibilities.

Hypochondriasis is a crippling preoccupation that one has or will develop serious illness despite medical examinations and reassurance to the contrary. To be diagnosed as hypochondriacal, the preoccupation must not be delusional in intensity or bizarre in character, be affected for obvious gain, limited to concerns about one's appearance, and have endured for no less than 6 months. These unfortunate persons have frequently seen multiple physicians, have received an array of diagnostic procedures and interventions, and are frustrated and angry at their doctors for not providing relief. Older persons may have a number of concerns about health, but it is the obsessive pursuit of examinations, practitioner attention, and anger that characterize hypochondriasis (Gurian, 1991).

Somatization disorder presents a history of multiple physical symptoms, usually beginning before age 30, in which pain from at least four different sites, in addition to two gastrointestinal, one sexual, and one neurological symptom, can be recounted over the course of the illness. In each instance either care was sought or there was substantial impairment in social function. The course is persistent but variable. Hysteria, neurasthenia, and Briquet's syndrome are the historical predecessors of somatization disorder. Conversion disorder represents a failure of voluntary motor or sensory function which is psychologically based but not consciously effected. This apparent loss of neurological function serves the purpose of protecting the patient from a conflicted situation, expectation, or overwhelming affect which preceded the onset of symptoms. There is usually someone in the patient's experience who has had similar signs or symptoms which serves as a model for mental conflict to be converted into physical incapacity. The patient, temporarily freed of the conflict, is less disturbed by the disability, but true indifference to the symptoms is rare.

DSM-IV criteria for pain disorder describe an entity in which pain is the most salient and disabling complaint even when anatomic findings are present. Psychological factors affecting the onset, persistence, or intensity of pain are present and need not be the sole cause of the pain. The symptoms are not feigned but the presence of pain and the personal functions it prevents serves a psychological purpose. Secondary gains from the receipt of formal or informal supports reinforce the disorder but are not the sole etiology.

Body dysmorphic disorder is an unrealistic, persistent preoccupation that some aspect of one's appearance is defective and substantially inhibits social or occupation performance. The affected individual may pursue surgical or dental procedures to correct the presumed deformity.

Treatment

The basic principles of treatment are similar across the somatoform disorders. The practitioner should seek to establish and maintain a supportive, empathic relationship through judicial use of physical exam and regularly scheduled rather than "as needed" appointments. Clear expectations with reasonable limits on phone contacts, emergency services, medications, and length of sessions will provide a structure that is both reliable for the patient and realistic for the practitioner (Fogel & Sadavoy, 1996). The promise of constancy is more important than cure when forging a therapeutic alliance. Even though the patient may see through the approach and disparage the provider, a sustained relationship is nonetheless possible which with time lends a sense of security and a reduction in both symptoms, hostility, and care seeking. This requires tact and tolerance on the practitioner's part and a genuine acknowledgment of the frustration engendered when a full remission of symptoms has not been achieved despite considerable effort and at times expense on the patient's part.

Unacknowledged depression should be identified and treated aggressively even though the somatoform disorder may not remit in every case with resolution of the depression (Kramer-Ginsberg et al., 1989; Abrams et al., 1994). Anxiety related to the stress of the disorder may be approached with cognitive therapy and relaxation training (Pasnau & Bystritsky, 1990). Dementia may also present as a somatoform disorder (Brown, 1991). Polypharmacy and use of excessive analgesics or sedatives should be addressed with either reduction in quantity or substitution with less harmful agents. Family therapy may also be indicated (Goldstein & Birnbom, 1976) to establish realistic goals and reinforce the treatment plan. And the family may need considerable support and information to accept the level of associated disability which will legitimately seem out of proportion and excessive (Kay & Bergman, 1966).

Referral to a pain specialist, physiatry, and occupational or physical therapy to reduce pain, increase mobility, and allow the resumption of regular exercise may also be critical to effective management. Once the practitioner has stabilized (not necessarily removed) the somatoform disorder he or she will have ample opportunities to demonstrate competence when episodes of acute physical illness arise and when health maintenance procedures are due. Protecting these patients from unnecessary invasive procedures and excessive use of family and health care resources are worthy goals whether or not the incapacity occasioned by a somatoform disorder can be reduced.

To avoid working at cross-purposes and becoming trapped in an unproductive power struggle, the practitioner should focus on a rehabilitative approach and reducing the disability rather than achieving insight and making the patient abandon the symptoms. Recall that somatic concerns in late life are the norm but can take on a life of their own and be transformed into a somatoform disorder. Helping patients worry less about their very real problem is the goal. And again the approach is psychological and behavioral but the focus is on the physical and functional (Abrams, 1995).

REFERENCES

Abrams, R. C. (1995) Personality disorders. In J. Lindesay (Ed.), *Neurotic disorders in the elderly*. Oxford, UK: Oxford University Press.

Abrams, R. C., Rosendahl, E., Card, C., et al. (1994). Personality disorder correlates of late and early onset depression. *Journal of the American Geriatrics Society, 42,* 727–731.

American Psychiatric Association. (1994). *Diagnostic and statistical manual of mental disorders* (4th ed.). Washington, DC: Author.

Barsky, A. J., Frank, C., Cleary, P., et al. (1991). The relation between hypochondriasis and age. *American Journal of Psychiatry, 148,* 923–928.

Bergman, K. (1971). The neuroses of old age. In D. W. K. Walk & A. Walk (Eds.), *Recent development in psychogeriatrics* (pp. 39–50). London: British Journal of Psychiatry Special Publications.

Brown, F. W. (1991). Somatization disorder in progressive dementia. *Psychosomatics, 32,* 463–465.

Burns, A., Bergman, K., Lindesay, J. (1988). Neurosis and personality disorder in old age. *International Journal of Geriatric Psychiatry, 13,* 199–202.

Busse, E. W. (1976). Hypochondriasis in the elderly: A reaction to stress. *Journal of the American Geriatrics Society, 24,* 145–149.

Costa, P., McCrae, R. (1987). Somatic complaints in males as a function of age and neuroticism: A longitudinal analysis. *Journal of Behavioral Medicine, 3,* 245–257.

Duberstein, P. R. (1995). Openness to experience and completed suicide across the second half of life. *International Psychogeriatrics, 7*(2), 183–198.

Fogel, B. S., Sadavoy, J. (1996). Somatoform and personality disorders. In J. Sadavoy, L. W. Lazarus, L. F. Jarvik, et al. (Eds.), *Comprehensive review of geriatric psychiatry—II* (pp. 637–658). Washington, DC: American Psychiatric Press.

Gabbard, G. O. (1997). Finding the "person" in personality disorders. *American Journal of Psychiatry, 154,* 891–893.

Goldstein, S. E., Birnbom, F. (1976). Hypochondriasis and the elderly. *Journal of the American Geriatrics Society, 24,* 150–154.

Gurian, B. (1991). Coping with hypochondriasis in older patients. *Geriatrics, 46,* 71–77.

Hori, A. (1998). Pharmacotherapy for personality disorders. *Psychiatry and Clinical Neuroscience, 52,* 13–19.

Kay, P. W. K., Bergman, K. (1966). Physical disability and mental health in old age. *Journal of Psychosomatic Research, 10,* 3–12.

Kellner, R. (1989). Somatoform and factitious disorders. In *Treatment of psychiatric disorders* (pp. 2119–2172). Washington, DC: American Psychiatric Association.

Kramer–Ginsberg, E., Greenwald, B., Aisen, P., et al. (1989). Hypochondriasis in the elderly depressed. *Journal of the American Geriatrics Society, 35,* 507–510.

Livesley, W. J., Jang, K. L., Jackson, D. N., et al. (1993). Genetic and environmental contributions to dimensions of personality disorder. *American Journal of Psychiatry, 150,* 1826–1831.

Lyness, J. M., King, D., Conwell, Y., et al. (1993). Somatic worry and medical illness in depressed inpatients. *American Journal of Geriatric Psychiatry, 1,* 288–295.

McCrae, R., Costa, P. (1988). Psychological resilience among widowed men and women: A 10-year follow-up of a national sample. *Journal of Social Issues, 44,* 129–142.

McCrae, R. R., Costa, P. T., Pedroso de Lima, M., et al. (1999). Age differences in personality across the adult life span: Parallels in five cultures. *Developmental Psychology, 35,* 466–477.

Molinari, V., Marmion, J. (1993). Personality disorders in geropsychiatric outpatients. *Psychological Reports, 73,* 256–258.

Oldham, J. M. (1994). Personality disorders: Current perspectives. *Journal of the American Medical Association, 272,* 1770–1776.

Pasnau, R., Bystritsky, A. (1990). Importance of treating anxiety in the elderly ill patient. *Psychiatric Medicine, 8,* 163–173.

Robins, L. N., Helzer, S. C., Weissman, M. M., et al. (1984). Lifetime prevalence of specific psychiatric disorders in three sites. *Archives of General Psychiatry, 41,* 949–958.

Sadavoy, J., Dorian, B. (1983). Management of the characterologically difficult patient in the chronic care setting. *Journal of Geriatric Psychiatry, 16,* 233–240.

Sadavoy, J., Fogel, B. S. (1992). Personality disorders in the elderly. In J. Birren, G. Sloan, G. Cohen (Eds.), *Handbook of mental health and aging* (pp. 433–462). New York: Academic Press.

Schneider, L. S., Zemansky, M. F., Berden, M., et al. (1992). Personality in recovered depressed elderly. *International Psychogeriatrics, 4,* 177–185.

Soloff, P. H. (1998). Symptom–oriented psychopharmacology for personality disorders. *Journal of Practical Psychiatry and Behavioral Health, 4,* 3–11.

Woods, R. T. (1995). Psychological treatments. I: Behavioral and cognitive approaches. In J. Lindesay (Ed.), *Neurotic disorders in the elderly* (pp. 125–137). Oxford, UK: Oxford University Press.

Yesavage, J. A., Karasu, T. B. (1982). Psychotherapy with elderly patients. *American Journal of Psychotherapy, 36,* 41–55.

7

Individual Psychotherapies for Older Adults

Older adults are particularly receptive to the short-term, focused psychotherapies developed in recent years. Both primary care and mental health specialists can acquire skills for the shorter-term more directive therapies, particularly for bereavement (Friedli & King, 1996). However, age-relevant adaptations in the therapist's technique are necessary to make the enterprise effective.

ARGUMENTS FOR PSYCHOTHERAPY IN LATE LIFE

Niederehe (1996), in his review of psychosocial treatments in late life, summarizes much of what is known about therapy with older persons. First, advanced age is not in itself an obstacle to therapy, nor does it predict less favorable outcome (Knight, 1988). Indeed, older adults who enter therapy may be more compliant, less prone to drop out, and more positive toward treatment than younger patients. Techniques with demonstrated effectiveness in youth can be effectively extended to old age. Second, age-related health problems, principally cognitive impairment and physical illness, make the conduct of therapy more difficult and the outcome less certain (Mossey et al., 1996). Similarly, severity of mental illness, presence of a personality disorder, lack of insight ("psychological mindedness"), low expectations for change, and poor quality of relationship with the therapist (mismatch) also predict less success.

Third, the choice of therapeutic techniques must be tailored to the older adult's cognitive capacity, flexibility, and preferences. Ongoing psychotherapy may augment the effects of antidepressants minimizing recurrence (Reynolds et al., 1994) yet some persons will prefer medication management only. Similarly, the person's circumstances regarding independent travel, physical mobility, or brief hospitalization may allow for few or infrequent visits, making psychotherapy too dilute to be effective. Conversely, sufficient numbers of geographically clustered nursing home residents and home-bound patients or those in retirement communities may make an out-of-office psychotherapy practice feasible. Evidence suggests that psychotherapy alone may be effective for milder disorders and has an important role, in conjunction with medication, in diminishing the recurrence of more severe conditions.

Fourth, because family members often bring the older adult into treatment, the role of family should not be underestimated. Family may help maintain regular visits and optimism for psychotherapy with which their older relative has little familiarity. Similarly, family are the sentinels for recurrent symptoms or flagging enthusiasm for maintenance medication. Other concerned parties such as the primary care provider, home care agency, senior citizen center, church, or synagogue may also play a role. Here the older adult's confidentiality is preserved by first gaining permission to communicate the therapist's name, numbers, and general treatment plan to the third party. Intimate or sensitive personal information need not be disclosed. Indeed, the most frequent criticism of psychiatrists is lack of communication with the primary care physician (Bartle et al., 1995). Older adults generally welcome the therapist's communication with family and they expect communication with the primary care provider. Collaboration between the professional and family caregivers is the modern meaning of interdisciplinary teamwork.

Fifth, although studies of psychosocial treatments in combination with medication are few, combined therapy is the rule rather than the exception in routine practice. And given the serious consequences of relapse in the elderly, the capacity of psychotherapy to sustain adherence to a regimen of medication may be adequate justification for periodic visits. Sixth, the goals of therapy should be considered more broadly than simply the reduction or the elimination of symptoms. Improved or restored social and family function, increased self-reliance, reduced use of primary care services, better health care planning, and therapeutic compliance are only some of the examples with tangible benefits. Perhaps the most obvious example is psychotherapy and counseling of family caregivers of persons with dementia. These caregivers provide the bulk of noninstitutional, informal (unpaid) dementia care. They are an immense public health resource who are burdened by an elevated risk of depression, loss of social ties, and poorer physical health than their noncaregiver counterparts. Therapy, which sustains the quality and life of their caregiving, has obvious social benefits. And the personal satisfaction family members take in being productive caregivers is equally important.

Finally, the scope of need and the possible benefits of psychosocial interventions in late life far exceed the scientific evidence of efficacy. Most studies are the work of academic mental health specialists with self-selected, relatively independent older adults for whom measures of benefit are narrowly defined in terms of reduced symptoms of mental illness. Findings are then generalized to the average patient in the more typical nonacademic setting. An individualized approach with clearly defined, realistic goals should be the target of any psychotherapy.

All therapies (see Table 7.1) share common themes of establishing a supportive optimistic relationship, examining distortions, addressing conflict and ambivalence, repairing interpersonal or intrapsychic deficits, and restructuring defenses. The goal of each is to change expressed behavior brought about by an individualized treatment (Karasu, 1986; Yesavage & Karasu, 1982). Presented next are brief therapies adapted to older adult needs. The focus is on functional outcome first with restoration of mood and control of counterproductive impulses seen as a means to an end. Each therapy seeks to define the

TABLE 7.1. Types of Psychotherapy for Older Adults

Therapy	Distinguishing attributes
Cognitive-behavioral	Directive, symptom focused, techniques practiced outside therapy, counters misperceptions, mistaken beliefs
Interpersonal	Exploratory, focused on interpersonal conflict, role change and deficits
Short-term psychodynamic	Problem focused, transference not examined
Life review, reminiscence	Recall of personal history to master one's present and future
Problem solving	Focused on change, narrow and pragmatic
Supportive	Meant to maintain present level of function or symptom control
Dementia caregiver counseling	Focused on the caregiver role, combines elements of cognitive-behavioral and interpersonal therapy
Bereavement therapy	Restructuring (not restoration) the experience of the lost loved one
Behavioral	Educational with focus directed at reducing negative and increasing positive experiences

problem from the patient's perspective and seeks to limit the field of therapeutic play to the pursuit of realistic outcomes. Thus the assessment carried out during the initial session is critical and time-consuming. Family members may be involved in the evaluation session and in some of the therapies are crucial to success. Confidentiality is important but less an absolute for most seniors whose family and other providers may be intimately involved in the request for therapy. However, it is critical to determine the extent to which patients and family members have congruent goals and motivations for treatment. Unrealistic or conflicting expectations should be identified at the outset.

ASSESSMENT FOR PSYCHOTHERAPY

Efficiency is critical to conducting psychotherapy in present care settings. Unfortunately, older persons, because of the complexity of their conditions and longer life histories, require more time and skill from the clinician. Particularly in the initial assessment, the clinician needs to be active, structured, and alert to emotionally charged comments. A missed opportunity to explore a sensitive statement can be repaired once the clinician recognizes the error: "You mentioned something a moment ago I would like to return to." Similarly, time allowed for exposition of a sensitive area can be limited more effectively if the initial inquiry is handled deftly: "The details of how you feel are important but we also need to reserve time for discussion of what to do." A more active, focused, directive approach is better suited to the practice style of a primary care provider as well as being more appropriate to the older person's needs. At the end of the more lengthy assessment visit, the clinician should prepare the patient for briefer more focused sessions to follow.

A review of the developmental milestones of late life will inform the practitioner of patterns of mastery or defeat and capacity for change. For the older person distressed by growing dependency and the burden placed on family, a brief review of the patient's experience with parents will illuminate expectations of care from the family as well as hopes and fears recalled from prior experience. Problematic self-defeating reactions may represent models of behavior learned from a previous generation. The senior's dissatisfaction with time and attention from adult children may be based in part on inability to accept differences imposed by life changes unanticipated with advanced age. Similarly, the aftermath of the loss of the patient's parent may inform the therapist's perspective for the senior who has recently lost a spouse. Responses to prior episodes of illness and hospitalization may also be informative. Did the person recover fully after stroke or myocardial infarction or was there a prolonged period of disability and distress? How were these earlier stresses managed? What resources did the older person marshal for support then? What is available now?

BRIEF PSYCHODYNAMIC VERSUS SUPPORTIVE THERAPY

Short-term psychodynamic therapy is indicated for older persons with adjustment disorders, grief reactions, and recent onset of traumatic stress disorders (Lazarus & Sadavoy, 1996). Setting a time limit of 15 sessions avoids excessive dependency. The patient is helped to reestablish a positive sense of self and mastery. Both conscious and unconscious themes emerge in the treatment. These include the wish that the therapist will overcome the patient's fears that age has made change or adjustment impossible. Support is also sought to resolve problems of survivor guilt and negative attitudes toward the self and aging. Most important, patients can achieve insight and successfully terminate treatment without requiring long-term supportive care. Although transference may not be interpreted in shorter-term psychotherapy, an awareness of transference and countertransference are important elements in any therapeutic relationship.

Transference

Transference is the psychological phenomenon whereby unconscious hopes, fears, and attitudes are evoked in the patient by the therapist. The patient reacts in a predetermined way to real-life contingencies brought about by the therapeutic interaction. Processes outside the immediate awareness of the patient distort the relationship with the therapist. Transference in late life evolves out of childhood relationships as well as significant adult ties but is provoked by stress or conflict. Certain transferences arise more frequently in late life as the older adult confronts the loss of goals and ideals, changes in family and intimate relationships, illness, disability, and mortality.

Lazarus and Sadavoy (1996) have summarized the literature on transference. Some older patients initially affect the status of mentor or parent seeking to assist the younger inexperienced therapist rather than settling into the more direct work of treatment. They may discount the therapist's capacity to understand or help so senior a citizen. However this "reverse transference" (Grotjahn, 1955) often hides deeper fears of decline, inferiority, and dependence and more often yields to a more productive, realistic alliance. Retired persons seeking to adjust to the loss of self-esteem and the rewards of competition in the workplace may experience the therapist as the domineering, rival sib who is privileged to win at work what the patient is losing at home. An angry, depressive response to the therapist as well as the frustrations of retirement emerges. The therapist who is unable to restore the damaged self-esteem immediately may be seen as a withholding or depriving parent. Other narcissistic insults such as loss of physical or verbal prowess, beauty, or stature may provoke an idealized, mirror, or magical transference. These patients unconsciously perceive themselves as the powerful, admired beings they envision their therapists to be.

Frail, dependent patients may also develop idealized transferences. In either case a desperate sense of inadequacy lies just below the surface. A minor disappointment on the therapist's part or a turn of events beyond the therapist's control may provoke rage, rejection, and exaggerated dependency as fantasies of rescue are replaced by reality and the need to adapt. Patients may also develop a spousal transference, particularly following bereavement. The unavailability of a sex partner and the perceived loss of physical attractiveness in contrast to the intimacy and privacy of the clinical setting may provoke a frankly erotic transference. Thus the initial warm rapport may decay into bitter feelings as the unconscious hopes for restored youth and sexuality are frustrated by the therapist.

However irrational transference may be, it is provoked by real events that have real consequences. As examples, the individual grieving the death of a spouse or reacting to nursing home admission has reason to be sad and angry. Yet it is the vehemence with which the patient reacts to the therapist that indicates the reality of transference. Transference is often described as resistance to treatment or a defense against fears that would overwhelm were they admitted to consciousness. Yet the skilled practitioner recognizes transference as a guide to building a more reality-based relationship. Having appreciated the transference elements at the outset will allow the practitioner to work more efficiently whether the task is psychotherapy, initiation of insulin treatment, or rehabilitation following stroke.

Countertransference

Practitioners self-select their level of comfort with older patients by the specialty or area of interest they choose. Lack of experience with older adults makes one more vulnerable to countertransference. And countertransference will rarely be a problem until treatment becomes complex or difficult. However, an awareness of countertransference will help practitioners, whether or not their practice is geriatric, understand the intense feelings that are routinely evoked in elder care. Lack of such awareness will lead to inefficiency for the practitioner and dissatisfaction for the patient and family.

Lazarus and Sadavoy's (1996) review of therapists' unconscious reactions to the older patient reveals several pitfalls that practitioners may encounter. Bringing these automatic, stereotypical reactions to the practitioner's awareness is meant to enhance rather than constrain the therapeutic task. First are ageist responses that seniors are lacking in appeal, productivity, and capacity for change and that physical morbidity and approaching mortality overshadow any novelty or reward that the practitioner might find in the work relationship. Unresolved conflicts over dependency, illness, parental rejection, or threatened engulfment may also be evoked in the practitioner. Unconscious avoidance and distancing are the result, truncating empathy and making the relationship "safe" but sterile. The practitioner may also idealize the patient and the relationship to counter latent hostile or sexual feelings toward parents or the threat of abandonment occasioned by the patient's frailty. An authoritarian, overmedicalized stance prevents both patient and therapist from exploring more genuine, deeper feelings. The practitioner may engage in ill-considered power struggles with family over control in a countertransference-driven sibling or Oedipal rivalry. Lost opportunities to encourage other attachments and activities outside the therapy, failure to terminate after treatment goals are clearly attained, and visits or phone calls that are overlong or indulgent are also examples of countertransference phenomena. (For greater depth on transference and countertransference, see Zarit & Knight, 1996.)

GENERAL PRINCIPLES OF COGNITIVE-BEHAVIORAL THERAPY

Cognitive-behavioral therapy (CBT) seeks to change thoughts, feelings, and action by focusing on erroneous perceptions and habitual behaviors which the individual can learn to change. It has been tailored to specific disorders including depression, anxiety, panic, agoraphobia, obsessive–compulsive, and sleep disturbances. The general approach is educational and directive, requiring the practice of self-help techniques and homework. The therapist is active and the sessions are structured and problem oriented, emphasizing the present and future rather than the past. The patient is trained to monitor the thoughts that accompany emotional, symptomatic episodes. The mediating effect that thoughts have on feelings and behavior is examined. The patient and therapist then question the validity and logic of these thoughts to identify cognitive distortions and misinterpretations. The patient is asked to query the evidence in support of the interpretations and to identify contrary or alternative explanations. Biases toward fatalism are identified and the patient is asked to consider more reality-oriented possibilities. Finally, the patient is taught to identify and change dysfunctional patterns of belief that predispose to distorted experience. Because of its mechanistic approach, CBT appears straightforward, but it requires experience and skill to serve severely ill patients.

Gallagher and Thompson (1982) suggest the following adjustments for CBT to be effective with older persons. First, the patient needs an orientation to the approach with the emphasis placed on mastering stress through active participation in the treatment. Second, learning habits need to be acquired to overcome difficulties accepting therapeutic suggestions. Third, termination is relative rather than absolute, allowing return to therapy if new problems emerge or old ones recur. Fourth, the number of sessions may need to be extended, particularly when the problems presented are long standing or complicated by personality disorder. Finally, improvement may be a more realistic if moderate goals are set for the older person with limited resources and difficult life circumstances. Greater activity and flexibility are necessary when working with persons with cognition impaired by stroke or other medical disorders or sensory impairments (Gallagher-Thompson & Thompson, 1995). The sessions may need to be recorded for playback at home. Written instructions and homework may need to be provided in lessons and reinforced before proceeding to the next assignment. Some patients will feel themselves too old to change or find the therapist too young to help. The potential limitations of both parties should be acknowledged but with the caveat that failure is certain only when treatment is never attempted. Older adults may also feel stigmatized by psychotherapy that they equate with insanity, institutionalization, or lasting dependency on the therapist. Education regarding the scientific basis of modern therapy, the goal of greater rather than less autonomy, and the confidential nature of the enterprise should be provided.

Cognitive-Behavioral Therapy for Late-Life Depression

Perhaps best developed for depression, CBT seeks to alleviate dysphoria by attacking what Beck (1976) called a "cognitive triad" of negativism toward the self, the environment, and the future. The triad is maintained by persistently distorted perceptions and beliefs. Depressed persons see themselves as deficient, incapable, unlovable. The present environment seems overwhelming, promising only continuous failure. And the future course of life is hopeless, immutable. For many physically ill older adults, the future may seem threatening. Yet most seniors manage to maintain their spirits and contribute to the well-being of family and community. In CBT, the therapist helps the patient to examine pointless self-criticism, loss of positive motivation and reward, indecisiveness, guilt, and shame and the tendency to view problems as overwhelming. This means changing the erroneous beliefs and bad habits as well as asking the patient to add more pleasurable activities.

The patient is asked to examine behaviors that perpetuate depression (e.g., withdrawal from family, friends, and religious or community support institutions). Several behavioral strategies are invoked. Activities leading to a sense of accomplishment and pleasure are scheduled rather than being left to impulse or to others' initiative. Keeping count and assessing the emotional effects of the activities measures progress. Pleasurable activities that the patient may have abandoned or never considered are included. Assertiveness rather than passivity is encouraged. For example, the older parent who seeks more time with family is asked to take the initiative, be direct, and state a specific preference rather than waiting to be invited or telling the family what they should do. Social skills are also emphasized. When suicidal thoughts are present, the therapist explores the motives in an effort to reduce hopelessness and to tip the balance toward survival. Here reasons for living such as family, faith, future goals modest as they may be, and previous demonstrations of resiliency are made more salient. Even if the patient feels "it's just going through the motions," the effect over time is to alleviate depression through reinforcing positive, rewarding experience and perception. Again, the approach is adapted to the realities of late-life losses and disability to reach realistic goals that offer a degree of improvement if not full recovery.

Behavioral Therapy for Depression

Behavioral therapy for depression emerges from Lewinshon's (1975) observations that depressed people both produce and engage in fewer pleasant activities. Lack of positive reinforcement leads to a downward spiral that takes on a life of its own, namely, a depressive disorder. Once made habitual, the depression is resistant to simple commonsense advice and requires a more systematic intervention. Gallagher-Thompson and Thompson (1995) adapted these insights to the treatment of late-life depression. There are several components to this purely behavioral approach. First, an active educational component informs the patients of the underlying theory of depression and identifies examples of both pleasant and unpleasant behaviors and events in the day-to-day experience. Reading assignments and educational materials reinforce the therapy (Burns, 1989). The patient assigns a value to each event to construct a hierarchy of targets for change. Second, a specific plan or contract specifying which aversive events can be realistically avoided and which pleasant events can be increased is worked out. Third, realistic frequencies of events or duration of behavior are agreed on and a performance log is constructed. For example, if the pleasant event is exercise, the patient might specify 20 minutes a day three times a week. Improved mood is not expected with the initial phase, only a new set of behaviors. Rather, graded improvement is anticipated as the pleasurable events are increased in time or amount. Fourth, the patient monitors mood with depression instruments or a simple linear scale from 1 (totally depressed) to 10 (totally happy). Thus, subjective experience is converted into a quasi-objective measure. As the patient becomes accustomed to self-monitoring, the array of pleasant and unpleasant events may be expanded and the contract advanced. As mood and self-assurance improve, more difficult, complex tasks are approached. Ultimately, the patient free of depressed mood abandons the recordkeeping and scheduling as the positive reinforcement becomes habitual. The simplicity of the theory, the commonsense quality to the intervention, and the mechanistic technique works well with older persons (Zarit & Zarit, 1998).

Cognitive-Behavioral Therapy for Late-Life Anxiety Disorders

Table 7.2 outlines the general principles of CBT for anxiety disorders. Whether for panic, agoraphobia, obsessive–compulsive disorder, or generalized anxiety, CBT, works by eliciting manifestations of the disorder under controlled conditions that lead to extinction of the symptoms (Sanderson & Wetzler, 1995). Older adults who have isolated themselves for years and have become psychiatric shut-ins may resist the effort, especially if supportive services from a visiting nurse and Meals on Wheels are in place. Nonetheless, offers to make them less agoraphobic with the help of friends and other providers should be discussed. It is important to add that frail persons of advanced age have realistic fears of being out of their homes alone.

The symptoms of panic and anxiety consist of emotional, cognitive, and somatic components. Once the symptoms reach diagnostic proportions, the components are so intertwined that a single feature is

TABLE 7.2. Guidelines for the Cognitive-Behavioral Treatment of Panic, Anxiety, and Agoraphobia in Late Life

1. Psychoeducation
   - Panic, anxiety, agoraphobia defined with symptoms shown to be physically harmless and possible to control
   - Fears of brain tumor, stroke, heart attack, fainting debunked
   - Avoidance behavior and anticipatory anxiety shown to be counterproductive
   - Written materials offered or referred to

2. Cognitive restructuring
   - Demonstration that certain thoughts provoke or accentuate panic and anxiety
   - Most recent attack of anxiety or panic reviewed to elicit the associated internal monologue and test reality
   - Thought record looking for evidence of jumping to conclusions
   - "Decatastrophize"

3. Respiratory control
   - Recognition of hyperventilation (rapid, shallow breaths with chest muscles)
   - Practice of diaphragmatic breathing (slow, regular abdominal breaths)

4. Relaxation training
   - Practice of progressive muscle relaxation (see Barlow & Craske, 1989)

5. Controlled provocation of anxiety and panic
   - Visualization and imagery exercises for inoculation
     - Anxiety-provoking situations (from least to greatest) progressively imagined and described in detail
     - Coping strategies subsequently imagined and applied
   - Exposure
     - Interoceptive: Hierarchy of fear-provoking sensations (dizziness, palpitations) described and rehearsed in therapy
     - Situational: Anxiety-provoking situations (from least to greatest) and coping responses rehearsed in therapy and enacted outside

Note. Data from Sanderson and Wetzler (1995) and Sanderson and McGinn (1997).

likely to trigger the total configuration. The goal is to counter the entire configuration of anxiety and panic. This will include the anticipatory anxiety ("fear of fear"), the agoraphobic avoidance of triggering situations and perceptions, and the despair that sets in once other symptoms have become persistent and disabling (Sanderson & Wetzler, 1995).

Sanderson and Weztler (1995) argue that medications interfere with the treatment of panic disorder. In theory, patients encounter their symptoms in therapy to learn how to extinguish them. By blunting the experience of symptoms, medications interfere with the programmatic de-escalation of the disorder to a trivial level of symptoms.

Their argument is especially compelling for older adults in whom the sedative effects of the benzodiazepines may be associated with impaired cognition or falls. Although medications may be required to give some patients enough relief to access psychotherapy (see Chapter 2), the gradual reduction if not elimination of antianxiety agents may be required for CBT to be fully effective. Thus for persons who are able to tolerate their disorder long enough to learn to lessen their symptoms through psychotherapy, medications may be avoided entirely.

The therapy is initiated with an orientation to the methods regarding teaching and training of coping techniques and a lesson plan focused on countering misapprehensions. Panic, anxiety, and agoraphobia are formally defined and shown to be physically harmless despite transient tachycardia, lightheadedness, palpitations, and pounding heart. Fears of brain tumor, heart attack, and fainting are debunked. Patients are also reminded that despite comorbid conditions, they have managed to survive the panic attacks to date.

The practitioner either calls the primary care provider or openly reviews with the patient the present treatment of any concurrent cardiovascular or pulmonary disease. This will assure both patient and therapist that complicating conditions are indeed stable. The physiology and psychology of fear and anxiety and the physiological consequences of overbreathing are reviewed. Increased aerobic exercise (see Chapter 15) and reduction in stimulant coffee and tea are also suggested. The patient's avoidance behavior and anticipatory anxiety are brought out and shown to be counterproductive and self-defeating. For example, the person who rarely leaves the house for fear of a heart attack is missing both the exercise and social interaction that have known cardioprotective effects. Written materials explaining the diagnosis, the treatment plan, homework assignments, and self-help tracts are offered or referred to. Bernstein and Borkovec's (1973) *Progressive Relaxation Training* and Barlow and Craske's (1989) *Mastery of Your Anxiety and Panic* are excellent resources for patient and family.

As the therapy progresses, cognitive restructuring is introduced. Based on patient history, the practitioner demonstrates that certain thoughts provoke or accentuate panic and anxiety. The most recent attack of anxiety or panic is reviewed to elicit the associated internal monologue (e.g., "My heart's racing so fast I'll have a heart attack if I don't get out of here I'll die."). The patient is instructed to keep a record of similar thoughts that either precede or accompany the panic or anxiety. The erroneous conclusions and assumptions of catastrophe that follow are also recorded. With the record in hand, the practitioner asks the patient to "decatastrophize." For example, patients who feel the beginnings of a panic attack if kept waiting more than 5 minutes in clinic would be asked to recall that anxiety is natural in such circumstances, that they have managed to survive repeated clinic visits, that worrying ahead of time about the anxiety only heightens it, and that there are several coping techniques which can be effectively utilized with practice.

Among these are respiratory control and the relaxation response. The patient is taught to recognize the signs of hyperventilation (rapid, shallow breaths with chest muscles). The practice of diaphragmatic breathing (slow, regular abdominal breaths) is introduced and reinforced by asking that it be practiced on a regular, scheduled basis. Relaxation training through the practice of progressive muscle relaxation is also introduced (see Barlow & Craske, 1989). Regular practice during periods of comfort is essential to confident application when a panic attack threatens. With practice, the duration and frequency of occurrences can be reduced. A log of attacks and near attacks is kept to monitor progress and reinforce practice.

Once the educational components are complete and the techniques for breathing and eliciting the relaxation response are mastered, controlled provocation of anxiety and panic may be approached. The hierarchy of fear-provoking sensations (dizziness, palpitations) is described and rehearsed in therapy. First, visualization and imagery exercises are introduced in the office to inoculate the patient against triggering events encountered outside therapy. Anxiety-provoking situations (from least to greatest) are progressively imagined and described in detail. The simple description often provokes mild anxiety, which is then extinguished with the breathing or relaxation techniques. Coping strategies are imagined and potential obstacles to their application explored. The practice generates a sense of mastery as well as a set of tools to attack the problems. The patient is then asked to purposefully and progressively seek out the anxiety-provoking situations, from least to most threatening, outside therapy and to implement the rehearsed coping responses. Once the prearranged termination goal has been achieved, the patients is inoculated against future failure with the instruction that recurrence under stress is not a catastrophe, only an indicator for a booster session or the need to redouble practice of techniques (Sanderson & McGinn, 1997).

Cognitive-Behavioral Therapy
for Obsessive–Compulsive Disorder

Obsessive–compulsive disorder originates less frequently in late life. It may be difficult to diagnose because the patient is reluctant to share the symptoms which are acknowledged as irrational or because depression is a more salient but masking disorder. Stressful events amplify the symptoms to disabling proportions. Older patients with the disorder are more likely to have sustained the symptoms without treatment for a longer time than younger patients. However, elders appear to respond as well as younger patients to treatment (Carmin et al., 1998). The treatment plan is based on an assessment of symptoms. Obsessions are recurrent unwanted impulses, ideas, images, or thoughts that increase anxiety. Common examples are fears of contamination (dirt or germs), having a serious illness, or an inability to discard objects that are clearly useless, worn out, and in the way. Overconcern for order, sameness, or symmetry may also occur. Irrational fears that one will be responsible for hurting a loved one are also common.

Compulsions are repetitive behavioral or mental rituals, which the patient may see as irrational but feels driven to carry out because they decrease anxiety. Hand washing, repetitive checking on household appliances or locks, mental counting, forced recitation of prayers, and constant need for reassurance are examples. The patient and therapist catalogue both symptoms and frequency to set the stage for baseline monitoring and subsequent reduction. Problems are weighted from most to least disruptive to prepare a therapeutic hierarchy. Triggers to anxiety from both the patient and the environment are listed. The feared consequences, both specific and otherwise, are noted. Maneuvers used to avoid or distract are described. Insight and mood are assessed to determine the presence of psychosis or depression, both of which will alter the approach substantially but not entirely. Most important is an assessment of impairments in daily functioning which will suggest a priority of targets for intervention as well as the end point of treatment.

The interventions are focused on symptoms or problems and include both psychological and pharmacological (see Chapter 2). Including the family as cotherapist may be essential to interrupt the cycle of obsessions and compulsions and for completion of homework. An educational discussion, self-help bibliography, and materials related to the diagnosis, interest groups, and organizations should be provided at the outset. The clinician should make clear that the goal is to break the linkage between the obsession and resultant thought or anxiety. Cognitive restructuring is used to examine any distorted beliefs. For specific fears the patient is asked to practice imagining the trigger object or thought beginning with the least threatening element or item. These items may be written on flashcards to facilitate practice. One item at a time is revealed and followed by a relaxation exercise rather than the obsession or compulsion. Self-monitoring is used to reinforce a sense of mastery over the provoked anxiety and ultimately to extinguish the response. The patient proceeds up the hierarchy until the most threatening item has become trivialized by practice. Termination is accomplished with the option for booster sessions should symptoms again become disabling. Transient emergence of symptoms under stress is to be expected and is not an indicator of recurrence.

INTERPERSONAL THERAPY
FOR LATE-LIFE DEPRESSION

Interpersonal therapy was been developed for the treatment of depression over 12 to 20 weekly sessions and successfully modified for use with older adults (Frank et al., 1993). Interpersonal psychotherapy is meant to elicit thoughts and feelings that cause distress and may be changed by examination (see Table 7.3). The therapist lends a sense of optimism and empathy that allows patients to express difficulties that may be out of their day-to-day awareness yet cause an undercurrent of distress. As in CBT, educating the patient about how treatment works is as important as establishing rapport. Although interpersonal therapy is less directive than cognitive-behavioral or problem-solving ther-

TABLE 7.3. Guidelines for Interpersonal Psychotherapy in Late-Life Depression

1. Attributes of the approach
   - Therapist is active, not neutral
   - Target is behavioral change in present interpersonal relations
   - The work area is interpersonal rather than intrapsychic
   - Focus is on short-term goals and problem resolution, not open ended

2. Typical problem life areas
   - Grief and bereavement (loss of spouse, siblings, adult children)
   - Role disputes (marital conflict, family dissension)
   - Role transitions (breadwinner to companion, homemaker to caregiver)
   - Interpersonal deficits (social isolation)

3. Therapist's adaptations for work with the aged
   - More directive—dependency needs addressed practically
   - More supportive—acceptance is often more realistic than change
   - More flexible with problems of transportation, finance, and health
   - Existential reality of loss, lifelong pathology, advanced age recognized
   - Unconscious meaning of the therapeutic relationship not interpreted

Note. Data from Miller and Markowitz (1999).

apy, the therapist working with physically disabled, medically frail older persons will not hesitate to provide advice and information (Miller & Silberman, 1996). Particularly with older adults, the therapist must be active rather than neutral, targeting issues, focusing on solutions, and pragmatic about what the patient should do. The target is behavioral change in present interpersonal relations rather than resolution of intrapsychic conflict. The focus is on short-term goals and problem resolution rather than an open-ended exploration of thoughts and feelings. The influence of past relationships on present problems is acknowledged but the work is focused on the present and future (Miller & Markowitz, 1999).

During the assessment phase the therapist will examine the important personal relations within the patient's life to determine where conflicts and problems lie. Relationships involved in the current and any previous episodes of depression will also be identified. The approach is explicitly time limited and not designed to alter personality traits or delusional material. There are four typical problem areas related to depression which interpersonal therapy is conceived to address: (1) grief and bereavement including loss of spouse, siblings, or adult children; (2) role disputes such as marital conflict and family dissension; (3) role transitions such as change from breadwinner to companion, homemaker to caregiver, employee to retiree; and (4) interpersonal deficits, which have lead to social isolation and difficulty accepting care and support. Here the patient may complain of loneliness, find it difficult to make new friends, or unwittingly drive acquaintances away (Zarit & Zarit, 1998).

Because of older adult realities, the therapist addresses the patient's dependency needs and limitations due to loss, lifelong psychopathology, and the existential realities of advanced age practically. Goals are kept modest and realistic. Reassurance and support are offered. Role play may be used to demonstrate or practice new interpersonal approaches or responses. More time and telephone accessibility are provided than would be expected with younger persons. Because the older adult may have limited options to develop new relationships or living situations, the patient is more often advised to tolerate rather than terminate problematic long-term relationships. This does not mean ignoring the problem but, rather, seeking other solutions. Greater flexibility toward the length of the sessions and missed appointments due to problems with transportation, health, and finances is extended. The unconscious meaning of the therapeutic relationship is generally not interpreted. Transference is not examined directly. Modest gifts can be accepted at termination or holidays with thanks rather than interpretation.

LIFE REVIEW OR REMINISCENCE THERAPY

Life review or reminiscence therapy has much to offer the older person who is struggling with troubling events and the realization of mortality (Butler, 1963). The therapist encourages a review of the past in an effort to help the patient find meaning in the present through partial resolution of conflict within the self or with others (Haight, 1992). As in CBT, homework may be assigned, such as review of memorabilia, photos, or journals, which may also be brought to the therapist. The patient may be asked to write an autobiography or reunite with friends or family. In addition to solving old problems, the patient may find an increased tolerance for conflict, a lessening of guilt and fears, enhanced creativity and a sense of giving, and acceptance of life circumstances (Butler & Lewis, 1982). This technique may be the treatment of choice for survivors of the Holocaust and others traumatized by overwhelming stress. Tauber's (1998) *In the Other Chair* and Novick's (1999) *The Holocaust in American Life* provide historical as well as emotional background to inform the therapist.

Clearly some persons need to keep old wounds covered (Kahana et al., 1988). More often they are responding to the unspoken preferences of others who would rather not be burdened or who trivialize the events with superficial identification (Tauber, 1998). Themes of survivor guilt, impotent rage and lasting resentment, alienation ("you can't understand if you weren't there"), cynicism, distrust, and the futility of suffering challenge the therapist's capacity to engage the patient. Recollections of betrayal, desecration, humiliation, and incomprehensible loss (e.g., the murder of one's child) threaten to overwhelm the therapist. Acts of desperation provoked by survival instinct, such as stealing a starving inmate's rations, may be difficult to confess (Bluhm, 1948/1999). And it may be easier to recall what was perpetrated than the thoughts and feelings that were evoked at the time. Family members may know considerable details of the atrocities but nothing about the survivor's reaction. However, one's willingness to listen if the patient is willing to talk is a powerful incentive as well as protection against damaging intrusion. Without question the therapist will never fully realize the patient's experience. Yet a meaningful degree of understanding for both parties is possible provided the patient is willing to recall and communicate. This understanding can be crucial to coping with life-threatening illness or injury, bereavement, or nursing home admission that may evoke recollections of catastrophic events. The need for and benefits of life review therapy remind one that "medically justified" treatment for human suffering goes beyond diagnostic nomenclature.

PROBLEM-SOLVING THERAPY

Problem-solving therapy is directive and brief, usually spanning six sessions. Written lists are generated in the therapy session and homework is prescribed. The patient is asked to specify and prioritize problems whether they are thoughts, feelings of fatigue, anxiety or depression, or interpersonal difficulties. The patient and therapist assess the circumstances surrounding the problem. The therapist urges the patient to formulate a feasible approach as well as to triage problems with less probability of change to a lower priority. Once a problem is identified and its determinants specified, a brief list of potential solutions is generated by patient and therapist. For each solution a set of pros and cons are drawn up which prioritize the solutions from most to least difficult to effect. Pessimism ("it hasn't worked before") and lack of motivation ("I forgot to practice") are addressed again by taking the problem-solving approach. However, the focus is kept purposefully narrow on the initial problem identified by the patient in order to minimize a diffusion of effort. The patient is also reminded that the number of sessions set aside may be specific to the identified problem and that additional problems may be beyond the scope of the present therapy. This is not to say that genuine problems do not arise during therapy or that they never displace the identified difficulty. However, the aim is to keep the patient and therapist on track, to focus the effort on realistic solutions.

TREATMENT OF CAREGIVER
BURDEN AND DEPRESSION

The overlapping roles of primary care practitioners and mental health specialists are nowhere more evident than in the needs of dementia caregivers. Family members remain the mainstay of dementia care in the community. Their caregiving burden has long been recognized as a major public health concern. A number of studies indicate that caregiver burden can be reduced and nursing home admission delayed by specific interventions (Mittelman et al., 1995; Whitlatch et al., 1995). With support and training, caregivers can reduce their depressive symptoms and those in their dementing relatives as well (Teri et al., 1997). Considerable attention has been devoted to the distress associated with caring for someone with dementia in the community (Cohen & Eisdorfer, 1988), but less has been directed to caregivers once their family member has been admitted to a nursing home. Efforts to contain Medicare and Medicaid expenditures for home care and nursing facilities threaten to increase the burden expected of family members. Their burdens are already substantial. Gallagher et al. (1989) found that 46% of caregivers seeking help met diagnostic criteria for depression; even among those not seeking help, 18% met criteria for depression.

Family assistance with activities of daily living may decline after nursing home admission without relieving the caregivers' burden (Light et al., 1994; Zarit & Whitlatch, 1992). Indeed, more than 80% of community caregivers do not relinquish the role once their relative is admitted (Kiecolt-Glaser et al., 1991). Although caregivers are accurate in assessing the level of impairment in their demented relative (Reifler et al., 1981), the severity of impairment does not explain the caregiver's burden or depressive symptoms (Zarit et al., 1980).

Conflicts and distorted beliefs over separation–individuation or "letting go" add to the burden of caregiving. Caregiver spouses may become "shadow residents" of the facility (Riddick et al., 1992), averaging more than 20 hours per week at the home (Zarit & Whitlatch, 1993). Caregivers may be likened to military wives whose husbands were declared missing in action. Preoccupation with the demented individual and confusion as to where the patient fits in the family predict caregiver depression (Boss et al., 1990).

Studies of therapeutic interventions regarding separation–individuation (Mittelman et al., 1995) have employed individual counseling and educational support groups to lessen burden and delay nursing home admission. However, these studies focus on negative end points rather than the broader purposes, outcomes, and positive personal meaning of caregiving (Nolan et al., 1996). Questions as to the relevance of caregiver burden after nursing home admission remain. Is excessive caregiver burden an indicator of untreated depression? If not, are family support groups in nursing homes sufficient (Toseland et al., 1992), or are mental health services necessary? Are there costs saved through family caregiving in the nursing home as well as in the community? Indeed, family involvement in nursing home care has been linked to improved quality of life for the demented resident. Nursing facilities are not staffed to provide mental health services to families whose distress is an obstacle to the residents' well-being (Robinson, 1990). If the expense of long-term care is capped, will the savings be realized through a transfer of costs to the "hidden victims" (Zarit et al., 1985) of dementia, the family members? Thus, both before and after nursing home admission, family caregivers (and indirectly the care recipients) are likely to benefit from therapy.

Zarit and Zarit (1998) have developed an assessment and intervention model to reduce caregiver burden and improve caregiver skills. The assessment entails; (1) characterization of problems emanating directly from the patient's needs and behaviors; (2) recognition of secondary stressors which add to caregiver burden but are not patient based; (3) estimating the network of support available from family, friends, and formal (purchased) support services; and (4) the presence of depression or an anxiety disorder. After assessment there is a three-part approach to intervention which involves (1) provision of information regarding the disease and course of illness via counseling and education, (2) specific problem solving through family meetings, and (3) support through individual or peer-group work. Chapter 3 details the educational material and the approach to problem patient behaviors. Here we focus on caregiver needs not covered elsewhere.

Semple (1992) suggests there are three typical conflicts that family will experience in dementia care (1) disagreements and uncertainty over the diagnosis and medical treatment; (2) conflict over the quantity and quality of care provided; and (3) discussions about who should provide care and to what extent it is a shared rather than delegated burden. Some families are vocal and assertive. Problems are routinely surfaced and negotiated to consensus or open impasse. However, other families expect needs to be met as a matter of entitlement rather than negotiated. Their style may require a more uncovering stance in which diagnosis and prognosis are shared via the authority of the practitioner's concern for the demented patient. The goal of the family meeting is to make explicit differing views and to gain consensus on interventions when possible. (See Chapter 8 on the conduct of a therapeutic family meeting.)

Some caregivers are reluctant to make their needs known to other family members or to accept assistance from a home care agency. They are afraid of rejection or admitting inadequacy. They fear loss of control or assume that no other person could provide adequate care or be accepted by the demented relative. The loss of privacy and the economic costs when paid companions enter the home are genuine concerns. In each instance the caregiver should be asked to consider a trial intervention with the caveat that the need for repeated trials or alternative companions is to be expected.

Zarit and Zarit (1998) note that caregivers usually seek help for their relative rather than themselves so that the initial assessment must begin with the identified patient but transition to the caregiver's needs. At times the caregiver comes prepared with extensive experience, background information, and family support. Others need time to realize their needs and express their preferences. The practitioner should anticipate the right pace of treatment and allow time for assimilation of new information and adjustment to new roles. Secondary stresses to the caregiving task need to be identified both to broaden the scope of potential intervention and to realize the limits of the person's circumstances. For example, is dementia caregiving eroding the caregiver's employment or other family roles? Are the caregiver's medical problems being neglected? Can an accumulation of stress be avoided by anticipation and prioritization? Is respite care in the home with another family member or a paid companion an option? Is a temporary stay in a nursing home financially feasible? What are the quality and extent of supportive relationships that can substitute for the caregiver or act as a buffer when stress becomes overwhelming? A family genogram with ages and geographic location may allow both the practitioner and the caregiver to identify untapped resources as well as clarify the limits.

Support for the caregiver is integral to each aspect of intervention. Peer support through dementia caregiver groups is available in community settings through contact with the local Alzheimer's association and at some nursing homes. Peer support will lessen the alienation and sense of inadequacy the caregiver feels. Caregiving tips and experience negotiating community agencies (and practitioners) may be voiced. The means of overcoming barriers both practical and emotional are shared. Because the task is one of support, relationships that extend beyond the group are encouraged. However, support groups are not available to, nor are they desired by, all caregivers. A support group in which all the caregivers have late-stage relatives will shock the person whose spouse or sibling is in the early stage of illness. A support group is no substitute for the ongoing care of the primary practitioner or mental health specialist.

Beyond the educational counseling, behavioral techniques, and problem solving, individual support for the caregiver should also focus on treatment of depression and anxiety with adequate attention to sleep disturbance and the potential for substance abuse. Medication may be a necessary adjunct to alleviate symptomatic impairment. On occasion the caregiver's failing cognition will become a focus of attention. Elements of cognitive-behavioral and interpersonal treatment may be included. Certainly in the initial and final phases of dementia, the caregiver is involved in a grief reaction for which elements of bereavement therapy are appropriate. However, what is different about treatment of caregivers is the ongoing and progressive nature of the stress. Some will master the task after brief individual intervention. Others will require a more prolonged effort in which family members, community agencies, and other providers will need to be engaged. Some will not be capable of change due to unrecognized mental disorder, substance abuse, lack of familiarity with medical care, or a developmental disorder. Depending on the locale, educated clergy may assist caregivers and can be a source of both therapeutic support and leverage. However, when psychosis, substance abuse, or suicidality is evident, referral to a mental health specialist is indicated.

In summary, a sophisticated, structured approach to the caregiver will delay the dementing person's entry into nursing home. The intervention need not increase caregiver burden. Many caregivers will cope with a minimum of support and information. Others will need referral to community agencies and peer support groups. However, a minority, which will grow in size as the prevalence of dementia increases, will require the assistance of a mental health specialist.

BEREAVEMENT THERAPY

Bereavement is a major, predictable life event among older adults and a frequent occurrence in geriatric care. With advanced age, fewer of the senior's friends and sibs remain. Spousal bereavement is more prevalent among older women whose survival advantage over their husbands is countered by a greater likelihood of disability, solitary living, and nursing home admission. Also, with increasing lifespans older adults will more frequently live through the loss of an adult child. And the death of a grandchild, particularly in large families, is not entirely remote. Most older persons will not perceive bereavement to be a problem that merits professional attention (Shuchter & Zisook, 1993). However, bereavement late in life has a demonstrable impact on mortality. Bereaved older adults are also more likely to develop a major depressive episode within the year of their loss than are younger persons (Zisook & Shuchter, 1996). As a result, the generalist practitioner should have the skills for the brief psychological treatment of the bereaved and to recognize cases in which grief is complicated by a major depressive disorder. This is especially important for the older patient who is of advanced age, lives alone, or has few social contacts.

In my experience, most older patients are not surprised by the emptiness, sadness, loneliness, and preoccupation with their lost loved one. And the hallucinated scent, sight, or feel of the deceased spouse that is common rarely provokes fears of insanity and may evoke comforting memories. However, the fatigue, anger, irritability, insomnia, and social isolation are unexpected and unwelcome. Ambivalent past relations fraught with unresolved resentments or episodes of abuse may lead to particularly complicated grief reactions. Childless older adults and older men dependent on their wives for a social life may find the isolation difficult to bear. Sudden unexpected death occurs with little time for the individual and his or her supportive relationships to prepare. Conversely, the death of an aged parent or spouse after prolonged dementia or other chronic illness may be followed by relatively brief period of mourning. In any event, the principles of therapy with the bereaved are straightforward and incorporate cognitive-behavioral and interpersonal elements. Although they apply to the loss of any family member or intimate friend, we will address the techniques for convenience sake as applying to spousal bereavement.

First the patient is offered a session to talk about feelings and coping with the loss. The circumstances of the spouse's death are elicited in an effort to alleviate the burden of grief but also to uncover doubts and ambivalence about what the spouse of other caregivers might have done to prevent the loss. Self-blame or resentment toward others needs to be explored and the reality of interpretations tested. Similarly, guilt over feeling relief at the passing of a difficult burden should be uncovered. The patient should be made aware that rich relationships are rich in feelings not all of which are pleasant. However, anger at the spouse for "going first, leaving me alone with all this" is not easily expressed initially. The intensity of resentment may frighten the person and threaten to breach the taboo of speaking ill of the dead.

For patients seen in referral by a mental health specialist and those in whom several sessions seem indicated, an interpersonal inventory of the bereaved will be helpful (Frank et al., 1993). To what extent was the deceased responsible for social and financial transactions and who will assist in his or her absence? What practical adjustments must be made to manage without the spouse? Has the survivor independent social or leisure pursuits or were they shared and dependent on the deceased? What were the circumstances of death? Was it sudden, expected, or suicidal? Was illness or death prolonged, financially and emotionally burdensome? Was the death seen as an exit from suffering? Was the marriage problematic or difficult? Did death bring freedom from ongoing marital conflict? Were there episodes of separation? What financial (last will and testament, insurance) preparations or discussions occurred in anticipation of death? Are there thoughts of future romance? Has a waiting period been consciously chosen? Were there extramarital affairs from either spouse about which the survivor has feelings? Are children and grandchildren a readily accessible and realistic source of support? Is relocation to the children's area being considered? What was the impact of losses earlier in life, especially the death of parents (Miller & Silberman, 1996)?

It is helpful to ask the patient to bring in old photos of the deceased spouse. These invariably evoke patient memories and spark the therapist's curiosity. Questions such as how the couple first met, what were shared leisure interests and life accomplishments, and what was the deceased's reaction to births of children serve to balance more negative feelings. Here the purpose is to give the therapist insight into the relationship as well as a more vivid picture of the lost spouse. For the patient, sharing positive memories reinforces the lasting value of the relationship as well as making it more acceptable to express less pleasant recollections.

Clichés such as "I know how you feel" or "With time you'll get over the loss" are rarely helpful and are more often perceived as insensitive. Similarly well-intended sharing of the therapist's reaction to personal loss of a spouse or parent detracts the focus from the patient. However, if the practitioner had a relationship with the deceased, shared recollections may be helpful if offered briefly and at the right time. The ultimate goal is to help the bereaved find comfort in the past relationship that will make the future separations possible to bear. The purpose is not to engender a new dependency but rather to demonstrate that existing relationships can be renewed or expanded.

Regarding behavioral advice, the patient should seek to reestablish life's routine and social rhythm. Regular sleep; exercise; attendance at church, synagogue, or senior center; volunteer organizations; and family affairs should be encouraged. The person who complains of being too sad to be with others is certainly too sad to be alone. This is not to underestimate the person's genuine vulnerability. It will be difficult initially to be around others who serve as a painful reminder of the loss. Yet it is better to confront painful moments in a context in which a more pleasant experience may follow than to be alone.

When the tears, sleep disturbance, weight loss, and helplessness are severe, persistent, or disabling, medication is indicated. The passive wish for death is not uncommon in bereavement, but intrusive thoughts of suicide or suicidal methods should be taken as signaling major depression. Increased alcohol intake, misuse of analgesics, or neglected life-saving medications (hypoglycemics, antihypertensives, antianginal, antiarrhythmics) approach criteria for major depression and call for a more aggressive intervention. Short-lived benzodiazepines (lorazepam, oxazepam) or zolpidem may be of considerable benefit, but a sedative antidepressant (nortriptyline, trazodone, nefazodone, mirtazapine) is better if the symptom profile approaches major depression criteria. Patients requiring a benzodiazepine for more than 2 weeks should be switched to an antidepressant. The bereaved patient's somatic preoccupation or fears of undetected illness do not necessarily indicate the emergence of psychosis. However, undue suspiciousness, refusal of companionship from family or friends, and extreme isolation suggest a paranoid reaction, particularly if frank delusions are in evidence. Without past history of similar episodes, the correct diagnosis may be brief psychotic reaction, and an antipsychotic should be prescribed with planned withdrawal within the coming months. It is important to recall that sleep deprivation can also precipitate brief psychosis.

SUMMARY

Individual psychotherapeutic interventions from different traditions offer benefits in older patient outcomes for a variety of indications. These include anxiety and depressive disorders, complicated bereavement, and caregiver burden. The differing psychotherapies for late-life depression share common elements that are easily adapted across techniques. These include a problem-focused, here-and-now approach with a distinct psychoeducational component. Homework may be assigned, faulty cognition confronted, and interpersonal changes suggested. For the motivated primary care practitioner, use of short-term psychotherapeutic techniques can enliven practice, lessen the need for referrals, and provide greater acceptance of mental health services for those patients who need specialist care. For mental health specialists accustomed to psychotherapy with younger persons, necessary adjustments in approach include allowances for sensory and cognitive impairments, greater collaboration with the patient's family and other care providers, and identification of improved function and symptom reduction as worthwhile goals. Despite advances in the choices and benefits of pharmacotherapy, familiarity with late-life psychotherapy will remain critical both for primary care and for specialists alike.

REFERENCES

Barlow, D. A., Craske, M. G. (1989). *Mastery of your anxiety and panic*. Albany, NY: Graywind.

Bartle, S. H., Aldin, P., Green, M. R., et al. (1995). Attitudes of physicians toward psychiatry: Some criticism which psychiatrists might modify. *Berkshire Medical Journal, 3,* 7–10.

Beck, A. T. (1976). *Cognitive therapy and the emotional disorders*. New York: International Universities Press.

Bernstein, T. A., Borkovec, T. D. (1973). *Progressive relaxation training*. Champaign, IL: Research Press.

Bluhm, H. O. (1999). How did they survive?: Mechanisms of defense in Nazi concentration camps. *American Journal of Psychotherapy, 53,* 96–122. (Original work published 1948)

Boss, P., Caron, W., Horbal, J., et al. (1990). Predictors of depression in caregivers of dementia patients: Boundary ambiguity and mastery. *Family Process, 29,* 245–254.

Burns, D. D. (1989). *The feeling good handbook: Using the new mood therapy in every day life.* New York: Morrow.

Butler, R. N. (1963). The life review: An intervention of reminiscence in the aged. *Psychiatry, 26,* 65–70.

Butler, R. N., Lewis, M. I. (1982). *Aging and mental health: Positive psychosocial and biomedical approaches.* St. Louis, MO: Mosby.

Carmin, C. N., Beck, J. G., Henninger, N. J. (1998). Obsessive–compulsive disorder: Cognitive-behavioral treatment of older versus younger adults. *Clinical Gerontologist, 19,* 77–81.

Cohen, D., Eisdorfer, C. (1988). Depression in family members caring for a relative with Alzheimer's disease. *Journal of the American Geriatrics Society, 36,* 885–889.

Frank, E., Frank, N., Cornes, C., et al. (1993). Interpersonal psychotherapy in the treatment of late-life depression. In G. L. Klerman & M. M. Weissman (Eds.), *New applications of interpersonal psychotherapy* (pp. 167–198). Washington, DC: American Psychiatric Press.

Friedli, K., King, M. (1996). Counseling in general practice: A review. *Primary Care Psychiatry, 2,* 205–216

Gallagher, D., Rose, J., Rivera, P., et al. (1989). Prevalence of depression in family caregivers. *Gerontologist, 29,* 449–456.

Gallagher, D. E., Thompson, L. W. (1982). Differential effectiveness of psychotherapies for the treatment of major depressive disorders in older adult patients. *Psychotherapy: Theory, Research, and Practice, 19,* 482–490.

Gallagher-Thompson, D. E., Thompson, L. W. (1995). Psychotherapy with older adults in theory and practice. In B. Bonger & L. Beutler (Eds.), *Comprehensive textbook of psychotherapy* (pp. 357–379). New York: Oxford University Press.

Grotjahn, M. (1955). Analytic psychotherapy with the elderly. *Psychoanalytic Review, 42,* 419–427.

Haight, B. K. (1992). Long-term effects of structured life review process in homebound elderly subjects. *Journals of Gerontology, Psychological Sciences, 47,* P312–315.

Kahana, B., Kahana, E., Harel, Z. (1988). Coping with extreme stress. In J. P. Wilson, Z. Harel, & B. Kahana (Eds.), *Human adaptation to extreme stress: From the Holocaust to Viet Nam.* New York: Plenum.

Karasu, T. B. (1986). The specificity versus nonspecificity dilemma: Toward identifying therapeutic change agents. *American Journal of Psychiatry, 143,* 687–695.

Kiecolt-Glaser, J. K., Dura, J. R., Speicher, C. E., et al.(1991). Spousal caregivers of dementia victims: Longitudinal changes in immunity and health. *Psychosomatic Medicine, 53,* 345–362.

Knight, B. (1988). Factors influencing therapist-rated change in older adults. *Journal of Gerontology, 43,* P111–112.

Lazarus, L. W., Sadavoy, J. (1996). Individual psychotherapy. In J. Sadavoy, L. W. Lazarus, L. F. Jarvik, et al. (Eds.), *Comprehensive review of geriatric psychiatry—II* (2nd ed., pp. 819–850). Washington, DC: American Psychiatric Press.

Lewinshon, P. M. (1975). The behavioral study and treatment of depression. In M. Hersen, R. M. Eisler, & P. M. Miller (Eds.), *Progress in behavior modification* (pp. 19–64). New York: Academic Press.

Light, E., Niederhe, G., Lebowitz, B. D. (Eds.). (1994). *Stress effects on family caregivers of Alzheimer's patients.* New York: Springer.

Miller, M. D., Silberman, R. I. (1996). Using interpersonal psychotherapy with depressed elderly. In S. H. Zarit & B. G. Knight (Eds.), *A guide to psychotherapy and aging* (pp. 83–100) New York: American Psychological Association.

Miller, N. L., Markowitz, J. C. (1999). Interpersonal psychotherapy of depressed patients. *Journal of Practical Psychiatry and Behavioral Health, 5,* 63–74.

Mittelman, M. S., Ferris, S. H., Shulman, E., et al. (1995). A comprehensive support program: Effect on depression in spouse-caregivers of AD patients. *Gerontologist, 35,* 792–802.

Mossey, J. M., Knott, K. A., Higgins, M., et al. (1996). Effectiveness of a psychosocial intervention, interpersonal counseling, for subdysthymic depression in medically ill elderly. *Journal of Gerontology, 51A,* M172–M178.

Niederehe, G. (1996). Psychosocial treatments with older depressed adults. *American Journal of Geriatric Psychiatry, 4*(Suppl. 1), S66–S78.

Nolan, M., Keady, J., Grant, G. (1996). Developing a typology of family care: Implications for nurses and other service providers. *Journal of Advanced Nursing, 21,* 256–265.

Novick, P. (1999). *The Holocaust in American life.* New York: Houghton Mifflin.

Reifler, B. V., Cox, G. B., Hanley, A. J. (1981). Problems of mentally ill elderly as perceived by patients, families, and clinicians. *Gerontologist, 21,* 165–170.

Reynolds, C. F., Frank, E., Perel, J. M., et al. (1994). Treatment of consecutive episodes of major depression in the elderly. *American Journal of Psychiatry, 151,* 1740–1743.

Riddick, C. C., Cohen-Mansfield, J., Fleshner, E., et al. (1992). Caregiver adaptations to having a relative with dementia admitted to a nursing home. *Journal of Gerontological Social Work, 19,* 51–76.

Robinson, G. K. (1990). The psychiatric component of long-term care models. In B. S. Fogel, A. Furino, & G. L. Gottlieb (Eds.), *Mental health policy for older Americans: Protecting minds at risk.* Washington, DC: American Psychiatric Association.

Sanderson, W. C., McGinn, L. A. (1997). Psychological treatment of anxiety disorder patients with comorbidity. In S. Wetzler & W. C. Sanderson (Eds.), *Treatment strategies for patients with psychiatric comorbidity* (pp. 75–104). New York: Wiley.

Sanderson, W. C., Wetzler, S. (1995). Cognitive behavioral treatment of panic disorder. In G. M. Asnis & M. H. van Praag (Eds.), *Pathogenetic mechanisms of panic disorder* (pp. 80–98). New York: Brunner/Mazel.

Semple, S. J. (1992). Conflict in Alzheimer's caregiving families: Its dimensions and consequences. *Gerontologist, 32,* 648–655.

Shuchter, S. R., Zisook, S. (1993). The course of normal grief. In M. S. Stroebe, W. Stroebe, & R. O. Hansson (Eds.), *Handbook of bereavement: Theory, research, and intervention* (pp. 23–43). Cambridge: Cambridge University Press.

Tauber, Y. (1998). *In the other chair: Holocaust survivors and the second generation as therapists and clients.* Jerusalem: Gefen.

Teri, L., Logsdon, R. G., Uomoto, J., et al. (1997). Behavioral treatment of depression in dementia patients: A controlled clinical trial. *Journal of Gerontology: Psychological Sciences, 52B*, P159–P166.

Toseland, R. W., Labrecque, M. S., Gooegel, S. T., et al. (1992). An evaluation of a group program for spouses of frail elderly veterans. *Gerontologist, 32*, 382–390.

Whitlatch, C. J., Zarit, S. H. (1995). Influence of the success of psychoeducational interventions on the course of family care. *Clinical Gerontologist, 16*, 17–30.

Yesavage, J. A., Karasu, T. B. (1982). Psychotherapy with elderly patients. *American Journal of Psychotherapy, 36*, 41–55.

Zarit, S. H., Knight, B. G. (Eds.). (1996). *A guide to psychotherapy and aging.* Washington, DC: American Psychological Association.

Zarit, S. H., Orr, N. K. Zarit, J. M. (1985). *The hidden victims of Alzheimer's disease.* New York: New York University Press.

Zarit, S. H., Peterson, K., Bach-Peterson, J. (1980). Relatives of impaired elderly: Correlates of feelings of burden. *Gerontologist, 20*, 649–655.

Zarit, S. H., Whitlatch, C. J. (1992). Institutional placement: Phases of the transition. *Gerontolgist, 32*, 665–672.

Zarit, S. H., Whitlatch, C. J. (1993). The effects of placement in nursing homes on family caregivers: Short- and long-term consequences. *Irish Journal of Psychology, 14*, 25–37.

Zarit, S. H., Zarit, J. M. (1998). Family caregiving. In *Mental disorders in older adults* (pp. 290–319). New York: Guilford Press.

Zisook, S., Shuchter, S. R. (1996). Grief and bereavement. In J. Sadavoy, L. W. Lazarus, L. F. Jarvik, et al. (Eds.), *Comprehensive review of geriatric psychiatry—II* (2nd ed., pp. 529–562). Washington, DC: American Psychiatric Press.

8

Adapting Principles of Marital, Group, and Family Therapy to the Needs of Older Patients

Burdens of illness, loss, and dependency are major interpersonal strains for the older individual. Family care is the rule rather than the exception in geriatric practice. Although many primary care providers have already developed an approach to the older couple or the family, there is an increasing body of literature available to enhance one's practice. For the mental health specialist, the use of therapeutic groups adapted to the older patient's needs is a closely related skill.

MARRIAGE OR COUPLE THERAPY WITH OLDER ADULTS

Aged marital and family relationships may be the new frontier for the therapist (Florie, 1989). But the dramatic increase in the number of elderly will mean that the marital and family therapists will be dealing with the problems of a population who have traditionally under-utilized the services of mental health specialists and who have often been viewed by them with a negative attitude. Thus the primary care provider will require greater skills to take full advantage of the couple as a health resource for the individual.

W. H. Auden considered a long happy marriage to be one of the most desirable of human conditions. In men's lives, a stable marriage may be synonymous with a life free from personal psychopathology

(Vaillant, 1977). Older couples who reach advanced age face an increasing risk that the caring bond will be diminished by adverse health and psychosocial events. The bond of a married couple can be particularly important in coping with the stresses of late life. There is a considerable literature on the importance of spouses to the well-being of persons with dementia (Cavanaugh et al., 1989; Coy et al., 1992). There is a similar body of writings regarding the "psychoeducational" approach to depression in which the family of the affected person receives information on the characteristics, course, and treatment of the illness (Hinrichsen et al., 1992; Papolos, 1994). However, published reports on the practices of primary care providers in geriatrics rarely identify the older couple as a therapeutic modality when one member of the pair is overwhelmed by illness. More important, interventions such as couple therapy which are thought of as the province of mental health specialists offer the promise of protecting or restoring the couple's equilibrium, provided they are adapted for the primary care setting.

Lewis (1998) working from an interpersonal perspective notes 10 basic relationship concepts which are used to assess difficulties among couples. These include (1) attachment and its centrality to the relationship; (2) connection and separation, the individual's need for both intimacy and independence; (3) negotiation which establishes the balance between intimacy and independence; (4) unconscious fears of connection and separation; (5) power to influence negotiations; (6) patterned, automatic maintenance of balance such that ongoing demands on the relationship do not disrupt the couple's equilibrium; (7) change and restoration of balance through negotiation of crisis and conflict; (8) health-facilitating balances which enhance personal mastery and growth; (9) the optimal balance which copes with external stressors such as illness but also promotes intimacy and individuality; and (10) values, shared beliefs, and attitudes about others and the world at large (e.g., outsiders can or cannot be trusted; the world is orderly or chaotic).

These 10 concepts help guide the practitioner to work with couples of diverse styles of relating. For example, couples vary on intensity of the connection, the importance they accord to sexuality, the extent to which work was an end in itself or a means to develop the relationship, and the importance of religion. However, well-functioning couples demonstrate common traits. First, the individuals share power to influence one another over a broad range of negotiations including sex, children, money, and dependency. Second, both connection and separateness are encouraged such that there is a high level of individuality and intimacy. Third, the partners respect each other's subjective

reality and are not preoccupied with the "truth" of personal perceptions unless the threat is concrete (e.g., malignancy). Fourth, emotions
are openly expressed, empathy is common, and feelings are free to
vary widely. Fifth, problem solving is highly developed with negotiation, compromise, and closure achieved through a variety of means
both within and outside the relationship. Sixth, conflict, as it arises,
does not become chronic and rarely escalates to crisis proportions
(Lewis, 1998).

MODELS

Marital adjustment is threatened by burdens of illness and age-related
problems. The weight of burden may not be explained simply by the
extent of concrete, instrumental caregiving (Beckman & Giordano,
1986; Bienenfeld, 1990; Draper et al., 1992; Gallagher et al., 1989;
George, 1984; Goldstein, 1996; Light & Lebowitz, 1989; Stone, 1989).
Yet Florie's (1989) study of the frequency with which the marital and
family process literature focused on problems associated with aging
families revealed virtually no coverage of later-life family care prior to
1985. Subsequently, a number of anecdotal reports have described the
needs of distressed older couples, the techniques of intervention, and
suggested areas for research. "Trouble in Paradise" cited marital crises
of midlife due to changes and heightened reflection of that period
(Maltas, 1992). Gilewski et al. (1985) discussed treatment extending
over 9 months to help a couple establish a better relationship after
long-standing marital conflict was exacerbated by retirement. Greenbaum and Rader (1989) emphasized how older couples negotiated life-
stage transitions at an earlier time. When long-standing marriages sud-
denly become conflicted, one precipitant may be the recent death of
the parent of one of the partners. The bereaved spouse may identify
with the deceased parent and cling to or withdraw from the partner.
Therapy can facilitate the bereaved partner's mourning, which, if unresolved may contribute to the breakdown of long-standing marriages
(Guttman, 1991). Psychoanalytic therapy has been suggested to help
patients transform the potential trauma of personal crises into the progressive developmental experience of transition (Bander, 1989; Brok,
1992).

Should the "complicated transition period" in the midlife phase of
marital relationships become conflicted, therapy termed "separation/
divorce initiation" can help couples overcome the traumatic effects of
impending disruption (Iwanir & Gyal, 1991). Gafner (1989) examined
premorbid behaviors and their antecedents in a case study in which

marital therapy was rejected when the therapist suggested separation. In another case report, marital separation was accepted after 50 years of marriage, resolving a conflicted relationship (Crose & Duffy, 1988). Klinnert et al. (1992) assessed areas of marital functioning to make a global judgment about the quality of the relationship, placing it on a 5-point scale from destructive to excellent. Mental health problems, including depression, of older couples were explored in individual case reports by Frey et al. (1989) and Gafner (1987).

Beckman and Giordano (1986) found that disabling illness or impairment in a spouse can result in a new caretaker role for the partner with resultant stress of that role producing "strong implications" for both partners. Depression, which proves resistant to antidepressant treatment, is a frequent cause of referral for marital or couple therapy (Lewis, 1998). Patient barriers to treatment included reluctance to admit responsibility for difficulties, preexisting marital conflict, the effects of health problems, and low income. Therapist barriers included personal anxiety generated by the work. Treatment techniques included behavioral approaches such as "contracting and relaxing techniques," conjoint marital therapy, and communication training. Wolinsky (1986) advocated four stages of treatment in long-standing marriages, including (1) a marital history and life-review process, (2) treatment techniques for support, (3) lifestyle changes, and (4) review of accomplishments and potential for growth. Subsequently, Wolinsky (1990) designed a developmental counseling model to encompass the emotional and psychological strengths and liabilities of an older population. Pertinent subjects included issues unique to the mature-stage marriage, marital life review, stress-reduction techniques, and improved drug therapies.

As to research, there are two major lines of inquiry, the social systems approach and lifespan development. There is a widening consensus for integration of these two lines, with the family life-cycle interview as the "basis of the scientific paradigm which focuses on the interface between the individual and the couple relationship" (Reiss, 1992, p. 119). Jacobson and Addis (1993) concluded that "behavioral couple therapy is the closest thing that couple therapy has to an established treatment" (p. 93). Less than satisfactory outcomes following behavioral couple therapy were found among the more severely disturbed couples, those of advanced age, the emotionally disengaged, and couples with marked gender role polarization.

> Given what researchers know about the predictors of success and failure for behavioral couple therapy, it makes sense that the problems would be easier to prevent than to modify after the fact. We think pre-

vention efforts should be expanded. Efforts to intervene at periods of the life cycle known to be at high risk for couple discord provides excellent opportunities to do preventative work. (p. 93)

Greenberg and Kennedy (1991) carried out therapy with 60 couples in a geriatric ambulatory practice in which psychiatric services were offered as part of a team approach. Common presenting issues focused on coping with loss and mastering change across several domains. In the psychological domain, the couples related (1) loss of independence, intimacy, and sexual activity; (2) inability of the marriage to meet the individual's need for companionship and emotional support; (3) role changes from provider or homemaker to caregiver; (4) fantasies about missed opportunities; and (5) fears about the future.

Economic issues included fixed income in the face of unanticipated costs of care and change in domiciliary needs. The couples also encountered physiologic problems of (1) both chronic and episodic illness, (2) temporary or progressive disability, and (3) treatments with unavoidable side effects such as steroids, hemodialysis, and prostatectomy. Social difficulties included shrinking vocational, religious, and recreational networks and the death and dispersal of friends and family. The assessment comprised (1) individual and marital life review; (2) focus on past separation–individuation issues, coping, and mastery; (3) partners' perception of the marital situation and the quality of the relationship; and (4) other family members' involvement. The therapists also searched for therapeutic motivators such as (1) a strong link between self-esteem and marital satisfaction, (2) obvious long-term investment, (3) children and grandchildren, and (4) financial interdependence. A key query in the assessment was, "How did the two of you first meet? How did you decide to marry?"

Therapeutic goals were established with the couples to (1) clarify values of the individual and the couple, (2) encourage independence and mastery, (3) increase self-esteem and mutual admiration, (4) reinforce emotional and physical intimacy, (5) redefine roles and reinforce role flexibility, (6) declare a truce on open hostilities, (7) mourn losses, (8) create a system for accurate and open communication and conflict resolution, (9) provide an explanation for life changes that maximize the sense of competency rather than vulnerability, (10) enhance historical link and use memory to consolidate rather than deplete, and (11) offer a model of behavior that alternates affective and instrumental roles.

Short-term conjoint therapy, crisis intervention, home visits, adjunctive individual psychotherapy, and pharmacotherapy made up the treament modalities. Psychotropic medications were prescribed most often for depression or for the agitation, sleep disturbance, or psychosis complicating dementia. Depression was a more frequent issue than dementia. More than half the couples had no grandchildren. Forty percent of cases required assistance with concrete social services including home health aide, day-center referral, and enriched housing referral.

The therapists required the flexibility to make home visits and provide adjunctive intervention to individual members of the couple. Issues of communication, intimacy, and individuation common to marital therapy among younger couples were present but could not be approached without attention to the individual member's need for concrete services or psychotherapeutic interventions, including medication. Although the service provided was highly specialized, the demand was manageable, acceptance of treatment was better than expected, interventions were generally short term, and outcomes appeared to be positive. Of the group, 14% did not require follow-up services, 10% entered nursing facilities or adult homes, and 6% either separated or divorced. Although depression and dementia were prominent issues, other illnesses, disabilities, and the complexity of treatments also required therapeutic attention. Marital therapy is feasible in the primary care setting but requires a flexible approach and interventions that may be viewed as beyond the traditional scope of practice by most of the primary care clinical disciplines.

GROUP THERAPY WITH OLDER ADULTS: GENERAL CONSIDERATIONS

Group therapy serves a variety of patient needs. In the nursing home, the group may be a sounding board used to adjust to the indignities of institutional living and to advocate for a greater stake in decision making (Burnside & Schmidt, 1994). In the outpatient setting it may range from psychodynamic or cognitive treatment of depression to maintenance of social interaction in cognitively impaired persons. But no matter what structure is used, the therapist's positive regard for each member, an air of optimism, and warmth and empathy are critical to success (Tross & Blum, 1988). Screening and preparation of patients for group work is critical. In each case the therapist will need to orient and instruct the patient prior to entry. The idea of therapy needs to be "demystified" for the older patient to reduce anxiety, establish a therapeutic alliance, clarify expectations regarding regular attendance, and ensure confidentiality. The group therapist's selection of the patient commits both the therapist and the group. And the patient needs to express a willingness to commit sufficient time and effort to a therapeutic trial. Patients who devalue other's participation, who blame others for their problems, who cannot or will not attend to the process, and who are too suspicious or depressed to share anything positive about themselves will do poorly. When group therapy is an adjunct to pharmacotherapy, it is essential that both the therapist and the prescribing provider communicate (Leszcz, 1996). An assessment of the individual's emotional, interpersonal, and cognitive capacity is critical to the work of any successful group (Radley et al., 1997).

Older adult groups need not be homogeneous with regard to age, gender, income, or marital status. However, differences in cognitive impairment, physical disability or frailty, hearing loss, and language will often prevent the development of cohesion and therapeutic success. Persons with these difficulties require a more rather than less homogeneous setting (Grant & Cassey, 1995). Patients in crisis or those who are actively suicidal should be excluded until their distress is in control through either individual attention or hospitalization. A mature, cohesive group can tolerate the addition of a problematic member. However, newly formed groups are particularly vulnerable when homogeneity is minimal.

Whatever the makeup of the group, positive outcome is correlated with a structured format (Scheidlinger, 1994). The structure will vary according to the problems addressed or the technique employed. Impaired patients may benefit more from an activity-oriented group than from a more verbal modality. Language skills vary more among older persons than among the young. Seniors' speech discrimination and immediate word recall decline and as a result comprehension may decrease. However, word recognition remains unchanged or increases as vocabulary expands such that sentences become more fluent and syntactically complex. The therapist must make allowances for failed communication and not hesitate to repeat or reinforce information, making sure that all group members get the intended message.

Positive reinforcement; initiating, activating, and closing the group; and ensuring that all members actively participate are the major activities of the therapist. Persons who tend to monopolize the time should be gently reminded that others need to speak. Members who seek to serve as self-appointed cotherapists will need redirection ("maybe you could share your experience rather than always giving advice") to avoid the group's wrath or ostracism. Building self-esteem and an expectation of benefit through the therapist fostering of group cohesion are critical (Gorey & Cryns, 1991; Snell, 1997). Leszcz (1996) suggests that group therapy be offered as a "buffet" of modalities that require flexibility on the leader's part and, depending on the size of the clinical population, may include a number of techniques. Use of a cotherapist ensures continuity across episodes of illness, professional leave, and vacation. To lessen the dropout rate, midmorning or early-afternoon groups are better suited for seniors. Examples of therapeutic structures follow.

Groups for Patients with Dementia

These groups include resocialization, remotivation, reality orientation, and activity or creativity components. Whatever the mix of modalities, the patients require more active support, direction and positive rein-forcement. Psychodynamic, cognitive-behavioral, goal-directed, or problem-solving formats are less beneficial. Psychodynamic interpre-tations and homework assignments are not used. Rather, efforts that focus on improved social skills and socialization, cognitive and sen-sory stimulation, reduced behavioral disturbance with secondary re-duction in caregiver burden, or staff distress are more realistic goals. Reminiscence and maintaining a sense of self-regard promote satisfac-tion and a sense of well-being. Reality orientation (e.g., "what's the next holiday") will help activate the group but will not carry forward unless reinforced at home or in the therapeutic milieu. The therapist must attend closely to difficulties with communication.

Patients may exhibit a lack of speech initiative or appropriate, timely responses. Word-finding difficulty may be marked and per-severation is frequent. Syntax may be disorganized and speech may be empty or noninformative. Some patients will have difficulty maintain-ing the flow of conversation. Others will not be able to stop. The thera-pist should speak more loudly, more slowly, and more intensely than in conversational speech. The therapist should cue individual open-ings and closures without hesitation. Topics of discussion and related vocabulary should be within the group members' grasp. Redundant categories of topics and direct association may assist failing memory. The flow of conversation should provide clues and cues for well-related responses. Tangential responses should not be amplified. Nei-ther should the therapist take on a pedantic stance. Patient errors should not be corrected. Rather, correct information should be stated with tact and sensitivity.

Relaxation exercises, in-chair range-of-motion practices, and dis-cussion of holidays and recent events are also useful. However, reflec-tion on the future is less beneficial. Transient improvement in verbal or physical skills may occur but will not persist. These groups have char-acteristics of both activity groups and conventional psychotherapy. Coordination with family caregivers is essential to arrange for attendance and feedback (Bonder, 1994; Josephson et al., 1993; Lantz et al., 1997).

Caregiver Support Groups

These groups are often used in parallel with group time for the patient with dementia. Here the focus is on a supportive relationship, problem solving, and coping strategies. Coping skills, information regarding nursing homes, power of attorney, and combating behavioral disturbances are shared (see Chapter 3). Depression, anxiety, and caregiver burden are reduced and the need for nursing home admission is delayed. Because the group may be more supportive than insight oriented, contact between individuals outside the group is not discouraged but is brought back for discussion. Support groups may be open ended and may sustain individuals beyond the death or nursing home admission of their family member. However, caregivers with long-standing marital conflict, personality disorder, substance abuse, or major depression are better served with individual treatment (Mittelman et al., 1995, 1996).

Psychodynamic Groups

There is an established literature on psychodynamic groups with older persons (Yalom, 1995). The narcissistic injuries of aging are the focus and the technique is meant to maintain a sense of self-efficacy and esteem in the face of age-related losses. The work is intrapsychic and interpersonal rather than behavioral. Increased insight and adjustment are the goals. The key elements revolve around transference to individual group members, the group as a whole, or the therapist and provide a sense of stability and renewal. Homework, skill acquisition, and education regarding care of others are not express goals or methods. Contact outside the group is discouraged to maximize the examination of individual reactions within the group. And it is important to emphasize the group as a means to an end rather than an end in itself (Phoenix et al., 1997). Caregivers of persons with dementia, Parkinson's disease, or stroke may be better served with a support group.

Reminiscence or Life-Review Groups

These groups assist patients in evaluating and reintegrating their past within the interpersonal sphere of the "here and now." Increased life satisfaction rather than improved social skills is the goal. However, in severely depressed persons, self-absorption and morbid preoccupation

with the past may occur. "Milestoning," the purposeful review of positive life events, may be emphasized to foster cohesion and to avoid
group anxiety or demoralization. More exploratory or uncovering approaches are appropriate depending on the setting purpose. Groups
may be conducted with nursing home residents but need to be tailored
to the cognitive and sensory capacities of the participants (Cook, 1998;
Burnside & Haight, 1994). In any event, the therapist emphasizes and
redirects the conversation back to the current interpersonal experience
of the individuals (Lesczc, 1996). Recollection of the past, both suc-
cesses and losses, is used to illuminate the future.

Cognitive-Behavioral Group Therapy

In cognitive-behavioral group therapy the emphasis is the achieve-
ment of mastery and a positive outlook (Leung & Ornell, 1993). The
therapist is directive rather than reflective. The treatment is time limited rather than open ended. The techniques focus on learning, adapting, the use of behavioral strategies, practicing alternative responses,
recognition, and rejection of negative thinking. Relaxation training,
breathing exercises, and guided imagery for the group as a whole may
be incorporated into the structure at either the opening or the closing
of the group session (Abraham et al., 1992). The therapist gives homework assignments, including log books focused on specific problem
thoughts or behaviors (see Chapter 7), but the psychoeducational lessons are evoked from the individuals within the group. Distorted notions of global negative outcomes (i.e., overarching pessimism) are
overcome with defocusing, depersonalizing, countering either/or
thinking, reframing (glass half empty vs. half full), and focusing on
small gains as evidence for the possibility of a positive outcome
(Thompson et al., 1991).

Group learning is achieved through individual example and the
participants' capacity to question distorted beliefs, self-defeating assumptions, perceived lack of alternatives, and social isolation. Role
play, education about symptoms and diagnoses, and focus on observ-
able behavior rather than motivation are key elements which make the
group a learning laboratory (Leszcz, 1996). The use of reminiscence,
psychodynamic interpretation, and alleviation of the narcissistic
wounds of old age are the focus of other modalities. The group may
not need to be diagnostically homogeneous. The overlapping symptoms of panic attacks, generalized anxiety, and depressive disorders
and the shared cognitive-behavioral approach to each facilitate a common effort. And in most settings, persons with obsessive–compulsive
disorder may be included due to the relative infrequency of their con-

dition. However, they may also require individual sessions for treatment to be efficient.

FAMILY WORK

The issues that most often bring families to seek therapy are centered on caregiving, which is covered for the individual in Chapter 7. Here we focus on the family as a more broadly defined source of support as well as locus of treatment. Sometimes the family is a cotherapist; other times the family is more of a "copatient." The clinician who neglects the family does so at the patient's expense.

The therapeutic approach begins with an effort to understand the family's dilemma from the family's perspective. The issues the family faces with a declining senior member are similar to the challenges of adolescence. The adolescent strives to establish autonomy within the context of depending on family for security and support. The older adult seeks to retain autonomy while increasing reliance on the family as caregivers. Zarit and Zarit (1998) describe five points regarding family caregiving. First, caregiving is stressful. Disability, brain disease, and mental illness are frightening and stigmatizing. The caregiving is time-consuming and the stress is chronic. Second, the sources of stress are multiple, arising from both the needs of the care recipient and the circumstances of the caregiver. Third, the family's adaptation to the stressors varies widely with the situation. Some find the opportunity to provide care rewarding. Others are crippled both at work and at home by demands that exceed capacities. Simple solutions rarely satisfy. Fourth, at least some of the factors associated with caregiver stress are modifiable but modification may not always be desirable. Nursing home placement may not be the cure for caregiver burden (Kiecolt-Glaser et al., 1991). Fifth, caregiving means both continuity and change.

Throughout the process there are three transitions: (1) the shift into the caregiving role, (2) transition from family and community care to reliance on agencies and ultimately institutions, and (3) bereavement, which may have started while the patient was still alive but completes the transition with death. In each instance crossing the boundary is likely to cause characteristic responses, which the alert practitioner can assist the family in weathering. Here the approach is individualized so that the clinician anticipates being ready to help the family adapt.

However, long-standing resentments, rivalries, power struggles, and shifts in allegiances or financial stakes can surprise even the best-prepared clinician. Family members may also disparage or undercut one another, leading to an atmosphere of demoralization and paralysis. From family systems theory a number of concepts emerge which can assist the practitioner (Minuchin et al., 1978). Some families are highly enmeshed, sustaining rather than resolving conflict in an inefficient pattern of preserving solidarity rather than achieving individual competence. Other families may be equally close but manage to work out conflict without subverting the individual. Certain families may be overprotective and rigid, prone to avoid conflict at nearly all costs. Family boundaries may be open or closed and yet still be effective in meeting the individual's needs for both support and autonomy.

Communication styles vary. In some instances everyone speaks at once. In other families there may be a care systems broker who is implicitly delegated the authority for decisions. Geography may complicate the brokering function if the designated family authority is distant from the problem ("The daughter from California syndrome"). Families may have "myths" about illness or obligations for support based on the experience of a previous generation. Financial dynamics are family dynamics such that the cost implications of caregiving need to be made explicit to the practitioner. Psychodynamic concepts are also informative. For example, the factors driving the motivation to provide or withhold caregiving may not be entirely conscious. Repressed hopes of reconciliation or fears of domination may not be clearly stated yet cause difficulties. Survivor guilt and identification with the aggressor may make a family member go to unreasonable lengths to meet the needs of the care recipient or the preferences of other potential caregivers. Character and coping styles differ from person to person and family to family. Some are characteristically contentious and circumspect. Others are too agreeable and lack the assertiveness necessary to achieve their legitimate needs.

Families may have distorted beliefs or false attributions, leading them to be pessimistic or cynical about assistance or the adaptability of a difficult situation. They may assume that nursing homes or homecare workers are uniformly untrustworthy or unfeeling. These distortions may be corrected by examination and practice. Ultimately, behavior is more important than motivation or style. Getting the job done is more important than how the work is accomplished.

How to Conduct a Therapeutic Family Meeting

Jarvik and Small (1988) enumerate six steps to improved relations between family members and older parents. These include (1) monitoring mood, (2) considering the intensity of reactions, (3) constructive planning, (4) reassessment of the situation, (5) listening then negotiating, and (6) compromise. The family meeting is the major source of intervention to achieve these steps. Zarit and Zarit (1998) describe the conduct of a therapeutic family meeting:

A single meeting with a telephone follow-up is often sufficient to provide information, orient to the prognosis and care needs, ensure future access to the clinician, and reduce misunderstandings and conflicts. However, adequate preparations are essential for a productive meeting, one that will not only express feelings but also voice solutions. Typically, the primary caregiver or one of the patient's children can provide a rough picture of the family structure. Who is more influential and who is less so. Who is the family mediator or care broker? Who characteristically leads and who follows? What were the patient's and caregiver's roles in the family before the onset of illness?

The clinician, patient, and primary caregiver decide who to invite to the meeting which may be held in the office but is more effective in the patient's home. The home meeting makes the family less defensive and the clinician less distant. Attention should be paid to the etiquette of the meeting. A period of introductions, identifying who is missing, who does the talking, and any difficulties encountered in arranging for the meeting is a prelude to addressing the agenda of the clinician, patient, and family. It is helpful for the clinician to state the general purpose of the meeting at the outset knowing that specifics will follow. The overall goals are to inform and to forge a better working alliance for the patient. Asking for questions from the outset will prepare the clinician for a more concise presentation of diagnostic and treatment issues as well as the transition to future care needs and the family's expectations. Although the patient and caregiver may have accepted the diagnosis and the limitations of treatment some time ago, the family may not have made the transition. Their questions as to what more the practitioner should do will need to be addressed before moving on to the more difficult task of what the family should do.

Once the family is satisfied that the clinician has addressed the patient's needs, the focus can shift to the caregiver and the family. Here the caregiver is asked to identify sources of stress and to specify areas in which help is needed. Most often one family member will take the lead in organizing a response and delegating authority for specific tasks. However, some families need time to absorb the news. Particularly when the caregiver played a dominant role in the family and has struggled not to burden others, the family may be surprised by the extent of distress.

The family plan that emerges should parcel responsibility broadly without rigidly allocating shares. Some will provide emotional support or backup; others will provide something more concrete but no less valuable. What is realistic and sustainable is more important than what is fair. Here the point is to begin a process of negotiating and contingency planning. Needs as well as limitations are expressed openly. Complete or even amiable consensus is not the point; planning is.

The typical family meeting runs smoothly and is remarkably efficient at achieving a realistic care plan. Yet at times the clinician may misperceive the family's agenda or misidentify the decision maker in the system. Here it is important to retreat to a position of assessing what the family needs and who makes the decision before offering a well-intentioned but off-the-mark suggestion. For example, caregiving agencies and regulations can seem insensitive and bureaucratic to families. Formal services are not always the solution. Indeed, having to relate to yet another set of strangers may be more burdensome than simply struggling through with conflict intact. Although the clinician may disagree, it is most often effective to work with the family on their terms by finding areas in which there is mutual motivation for change. When the relationship with the family becomes adversarial, an outside consultant should be called in to mediate the conflict and restore a working equilibrium.

WORK WITH ETHNIC ELDERS, ÉMIGRÉS, AND RELIGIOUS MINORITIES

In work with ethnic or religious minority families, it is important to acknowledge cultural differences before proceeding to treatment. Given the wide diversity of older patients and younger providers, sensitivity to the culture of the patient is a more realistic goal than cultural competence. Although DSM-IV provides a glossary of culture-bound syndromes and distress idioms, the context of both illness and treatment will vary for each individual. Thus the "contextualization" approach is critical (Mezzich et al., 1999). A simple "what can I do to help?" will keep the clinician from false assumptions about the patient's needs. Kleinman et al. (1978) suggest a number of other questions that will illuminate the patient's context: What does the patient call the sickness and what caused it? Why did it start when it did and how does it cause damage? How serious is the illness and will it be short or long? What steps do the patient or family think should be taken to remedy the sickness, and what are the most important results to be obtained? What are the major problems the illness has caused and what is feared the most? Has a similar problem ever occurred to other family members of friends? If yes, who was consulted, what treatment was provided, and what was the outcome? Are there important religious or spiritual issues that should be considered? Answers that may seem bizarre or irreconcilable with Western biomedicine require a stance of mediation and negotiation. Also willingness to prioritize and compromise will more effectively lead to satisfactory treatment than an ill-considered attempt to coerce or intimidate.

Immigrant families with a senior member in need of care may be confused about different professionals and roles of social agencies. They may delay seeking help because of their reluctance to ask for advice outside the ethnic group or fear of misdiagnosis and prejudice on the part of professionals. The stigma of mental illness may be exceptionally acute for groups who see the moral secularism of mental health care as inimical to their religious absolutism (Essau, 1998; Margolese, 1998). Thus a request for services may mean that the situation is desperate and all else has failed. Intergenerational differences in acculturation, assimilation, personal identification with the subculture, and the need to include extrafamily sources of support in the extended social network will complicate the process for the family and the provider. And the religious authority from the patient's community may need to be consulted to further the work. The practitioner also needs to be aware of differences in coping styles that may be less action oriented, as well as differences in beliefs about causality.

Differences in language, communication styles, and expectations of communications often dictate a more family- or dyad-oriented approach, rather than what is often the traditional Western individualism of the clinician. In some cultures husband and wife form the dominant dyad, while in others the dyad may be intergenerational (Falicov, 1995). A lack of "sympathetic" interest in or curiosity about the patient's culture on the part of the provider is a substantial obstacle to successful and efficient care. Rather, curiosity is the antidote to naiveté about other cultures (Dyche & Zayas, 1995). Simply learning the greeting and farewell in the patient's language, even if the pronunciation is imperfect, can break the ice and solidify trust. An awareness of major holidays will also demonstrate cultural sensitivity. Ultimately, caring for persons of a different ethnic or national origin can be rewarding provided the clinician is prepared to spend the necessary time. Allotting the extra time necessary for better communication will prevent the frustration of misunderstanding and difficulties with compliance (Sakauye, 1989).

PREPARING FOR GENETIC COUNSELING

The diagnosis of serious illnesses in the era of the Human Genome Project will increasingly have implications for the family (Papolos, 1994). Although genetic testing for the most common form of dementia is not reliable at the time of this writing, practitioners will encounter the testing dilemma before the end of the decade if not earlier (Cummings & Jeste, 1999). Indeed, in the handful of families with early onset, autosomal dominant familial Alzheimer's disease, the problem is already at hand. The literature on psychological consequences of testing for Huntington's disease provides an orientation. Wiggins et al. (1992) described the psychological consequences of predictive testing for Huntington's disease. For those identified at low risk there was an overall positive immediate and longer-term response. Uncertainty was reduced, allowing a more informed life plan. However, 10% of the group was unsettled by the news. Their new choices meant a loss of plans and a new identity. In the increased risk group, individuals experienced increased concerns about present physical symptoms that were clearly unrelated to Huntington's disease. There was also a tendency to see elevated risk as being synonymous with disease and an expressed need for counseling (Wiggins et al., 1992). Some individuals choose to withhold the information from their primary care provider to avoid difficulties with insurance or employment. A clear picture of what is motivating the requests for testing is thus important. Pre- and posttest counseling may need to be transformed to psychotherapy for some persons even when the results seem desirable (Nance, 1998; Williams et al., 1999). Once either genetic or other biological markers of premorbid risk for Alzheimer's disease risk become available, similar issues can be expected.

SUMMARY

The challenge of making care both efficient and fully effective requires the field of action to go beyond the individual patient and provider. Facility with couples, families, and group therapy techniques will expand the practitioner's options and the patient's opportunities.

REFERENCES

Abraham, I. L., Neundorfer, M. M., Currie, L. J. (1992). Effects of group interventions on cognition and depression in nursing home residents. *Nursing Research, 41,* 196–202.
Bander, F. M. (1989). Marital conflict and psychoanalytic therapy in the middle years. In J. M. Oldham & R. S. Liebert (Eds.), *The middle years: New psychoanalysis perspectives* (pp. 160–175). New Haven, CT: Yale University Press.
Beckham, K., Giordano, J. (1986). Illness and impairment in elderly couples: Im-

plications for marital therapy. *Family Relations Journal of Applied Family and Child Studies, 35,* 257–264.

Bienenfeld, D. (Ed.). (1990). *Other psychotherapies: Verwoerld's clinical geropsychiatry.* Baltimore, MD: Williams & Wilkins.

Bonder, R. R. (1994). Psychotherapy for individuals with Alzheimer's disease. *Alzheimer's Disease and Related Disorders, 8*(Suppl. 3), 75–81.

Brok, A. J. (1992). Crises and transitions: Gender and life stage issues in individual, group, and couples treatment [Special issue]. *Psychoanalysis and Psychotherapy, 10*(1), 3–16.

Burnside, I., Haight, B. (1994). Reminiscence and life review: Therapeutic interventions for older people. *Nurse Practitioner, 19,* 55–61.

Burnside, I., Schmidt, M. G. (1994). *Working with older adults group process and techniques* (3rd ed.). Boston: Jones & Bartlett.

Cavanaugh, J. C., Dunn, N. J., Mowery, D., et al. (1989). Problem-solving strategies in dementia patient–caregiver dyads. *Gerontologist, 29,* 156–158.

Cook, E. A. (1998). Effects of reminiscence on life satisfaction of elderly female nursing home residents. *Health Care of Women International, 19,* 109–118.

Coy, B., Kinney, J. M., Cavanaugh, J. C., et al. (1992, November 18–22). *Marital quality, daily, hassles, and depressive symptoms among spousal caregivers of Alzheimer's patients.* Paper presented at the annual meeting of the Gerontological Society of America, Washington, DC.

Crose, R., Duffy, M. (1988). Separation as a therapeutic strategy in marital therapy with older couples. *Clinical Gerontologist, 8,* 71–73.

Cummings, J., Jeste, D. (1999). Alzheimer's disease and its management in the year 2010. *Psychiatric Services, 30,* 1173–1177.

Draper, B. M., Pouols, C. J., Cole, A. A., et al. (1992). A comparison of caregivers for elderly stroke and dementia victims. *Journal of the American Geriatrics Society, 40,* 896–901.

Dyche, L., Zayas, L. H. (1995). The value of curiosity and naiveté for the cross-cultural psychotherapist. *Family Process, 34,* 389–399.

Esau, T. G. (1998). The evangelical Christian in psychotherapy. *American Journal of Psychotherapy, 52,* 28–36.

Falicov, C. (1995). Training to think culturally: A multidimensional framework. *Family Process, 34,* 373–388.

Florie, D. F. (1989). The prevalence of later life family concerns in the marriage and family therapy journal literature (1976–1985): A content analysis. *Journal of Marital and Family Therapy, 15,* 289–297.

Frey, J., Swanson, G. S., Hyer, L. (1989). Strategic interventions for chronic patients in later life. *American Journal of Family Therapy, 17,* 27–33.

Gafner, G. (1987). Engaging the elderly couple in marital therapy. *American Journal of Family Therapy, 15,* 305–315.

Gafner, G. (1989). Marital therapy with an old-old couple. *Clinical Gerontologist, 8,* 51–53.

Gallagher, D., Rose, J., Rivera, P., et al. (1989). Prevalence of depression in family caregivers. *Gerontologist, 29,* 449–456.

George, L. K. (1984, December). *The dynamics of caregiver burden.* Final report submitted to the Andrus AARP Foundation, Chicago.

Gilewski, M. J., Kuppinger, J., Sarit, S. H. (1985). The aging marital system: A case study in life changes and paradoxical intervention. *Clinical Gerontologist, 3,* 3–15.

Goldstein, M. (1996). Families of older adults. In J. Sadavoy, L. W. Lazarus, L. F. Jarvik, et al. (Eds.), *Comprehensive review of geriatric psychiatry—II* (2nd ed., pp. 881–906). Washington, DC: American Psychiatric Press.

Gorey, K. M., Cryns, A. G. (1991). Group work as interventive modality with the older depressed. *Journal of Gerontological Social Work, 16,* 137–157.

Grant, R. W., Cassey, D. A. (1995). Adapting cognitive behavioral therapy for the frail elderly. *International Psychogeriatrics, 7,* 561–571.

Greenbaum, J., Rader, L. (1989). Marital problems of the "old" elderly as they present to mental health clinic. *Journal of Gerontological Social Work, 14,* 111–126.

Greenberg, D., Kennedy, G. J. (1991). Till death do us part: Marital therapy in geriatric ambulatory practice. *Gerontologist, 31,* 118.

Guttman, H. A. (1991). Parental death as a precipitant of marital conflict in middle age. *Journal of Marital and Family Therapy, 17,* 81–87.

Hinrichsen, G. A., Hernandez, N. A., Pollack, S. (1992). Difficulties and rewards in family care of the depressed older adult. *Gerontologist, 32,* 486–492.

Iwanir, S., Ayal, H. (1991). Midlife divorce initiation: From crisis to developmental transition. *Contemporary Family Therapy: An International Journal, 13,* 609–623.

Jacobson, N. S., Addis, M. E. (1993). Research on couples and couple therapy: What do we know? Where are we going? *Journal of Consulting Clinical Psychology, 61,* 85–93.

Jarvik, L., Small, G. (1988). *Parent care.* New York: Crown.

Josephson, S., Beckman, L., Borell, L., et al. (1993). Supporting everyday activities in dementia: An intervention study. *International Journal of Geriatric Psychiatry, 8,* 395–400.

Kiecolt-Glaser, J. K., Dura, J. R., Speicher, C. E., et al. (1991). Spousal caregivers of dementia victims: Longitudinal changes in immunity and health. *Psychosomatic Medicine, 53,* 345–362.

Kleinman, A., Eisenberg, L., Good, B. (1978). Culture, illness, and care: Clinical lessons from anthropologic and cross-cultural research. *Annals of Internal Medicine, 88,* 251–258.

Klinnert, M. D., Mrazek, P., Mrazek, D. A. (1992). Quality of marital relationship: A clinical rating scale. *Psychiatry, 55,* 132–145.

Laham, J. W. (1990). Family of origin intervention: An intergenerational approach to enhancing marital adjustment. *Journal of Contemporary Psychotherapy, 20,* 211–222.

Lantz, M. S., Buchalter, E. N., McBee, L. (1997). The wellness group: A novel intervention for coping with disruptive behavior among elderly nursing home residents. *Gerontologist, 37,* 551–556.

Leszcz, M. (1996). Group therapy. In J. Sadavoy, L. W. Lazarus, L. F. Jarvik, et al. (Eds.), *Comprehensive review of geriatric psychiatry—II* (2nd ed., pp. 851–879). Washington, DC: American Psychiatric Press.

Leung, S. N. M., Orrell, M. W. (1993). A brief cognitive behavioral therapy group for the elderly: Who benefits? *International Journal of Geriatric Psychiatry, 8*, 593–596.

Lewis, J. M. (1998). For better or worse: Interpersonal relationships and individual outcome. *American Journal of Psychiatry, 155*, 582–589.

Light, E., Lebowitz, B. D. (Eds.). *Alzheimer's disease treatment and family stress: Directions for research.* Rockville, MD: National Institute of Mental Health.

Maltas, C. (1992). Trouble in paradise: Marital crises of midlife. *Psychiatry, 55*, 122–145.

Margolese, H. C. (1998). Engaging in psychotherapy with the orthodox Jew: A critical review. *American Journal of Psychotherapy, 52*, 37–53.

Mezzich, J. E., Kirmayer, L. J., Kleinman, A., et al. (1999). The place of culture in DSM-IV. *Journal of Nervous and Mental Disease, 187*, 457–464.

Minuchin, S., Rosman, B. L., Baker, L. (1978). Strategies for change. In *Psychosomatic families: Anorexia in context* (pp. 92–107). Cambridge, MA: Harvard University Press.

Mittelman, M. S., Ferris, S. H., Shulman, E., et al. (1995). A comprehensive support program: Effect on depression in spouse-caregivers of Alzheimer's disease patients. *Gerontologist, 35*, 792–802.

Mittelman, M. S., Ferris, S. H., Shulman, E., et al. (1996). A family intervention to delay nursing home placement of patients with Alzheimer's disease. *Journal of the American Medical Association, 276*, 1725–1731.

Nance, M. A. (1998). Huntington disease: Clinical, genetic, and social aspects. *Journal of Geriatric Psychiatry and Neurology, 11*, 61–70.

Papolos, D. F. (1994). The family psychoeducational approach: Rationale for a multigenerational treatment modality for the major affective disorders. In D. F. Papolos & H. M. Lachman (Eds.), *Genetic studies in affective disorders: Overview of basic methods, current directions, and critical research issues* (pp. 119–145). New York: Wiley.

Phoenix, E., Irvine, Y., Kohr, R. (1997). Group therapy with elderly depressed women. *Journal of Gerontological Nursing, 23*, 10–15.

Radley, M., Redston, C., Bates, F., et al. (1997). Effectiveness of group anxiety management with elderly clients of a community psychogeriatric team. *International Journal of Geriatric Psychiatry, 12*, 79–84.

Reiss, D. (1992). Marriage: The whole and its parts. *Psychiatry, 55*, 119–121.

Sakauye, K. M. (1989). Ethnic variations in family support of the frail elderly. In M. Z. Goldstein (Ed.), *Family involvement in the treatment of the frail elderly* (pp. 63–107). Washington, DC: American Psychiatric Press.

Scheidlinger, S. (1994). An overview of nine decades of group psychotherapy. *Hospital and Community Psychiatry, 45*, 217–225.

Snell, F. L. (1997). Group treatment of older veterans with post-traumatic stress disorder. *Journal of Psychosocial Nursing and Mental Health Services, 35*, 10–16.

Stone, J. D. (1989). Marital and sexual counseling of elderly couples. In G. R. Weeks & L. Hof (Eds.), *Integrating sex and marital therapy: A clinical guide* (pp. 221–244). New York: Brunner/Mazel.

Thompson, L. W., Gantz, F., Florsheim, M., et al. (1991). Cognitive-behavioral therapy in affective disorders in the elderly. In W. A. Myers (Ed.), *New tech-*

niques in the psychotherapy of older patients (pp. 3–19). Washington, DC: American Psychiatric Press.

Tross, S., Blum, J. E. (1988). A review of group therapy with the older adult: Practice and research. In B. W. MacLennan, S. Saul, E. Bakur, et al. (Eds.), *Group psychotherapies for the elderly* (pp. 3–29). Madison, CT: International Universities Press.

Vaillant, G. E. (1977). *Adaptation to life.* Boston: Little, Brown.

Wiggins, S., Whyte, P., Huggins, M., et al. (1992). The psychological consequences of predictive testing for Huntington's disease. *New England Journal of Medicine, 327,* 1401–1405.

Williams, J. K., Schutte, D. L., Evers, C. A., et al. (1999). Adults seeking presymptomatic gene testing for Huntington disease. *Image: The Journal of Nursing Scholarship, 31,* 109–114.

Wolinsky, M. A. (1986). Marital therapy with older couples. *Social Casework: The Journal of Contemporary Social Work, 67,* 475–483.

Wolinsky, M. A. (1990). *A heart of wisdom: Marital counseling with older and elderly couples.* New York: Brunner/Mazel.

Yalom, I. (1995). *The theory and practice of group psychotherapy* (4th ed.). New York: Basic Books.

Zarit, S. H., Zarit, J. M. (1998). Family caregiving. In *Mental disorders in older adults* (pp. 290–319). New York: Guilford Press.

9

Sexuality

As the proportion of older adults in the population increases, greater numbers of persons over the age of 65 will seek assistance for sexual dysfunction. Advanced age is associated with a slowing in sexual response, along with changes in relationships, health, and physical capacities. The loss of desire that results from abandoned sexual activity may relieve some older adults who cannot surmount the obstacles of illness, disability, lack of a partner, or personal inhibitions. Aging alone, however, does not abolish sexual desire or functioning. When the expectation is intimacy rather than intercourse or orgasm, many older persons can lead satisfying sexual lives to the end of their lifespan. Optimism is critical to address late-life sexual concerns. An awareness of the interactions between myth, biology, social expectations, personal history, and domestic circumstances is required for realistic treatment. Practitioners can improve the well-being of older adults by addressing their sexual concerns with skill and compassion.

The idea of lifelong sexual practice is contrary to the thinking of some older persons, their children, and their physicians. As a result, older adults may be reluctant to admit to erotic aspirations. Their children may resent a widowed parent's strivings for romance. Physicians often avoid questions of sexual health or history for fear of embarrassing the patient. Nonetheless, old age need not be devoid of sexual pleasures. There are a number of persistent myths about sex and aging (Dagon, 1989). Clinicians who are not aware of these myths will find it difficult to treat sexual problems in the aged.

MYTHS ABOUT SEX AND AGING

The "chronology" and "tranquillity" myths argue that older persons have escaped the tyranny of desire. In the Victorian myth of guilt and shame women may submit but are forbidden to enjoy and masturbation is harmful to body and soul. Rigid, traditional sex-role stereotypes and the myth that "ignorance is bliss" impair communication of needs as well as awareness of age-related changes in sexual response. In the "second class" myth, sex therapy is for the young because older persons are not "treatment responsive." The "frugality" myth suggests that sexual practice be limited to preserve performance whereas, in truth, practice and positive reinforcement are essential to maintenance of sexuality. In the menopausal and "dirty old man" myths, older women lose interest in sex and older men who have not become impotent are indiscreet and predatory. The opposite is true. Women experience greater sexual interest and men become more nurturing and less aggressive with age. In the "chronic" and "terminal illness" myths older persons are thought to have lost interest in sexual pleasure as a result of disability, disease, or fatal prognosis. Also, notions that homosexuality is a youthful indulgence incompatible with mature intimacy and that sex is only for procreation do not conform to clinical experience (Dagon, 1989).

Finally, there are the myths that older adults are not at risk for AIDS and need not use condoms. At age 50 close to 10% of Americans have at least one risk factor for HIV infection and the aged are less likely to use condoms. AIDS in the elderly will increase from current low prevalence of 3%. Particularly as survival rates increase, greater numbers of older persons will be represented in the prevalence of AIDS and HIV-positive individuals. Due to age-related changes in immune function and other factors, AIDS-related dementia complex is more rapidly progressive in the aged (Patterson et al., 1995).

REALITIES

The availability of a sexual partner becomes a problem in late life. Women increasingly outnumber men as age advances. At age 80 there are four women for every man. Most women over the age of 65 are widowed; most men are married (Butler & Lewis, 1990). Because religious institutions are a major source of meaning and support for the aged, religious prohibitions about sexual techniques and partners may be particularly acute for the present cohort of older adults.

The continuance of sexual activity into late age depends on the life pattern of each person. Persons with the highest level of sexual activity in middle age show the least decline in old age (Bretschneider & McCoy, 1988). The determinants of late-life sex drive extend well beyond biological factors. Gender differences in sex drive and personality traits tend to favorably synchronize with age, as shown in Table 9.1. But when one partner loses interest or is incapacitated, the other may simply accept the loss as inevitable. Mutually reinforced sexual abstinence can lead to atrophy of libido and sexual anatomy for both partners. Lack of privacy due to the ambiance of the nursing home and the presence of home health aides or family caregivers may also extinguish desire. And when the older lover assumes the role of caregiver for a demented or physically disabled partner, erotic perceptions and romance may suffer (Butler & Lewis, 1990). A "widower's syndrome" develops following bereavement; some individuals experience guilt over "betraying" the deceased spouse or anxiety over a new partner after years of monogamy (Dunn, 1988).

Table 9.2 summarizes age-related changes in sexual physiology, anatomy, and the stages of sexual response. These changes have an abrupt onset in women but occur more gradually in men. Estrogen and progesterone continue to decline after menopause whereas follicle-stimulating and luteinizing hormones increase. The size of the cervix, uterus, and ovaries decreases. Elastic tissue in the female breast is diminished but the nipple erectile repose is not eliminated. With the loss of estrogen there is a decline in vaginal thickness and elasticity. Fertility ceases. The excitement stage of the sexual response cycle is slowed; vasocongestion and lubrication are lessened. During the plateau stage the clitoral response remains but there is a reduced vaginal response. Uterine elevation is reduced; the labia majora may not elevate. Orgasm is briefer; the contractions are fewer and less intense.

TABLE 9.1. Synchronization of Sexual Response across the Life Cycle

Men	Women
Adolescence	
Predominant (intense)	Not fully developed
Remarkable biological drive	Less intense biological drive
Adulthood	
Declining biological component	Increasingly intense sexual drive
Advanced age	
Enhanced psychological aspect of sexuality	
Congruent expectations	
Decline in biological imperative	
Complementary nature of relationships	

TABLE 9.2. Impact of Aging on the Anatomy, Physiology, and Stages of Sexual Response

Men	Women
↓ Nocturnal penile tumescence	↓ Vaginal thickness and elasticity
↓ Testosterone and spermatogenesis	↓ Estrogen and progesterone, ↑ FSH and LH
↓ Size of testes, ↑ size of prostate	↓ Size of cervix, uterus, ovaries
Fertility declines, but may not cease	Fertility ceases with menopause

Excitement stage

Slowed response	Slowed response
Lessened tumescence	Vasocongestion reduced
Penile stimulation for erection	Reduced lubrication

Plateau stage

Prolonged	Vaginal response reduced, clitoral intact
Absence of pre-ejaculatory fluid	Uterine and labial elevation reduced

Orgasm stage

Shorter duration	Shorter duration
Contractions weaker, fewer	Contractions weaker, fewer
Ejaculate reduced	

Resolution stage

Rapid return to prestimulatory state	Rapid return to prestimulatory state
Refractory period increased	Multiorgasmic capacity retained

Note. Data from Kennedy et al. (1997).

There is a more rapid return to the prestimualtory state. However, the capacity for multiple orgasms may be retained (Zeiss et al., 1991).

Testosterone levels decline in men, but the diurnal elevation seen in the morning hours may remain. Nocturnal penile tumescence and testicular size decline while the prostate size increases. Spermatogenesis declines but fertility may continue to age 90 and above. However, the prevalence of erectile dysfunction increases from 25% at age 65 to 50% at age 75 (Rousseau, 1986). Regarding the stages of sexual response, the excitement stage is slowed and is accompanied by less firm erection. More prolonged and vigorous penile stimulation is required to achieve and sustain effective tumescence. Fantasy and verbal or visual stimulation alone may be insufficient. Similarly, the plateau stage is prolonged. There is a loss of preejaculatory fluid emission. The duration of orgasm is less, the contractions are fewer and less intense, and the volume and viscosity of the ejaculate are reduced. The refractory period is increased in the resolution stage, but there is a more rapid return to prestimulatory state (Zeiss et al., 1991).

THE GENESIS OF LATE-LIFE SEXUAL DYSFUNCTION

Table 9.3 summarizes common contributors to late-life sexual dysfunction. With older patients, comorbid physical and mental disorders are the norm rather than the exception. And the causes of functional decline, both sexual and otherwise, are usually several and interrelated. Although physical problems may account for the origin of most complaints, the extent of dysfunction is rarely wholly explained by physical factors (Wise et al., 1984). Lack of openness or information or about sex can prevent couples from mastering age- or illness-related changes in the sexual response. Rigid upbringing or mores may have less to do with the couple's failure to arrive at sexual satisfaction than do hidden resentments. Hostility may be expressed directly through sexual indifference and silence or indirectly through neglect for one's appearance, attractiveness, or availability.

Although men become more dependent on their partner's foreplay to achieve and sustain erections, premature ejaculation is less of a problem. As a result of the prolonged refractory period, men without oral or manual skills in their sexual repertoire may leave their partners who are dependent on intercourse unsatisfied. Women may feel that they have lost the sexual bloom of youth after menopause or mastectomy (Butler & Lewis, 1990). They may be unaware that male arousal is now more than ever dependent on their actions rather than their appearance. However, older women may not be entirely comfortable as-

TABLE 9.3. Common Factors in the Genesis of Late-Life Sexual Dysfunction

Pharmacological	Antihypertensives, psychotropics, cardiovascular agents, alcohol, nicotine, analgesics
Endocrine	Diabetes, thyroid disease, hypogonadism, tumors
Neurological	Stroke, peripheral or autonomic neuropathy, dementia, Parkinson's disease
Psychosocial	Bereavement, depressive disorder, lack of partner, lack of privacy, attitudes and expectations, disuse
Chronic illness	Degenerative joint disease, COPD, angina, chronic renal failure, other vascular disease
Surgery	CABG, prostatectomy (perineal > retropubic > TUR), mastectomy, hysterectomy, rectal surgery (dysfunction greater in men than women)

Note. CABG, coronary artery bypass graft; TUR, transurethral resection; COPD, chronic obstructive pulmonary disease.

suming the more assertive sexual role their partners require. The sharing of erotica or sex fantasies may be out of character for both.

Among pharmacological offenders, cardiovascular, antihypertensive (Hsueh, 1988), and antidepressant (Balon, 1995) agents are the most prominent. Of the antihypertensives, the angiotension-converting enzyme inhibitors enalapril (Vasotec) and lisinopril (Privinil) and the calcium channel blockers amlodipine (Norvasc) and verapamil (Calan) are the least likely offenders. The SSRIs may delay or prevent orgasm through their 5-HT2 serotonergic receptor activity (Segraves, 1995). However, over-the-counter medications, botanicals, and substances that might be abused, including alcohol, nicotine, and analgesics, can cause problems. Also, older persons are more sensitive to the effects of alcohol and may be unaware that even modest consumption may impair sexual performance.

Estrogen deficiency is the most common endocrine cause of sexual dysfunction among women; diabetes is more often the problem for men. Vulvovaginal dryness and atrophic vaginitis lead to a decreased vaginal response as a direct result of estrogen deficit. Painful intercourse is the result. Hypogonadism, tumors and deficiencies in gonadotropins and testosterone are less frequent. Loss of testosterone in older women may contribute to decreased libido as well. Diseases of the central and peripheral nervous system, which have their peak incidence in old age, are also associated with dysfunction. These include dementia, stroke, Parkinson's disease, and the peripheral and autonomic neuropathies (Mulligan et al., 1988). Pathological sexuality, including indiscreet, indiscriminate, self-mutilating, or aggressive sex acts are associated with frontal lobe degeneration of Pick's disease but may also appear with stroke, traumatic brain injury, vascular dementia, and Alzheimer's disease. Conversely, an increased interest in sex may occur in some demented persons, not always unwelcome by their spouses (Kennedy, 1995). Spouses may report difficulty with their partner's sequencing the sexual steps but value the affection and intimacy nonetheless (Redinbuagh et al., 1997).

Physical illness may also impair sexuality by degrading the muscle strength, endurance, and flexibility necessary for robust sexual performance. Surgical procedures that alter the person's appearance or change cardiovascular function may also be associated with sexual dysfunction. However, cardiac surgery and cardiac pacemakers, including the implantable cardioverting devices, are not incompatible with sexual activity, including orgasm (Kennedy et al., 1997). Modern microsurgical techniques promise that erectile dysfunction following perineal prostatectomy may approach the lesser prevalence observed with the transurethral approach. Retrograde ejaculation of semen into the bladder, which will cloud the urine, should not be cause for alarm following prostatectomy. Hysterectomy removes the uterus from the orgasmic platform and may change the perception of orgasm but not necessarily reduce the pleasure. Breast reconstruction following mastectomy may have significant benefits for sexual expression even without the restoration of erogenous sensitivity (Butler & Lewis, 1990).

EVALUATION

An evaluation of sexual dysfunction in the older adult should include a comprehensive assessment, sexual history, and treatment plan that will usually be shared with the partner. When the chief complaint is loss of libido or arousal, thyroid function studies, testosterone, prolactin and luteininzing hormone may be helpful to detect a primary endocrine cause of sexual dysfunction. Because testosterone secretion in men is pulsitile rather than continuous, three samples should be collected 30 minutes apart in the early morning. For laboratory work-up of erectile dysfunction, lipid profile and hemoglobin A1c should also be obtained. An intercavernosal injection of either papaverine or prostaglandin E_1 that produces a full erection makes the diagnosis of vascular etiology unlikely and suggests either neurogenic or psychogenic cause. Vascular followed by pharmacological causes are the most frequent etiologies of erectile dysfunction. Ejaculatory dysfunction (premature ejaculation or too rapid detumesence) should be differentiated from erectile problems. The penis should be examined for fibrous plaques associated with Peyronie's disease. Cremasteric reflex and evidence of orthostatic hypotension should also be sought. Loss of pubic hair, gynecomastia, and atrophic testes may suggest hypogonadism. A functional history including capacity to ambulate, climb stairs, and carry out household chores and review of systems with particular emphasis on the cardiovascular and musculoskeletal should be completed. Loss of stamina, strength, and flexibility may be due to inactivity as much as to medical conditions. The character of sleep-associated erections should be queried but may not be an adequate indicator of therapeutic potential (Godschalk et al., 1997). The pelvic exam may demonstrate erythema of the entroitus, suggesting atrophic changes. Cystocoele or rectocoele should also be readily apparent.

Mental status examination including a brief cognitive screening exam should be conducted. The detection of depression, anxiety, and psychotic disorders should be actively pursued. The clinician should not dismiss emotional distress as simply the result of sexual dysfunction or comorbid physical illness (Kennedy et al., 1997).

Taking a sexual history from an older adult requires tact and sensitivity. It is important that the interviewer indicate a sense of comfort, which is acquired with practice. Younger examiners may be reluctant to explore the sexuality of persons of their grandparent's age. They will be pleasantly surprised at the relief the older patient will express as a result of the inquiry. Shy examiners may desensitize themselves by rehearsing questions with their intimate partners. The history may also be facilitated by phrases such as "As people (age, retire, get sick or depressed) they often experience changes in their sex life. How has sex changed for you since . . . ?" (Cohen & Alfonso, 1997). An open-ended question is more likely to induce a discussion rather than a disclaimer. Inquiries that are detailed and specific as to sexual orientation, frequency of encounters across the lifespan, erectile dysfunction in men and discomfort in women, sexual techniques, sex after retirement, menopause, bereavement, or surgery set the stage for less inhibited communications between partners.

The domestic setting (availability and acceptance of partners, privacy) should be characterized. An inquiry into personal preferences and marital circumstances (widowhood, religious prohibitions, cultural sanctions, aging gays and lesbians) should be completed. Practices not compatible with the person's religious beliefs or personal mores should be deferred with respect. The patient's partner should be interviewed to assess compatibility and capacity to engage in therapeutic maneuvers. Both partners will need reassurance regarding the safety of sexual relations after surgery, stroke, and heart attack. Pain due to arthritis may be combated with analgesics and a warm bath prior to lovemaking. Side-by-side, back-to-belly, or the cross-wise sex position with one partner supine and the other on his or her side requires less flexion at the knee and hip and eliminates the pressure of body weight associated with the missionary position (Steege, 1986). Anti-angina agents may also be taken before sex to minimize discomfort for persons with coronary artery disease.

MANAGEMENT OF SEXUAL DYSFUNCTION

Treatment proceeds from multiple vantages with the aim of returning the person to optimum function through both the removal of obstacles such as medications and ill-informed attitudes and the introduction of pharmacological and behavioral adjuncts to sexual enjoyment. The patients will set the pace and intensity of treatment once the practitioner has conveyed a sense of optimism and confidence in the effort. The basic techniques and precepts of sex therapy (see Table 9.4) are the same

TABLE 9.4. Treatment of Late-Life Sexual Dysfunction

• History—physical	Diagnoses and personal/cultural expectations and preferences, functional capacity.
• Psychotherapy—education	Address covert hostility, major mental illness, inhibited communication. Counter myths and ignorance of age-related changes in sexual response and gender differences. Counseling regarding sexually transmitted diseases. Provide educational materials. Teach relaxation techniques.
• Behavioral	Focus on pleasure and intimacy rather than performance. Give permission (instruction) for manual and oral techniques, use of erotica and fantasy. Physical exercise to improve strength, endurance, flexibility. Graded sexual exercises (homework) to facilitate excitement rather than achieve intercourse or orgasm. Condom use.
• Pharmacological	Reduce polypharmacy, switch to calcium channel blockers or angiotensin converting enzyme inhibitors. Replacement therapy for primary and secondary hypogonadism. Sildenafil (Viagra) p.r.n.
• Surgical, mechanical	Refer to urologist, gynecologist.
• For sexual disinhibition in dementia	Open staff discussion; they should anticipate repetition, set limits, reinforce positive behaviors, define staff role, define problem for the patient while it is occurring; use redirection, alternatives.

in both youth and old age but are modified to conform to the physical capacity, social circumstances, and personal preferences of the parties involved. Following the comprehensive assessment, the partners are given permission to be more sexual, to shed inhibitory myths, and to restructure sexual attitudes. They are advised not to be "self-observers" or sexual spectators in order to refocus their lovemaking on release and pleasure rather than performance. To reduce fear of rejection, obsessive concern for the partner, and guilt, each individual is given permission to be selfish in sexual enjoyment. Options for increasing sexual attractiveness, eroticism, and fantasy life are explored. They are reminded that arousal begets arousal. Educational materials, progressive exercises to increase arousal and pleasure without requiring intercourse or orgasm, and informed techniques of foreplay are provided.

Sensate focus (SF), or nondemand pleasuring, is used to bring the couple together to restore intimacy through relaxed touching. For erectile dysfunction a ban on intercourse is prescribed to take away the demand to perform and to allow graded SF exercises to rebuild confidence. At the initial level, SF-1, the couple is instructed to caress one another anywhere but the genitals. They may proceed to SF-2 with genital pleasuring and the "start–stop technique." As arousal occurs, the pair are instructed to stop pleasuring, allow arousal to wane, and then to start again. The purposeful pattern of arousal and rearousal builds optimism that erections and pleasure can occur without the pressure to perform. At SF-3, penetration may occur but should not progress to intercourse until the therapist removes the ban.

Treatment resistance may take several forms indicating that problem dynamics (hostilities) within the marriage need to be addressed and a more direct style of communication encouraged. Some individuals will refuse or fail to complete the exercises. They may not find the time or complain that somatic concerns or mental symptoms preclude even the least demanding component of SF. Increased arguments with the partner or inability to adopt a more open, explicit style of communication may emerge. The couple is reminded that they cannot be expected to know what is pleasurable or how to resolve hostile feelings without communicating (Sviland, 1978).

Pharmacological and Mechanical Treatments

Changes in body composition (decreases in muscle mass, increase in body fat) are associated with the parallel decreases in testosterone and dehydroepiandrosterone (DHEA). Testosterone levels in older men relate to body weight, but the use of diet or exercise to increase testosterone remains hypothetical (Mazur, 1998). Oral testosterone preparations cause hepatic toxicity and are not prescribed. Side effects of intramuscular injections and transdermal patches include polycythemia, fluid retention, gynecomastia, and hepatic dysfunction. Most men prefer the injection rather than tolerate the rash so frequently seen with the patch therapy. Prostatic enlargement may also result, but there appears to be no promotion of malignant transformation. However, the effect of testosterone on the older male's prostate is unpredictable (Lamberts et al., 1997). Data on longer-term effects on the prostate, cardiovascular disease, and lipid risk factors are not available. Hypogonadism is a clear indication for a trial of testosterone, but not all men experience a return of libido. Thus in the absence of large-scale human trials, the National Institute on Aging (1997) cautions against the use of testosterone or DHEA in any routine way.

Both paroxetine and sertraline have been shown to reduce problems of premature ejaculation. However, the SSRIs, including venlafaxine, are also implicated in either erectile dysfunction or anorgasmia.

The interaction of decreased libido due to depression with drug-induced sexual side effects makes treament difficult. Women appear to recover from depression associated difficulties with desire and psychological arousal when treated with an SSRI, whereas orgasmic dysfunction seems to be drug related in men (Piazza et al., 1997). Men who are experiencing sexual difficulties with an SSRI may be switched to bupropion or nefazodone rather than withdrawn from antidepressant treament. Mirtazapine also shows promise in this regard. This substitution regimen is also advised for persons with an incomplete antidepressant response. For patients whose depression has remitted with an SSRI, the addition of another medication rather than withdrawal of antidepressant should be recommended. Coadministation choices include 75 mg bupropion, 20 mg dextroamphetamine, or 18.75 mg pemoline daily (Segraves, 1995).

Intercavernosal injection of prostaglandin E1 is FDA approved for erectile dysfunction and typically results in full erection of sufficient duration. However, only a minority of men find the route of delivery acceptable due to bleeding, bruising, and loss of spontaneity. Vacuum tumescent devices may be effective for a number of older men. The device consists of a vacuum cylinder, which causes the penis to engorge with blood; an elastic band is used to sustain the tumescence. Bruising may result (National Institutes of Health Consensus Development Panel on Impotence, 1993).

A variety of medications are reported to improve erectile dysfunction, including trazodone, vitamin E, yohimbine, and others (Godschalk et al., 1997). However, their efficacy is not impressive and the introduction of sildenafil (Viagra) seems likely to supplant their use entirely. Sildenafil citrate promotes erection in response to sexual stimulation by blocking phosphodiesterase 5 (PDE5), which degrades cyclic guanosine monophosphate (cGMP), a vasodilator generated in the penis. Sexual excitement releases nitric oxide that results in the generation of cGMP (Godschalk et al., 1997). Some 70% of men will respond to sildenafil. Patients should be informed that other treatments are available should the medication not prove helpful. With men who have not had sexual relations for some time, it is important to ask why the request is being made now. The importance of lovemaking to patient and partner should be assessed before a treatment plan or prescription is provided.

Sildenafil is most effective when the etiology of erectile dysfunction is psychological, less so for the neurogenic impotence of diabetes or following surgery for prostate cancer. Sildenafil (25, 50, or 100 mg) is taken once daily, usually an hour before intercourse with effects lasting up to 12 hours in some men. Mobley and Baum (1999) advise beginning the patients on 50 mg. If the dose is satisfactory after two attempts, it may be halved. If 50 mg is not sufficient, 75 mg then 100 mg may be used again, allowing two trials before escalating. There are no benefits beyond 100 mg. Because PDE5 appears to be generated only in the penis, systemic side effects seemed unlikely initially. However, sildenafil has mild systemic vasodilatory activity and may potentiate effects of nitrates. Cardiovascular deaths have been reported among men taking nitrates. As a result, sildenafil and should not be prescribed to patients taking nitrates and to those with congestive heart failure or unstable angina. Potent cytochrome P450 3A4 inhibitors (erythromycin) may elevate plasma levels of sildenafil and should not be taken after an alcoholic beverage. Transient headache, gastrointestinal symptoms, and blue green aura around bright lights are the most frequently reported difficulties. Priapism, which has been reported with prostaglandin injections, is unlikely. Because the mechanism of action is local and vascular, sildenafil should not enhance libido or sensation. Nonetheless, better sexual function is likely to have a halo of effects not explained by the pharmacology of the drug. The older person may require a prolonged therapeutic trial before rejecting therapy as ineffective. Partial return of function and satisfaction is frequently a more realistic goal than complete recovery (Kennedy et al., 1997).

Estrogen Replacement Therapy

The original indication for estrogen replacement was the relief of vulvovaginal atrophic changes, osteoporosis, and vasomotor disturbances—hot flashes and insomnia. Women receiving estrogen have lower risk of myocardial infarction, stroke, and cardiovascular death. Estrogen slows the loss of bone mass and resultant osteoporosis and reduces the risk of hip and vertebral fracture, thus limiting one of the main causes of incapacitation in the elderly. Although the postmenopausal decline in women's sexuality is only partially explained by physiological changes, estrogen may enhance sexual drive in postmenopausal women (Belchertz, 1994).

A number of studies suggest that estrogen replacement might affect the central nervous system. Some show that Alzheimer's disease may be related to estrogen deficiency and that estrogen replacement with or without cholinesterase inhibition may be useful to prevent or delay the progression of dementia (Kampen & Sherwin, 1994; Schneider et al., 1997). An additional benefit of long-term hormonal replacement may also be a decreased risk of depressive symptoms after age 60 (Palinkas & Barret-Connor, 1992). However, these suggestions are not well substantiated by randomized clinical trials. Thus the use estrogen as adjunctive treatment when antidepressants are prescribed for the depressed or demented older woman without estrogen risk factors seems reasonable yet untested (Seeman, 1997). Young et al.'s (1997) report of mania provoked by estrogen replacements further argues for caution. The Women's Health Initiative is presently testing these hypotheses using 0.625 mg of conjugated estrogens with 2.5 mg of medroxyprogesterone among women who have not had a hysterectomy. Those who underwent hysterectomy received estrogen only (Jones, 1998). The most frequently cited botanical alternative to estrogen is black cohosh (*Cimicifuga recemosa*). One double-blind, randomized trial with the commercial black cohosh preparation Remifemin, at doses ranging from 40 to 200 mg daily, demonstrated reductions in both physical and mental menopausal symptoms that were superior to both estrogen and placebo (Wong et al., 1998). In summary, if there is no absolute contraindication, the potential benefits of estrogen replacement may well outweigh the risks (see Table 9.5). However, the acceptance of risk remains the individual woman's choice (Belchetz, 1994).

TABLE 9.5. Benefits and Contraindications of Estrogen Replacement

Benefits
- Relief of postmenopausal vasomotor disturbances, insomnia
- Alleviation of urogenital atrophic symptoms
- Preventing, slowing osteoporosis
- Reduced morbidity and mortality
  Decreased incidence of stroke
  Preventing or slowing the progression of cardiovascular disease
  Reduction in fractures and disability
- Effect on the central nervous system
  Decrease in postmenopausal depressive symptoms
  Hypothetical role in slowing or preventing dementia
  Enhanced verbal memory

Relative contraindications
- Endometriosis
- Uterine myomata
- Fibrocystic breast disease, family history of breast or endometrial cancer
- Severe hypertriglyceridemia
- Chronic liver disease

Absolute contraindications
- Undiagnosed vaginal bleeding
- Active liver disease
- Recurrent thromboembolic disease
- Breast cancer, endometrial cancer

Note. Data from Palinkas and Barret-Connor (1992); Paganini-Hill and Henderson (1994); Kampen and Sherwin (1994); Belchetz (1994); and Kennedy et al. (1997).

SEX IN THE NURSING HOME

Most nursing home staff have had little education regarding sexuality in health care settings. They will encounter sexual activity of three sorts; consenting, willfully indiscreet, and disinhibited. First, most sexual activity among nursing home residents is neither pathological nor "acting out." The consultant should be prepared to dispel myths and educate staff (and families) about the rights to privacy that competent, sexually consenting adults retain as residents of nursing homes (Kennedy et al., 1997). Nursing home residents who are capable of consensual sex and free from threats of exploitation exhibit three characteristics.

1. They can identify their desired partner.
2. They can express the degree of intimacy they prefer.
3. Their sexual history is consistent with present behavior (Lichtenberg & Strezpek, 1990).

To address the sexual disinhibition of demented or brain-damaged residents of nursing homes requires an open staff discussion with a knowledgeable consultant. The behavior that staff identify as "inappropriate" needs to be carefully examined. Climbing into the wrong bed, displaying exposed genitals through open blouse or trousers, and touching staff about the breasts or hips may be nothing more than confusion. Staff need to be informed about the behavioral consequences of frontal-lobe degeneration. The results are a loss of social judgment, impulse control, and appreciation for the consequences of sexual acts rather than willful "acting out," mischief, or malice. Whether the activity is willful or disinhibited, staff should avoid a punitive attitude but anticipate repetition, set limits, and reinforce positive behaviors. The problem should be identified for the patient while it is occurring. Staff should use redirection alternatives such as recreational activities or snacks to satisfy the patient's need for stimulation (Kaiser & Morely, 1994). Antipsychotics, mood stabilizers, serotonergic reuptake inhibitors, and hormonal treatments (Kyomen et al., 1991) may be considered, but the management of problematic staff and patient behaviors will be required.

SUMMARY

With relief from childrearing, the workplace, and the reproductive imperative to achieve intercourse, older couples may relax and enjoy sex as never before. Indeed, changes in the stages of sexual response allow the physical demands of sex to be less taxing. Gender differences in drive, character style, and foreplay needs may become better synchronized in old age. And the diminished desire that results from disuse may be a blessing to persons who cannot surmount the obstacles of illness, disability, lack of a partner, or personal inhibitions. But as the proportion of older adults in the population increases, greater numbers of persons over the age of 65 will seek assistance with sexual dysfunction. Practitioners can improve the well-being of older adults by addressing their sexual concerns with skill and compassion.

SUGGESTED READING FOR PATIENTS

Butler, R. N., Lewis, M. I. (1986). *Love and Sex after 40: A Guide for Men and Women for their Mid and Late Years.* New York: Harper & Row.
Goodwin, A. J., Agronin, M. (1997). *A Woman's Guide to Overcoming Sexual Fear and Pain.* Oakland, CA: New Harbinger.

REFERENCES

Balon, R. (1995, September). The effects of antidepressants on human sexuality: Diagnosis and management. *Primary Psychiatry*, pp. 46–51.
Belchetz, P. E. (1994). Hormonal treatment of postmenopausal women. *New England Journal of Medicine, 330,* 1062–1069.
Bretschneider, J. G., McCoy, N. L. (1988). Sexual interest and behavior in healthy 80–102-year-olds. *Archives of Sexual Behavior, 17,* 109–129.
Butler, R. N., Lewis, M. (1990). Sexuality. In W. B. Abrams, R. Berkow, & A. J. Fletcher (Eds.), *The Merck manual of geriatrics* (pp. 631–644). Rahway, NJ: Merck, Sharp and Dohme Research Laboratories.
Cohen, M. A. A., Alfonso, C. (1997). A comprehensive approach to sexual history-taking using the biopsychosicial model. *International Journal of Mental Health, 26,* 3–14.
Dagon, E. M. (1989). Sexuality and sexual dysfunction in the elderly. In L. Lazarus, L. F. Jarvik, J. R. Foster, et al. (Eds.), *Essentials of geriatric psychiatry* (pp. 41–64). New York: Springer.
Dunn, M. E. (1988). Psychological perspectives of sex and aging. *American Journal of Cardiology, 61,* 24H–26H.
Godschalk, M. F., Sison, A., Mulligan, T. (1997). Management of erectile dysfunction by the geriatrician. *Journal of the American Geriatrics Society, 45,* 1240–1246.
Hsueh, W. A. (1988). Sexual dysfunction with aging and systemic hypertension. *American Journal of Cardiology, 61,* 18H–23H.
Jones, B. (1998, March). *WHIMS: Women's Health Initiative Memory Study.* Paper

presented at the meeting of the American Association for Geriatric Psychiatry, Miami, FL.

Kaiser, F. E., Morely, J. E. (1994). Sexuality and dementia. In J. C. Morris (Ed.), *Handbook of dementing illnesses* (pp. 539–548). New York: Marcel Dekker .

Kampen, D. L., Sherwin, B. B. (1994). Estrogen use and verbal memory in healthy postmenopausal women. *Obstetrics and Gynecology, 3*, 979–983.

Kennedy, G. J. (1995). Treatment of behavioral problems in Alzheimer's disease. *Resident and Staff Physician, 41*, 26–30.

Kennedy G. J., Haque, M., Zarankow, B. (1997). Human sexuality in late life. *International Journal of Psychiatry, 26*, 35–46.

Kyomen, H. H., Nobel, K. W., Wei, J. Y. (1991). The use of estrogen to decrease aggressive physical behavior in elderly men with dementia. *Journal of the American Geriatrics Society, 39*, 1110–1112.

Lamberts, S. W., van den Beld, A. W., vander Lely, A. J. (1997). The endocrinology of aging. *Science, 278*, 419–424.

Lichtenberg, P., Strezpek, D. (1990). Assessments of institutional dementia patient's competencies to participate in intimate relationships. *Gerontologist, 30*, 117–120.

Mazur, A. (1998). Aging and endocrinology. *Science, 279*, 305–306.

Mobley, D. F., Baum, N. (1999). Sildenafil in elderly men: Advice and caveats. *Clinical Geriatrics, 7*, 34–41.

Mulligan, T., Retchin, S. M., Chinchilli, V. M., et al. (1988). The role of aging and chronic disease in sexual dysfunction. *Journal of the American Geriatrics Society, 36*, 520–524.

National Institute on Aging. (1997). *Pills, patches, and shots: Can hormones prevent aging?* Bethesda, MD: Author.

National Institutes of Health Consensus Development Panel on Impotence. (1993). *Journal of the American Medical Association, 270*, 83–90.

Paganini-Hill, A., Henderson, V. W. (1994). Estrogen replacement and risk of Alzheimer's disease in women. *American Journal of Epidemiology, 140*, 256–261.

Palinkas, L. A., Barret-Connor, E. (1992). Estrogen use and depressive symptoms in postmenopausal women. *Obstetrics and Gynecology, 80*, 30–35.

Patterson, J., Nagel, N., James. E., et al. (1995). Basic and clinical considerations of HIV infection in the elderly. *Clinical Geriatrics, 3*, 21–34.

Piazza, L. A., Markowitz, J. C., Kocsis, J. H., et al. (1997). Sexual functioning in chronically depressed patients treated with SSRI antidepressants: A pilot study. *American Journal of Psychiatry, 154*, 1757–1759.

Redinbaugh, E. M., Zeiss, A. M., Davies, H. D., et al. (1997). Sexual behavior in men with dementing illnesses. *Clinical Geriatrics, 13*, 45–50.

Rousseau, P. C. (1986). Sexual changes and impotence in elderly men. *American Family Physician, 34*, 131–136.

Segraves, R. T. (1995). Antidepressant-induced orgasm disorder. *Journal of Sex and Marital Therapy, 21*, 192–201.

Schneider, L. S., Small, G. W., Hamilton, S. H., et al. (1997). Estrogen replacement and response to fluoxetine in a multi-center geriatric depression trial. Fluoxetine Collaboration Study Group. *American Journal of Geriatric Psychiatry, 5*, 97–106.

Seeman, M. V. (1997). Psychopathology in women and men: Focus on female hormones. *American Journal of Psychiatry, 154*, 1641–1647.

Steege, J. F. (1986). Sexual functioning in the aging woman. *Clinical Obstetrics and Gynecology, 29*, 462–469.

Sviland, M. (1978). A program of sexual liberation and growth in the elderly. In R. Solnick (Ed.), *Sexuality and aging.* San Diego: University of Southern California Press.

Wise, T. N., Rabins, P. V., Gahnsley, H. (1984). The older patient with a sexual dysfunction. *Journal of Sex and Marital Therapy, 10,* 117–121.

Wong, A. H. C., Smith, M., Boon, H. S. (1998). Herbal remedies in psychiatric practice. *Archives of General Psychiatry, 55,* 1003–1044.

Young, R. C., Moline, M., Kleyman, F. (1997). Estrogen replacement therapy and late-life mania. *American Journal of Geriatric Psychiatry, 5,* 179–181.

Zeiss, R. A., Delmonico, R. L., Zeiss, A. M., et al. (1991). Psychologic disorder and sexual dysfunction in elders. *Clinics in Geriatric Medicine, 7,* 133–151.

10

Elder Abuse, Neglect, and Self-Injurious Behaviors

Identification of elder abuse, neglect, and self-injurious behaviors is a major public health problem but receives little emphasis in health care curricula. For every case identified by community agencies, as many as 14 go undetected (Benton & Marshall, 1991). The elevated mortality associated with abuse and self-neglect cannot be explained by other sociodemographic or biomedical characteristics (Lachs et al., 1998). Specialists and generalists alike need added information to recognize the warning signs and institute preventive measures. Knowledge of available services will help practitioners avoid rage and despair when they encounter this most unsettling of late-life health problems.

DEFINITIONS

The term "mistreatment" is used to encompass both neglect and abuse. Although mistreatment may take the form of domestic violence (Brenneman & Lucey, 1996), neglect is more frequent than physical aggression. The Elderly Abuse Reporting Act (U.S. House of Representatives, 1981) defines abuse as an act or failure to act which harms or threatens to harm the health or well-being of an older adult. Detailed descriptions of the seven kinds of elder mistreatment are listed in the appendix. Acts of abuse include mental or physical injury; sexual aggression; and withholding food, clothing, or medical or supportive care necessary to meet the health needs, both mental and physical, of the older person. Perpetrators are those who have abrogated their responsibility for the care or fiduciary needs of the victim. Although there are well-established physical findings indicative of child abuse, evidence of abuse among the elderly is more subtle (Block & Sinnott, 1979). Also, unlike child abuse there is little legal uniformity among the states regarding mandatory reporting of suspected elder abuse. The first mandatory elder abuse reporting law with an ombudsman appointed to verify allegations dates to 1978 (Lachs et al., 1998). Today, most states do not have mandatory reporting. Without a formal network of services and procedures mandated by law, the only protection to the older victim may be that accorded by the examining clinician (Tatara, 1995).

PROBLEMS WITH REPORTS
OF ELDER MISTREATMENT

Because abuse, neglect, and exploitation of elders is always objectionable and often criminal, it is not surprising that reliable, methodologically sound data on the phenomena remain scarce. Lack of professional training, public awareness, and funding for protective services add to the underreporting. Victims are most often reluctant to report the perpetrators for fear of retribution or being "rescued" from the home only to be institutionalized. Embarrassment, denial, and a wish to protect abusive family members and physical or financial reliance on the abuser are added incentives not to report. Finally, cognitive impairment may effectively prevent the accusation of abuse or reduce its credibility (Fulmer et al., 1992).

There are also methodological problems in reporting abuse and mistreatment (Lehtonen & Pahkinen, 1996). Civil or criminal sanctions related to mandatory reporting complicate the willingness of perpetrators to divulge the information even in confidential interviews. Definitions of abuse and neglect are difficult to apply with certainty in the older adult due to the confounding influence of normal aging and frailty on physical signs of maltreatment (Sengstock & Liang, 1982). More than half of all elder maltreatment reports are made by social service or home care providers, landlords, utility workers, or law enforcement. Health care professionals and family members account for a third of the reported cases (Tatara, 1989).

Prevalence Estimates

Estimates of the number of older Americans who are abused or neglected in the 1980s ranged from 1 million (Pillemer & Finkelhor, 1988) to 2.5 million (Steinmetz, 1981). A more conservative estimate suggests that at least three-quarters of a million seniors are mistreated, with a lesser number seriously neglecting themselves (Tatara, 1993), a condition known poetically as the Diogenes syndrome. Random samples indicate that close to 3% of community residents experience mistreatment (Pillemer & Finkelhor, 1988). Surveys of police and health and social service providers put the figure closer to 5% (Tatara, 1993). Men are slightly more likely to be the perpetrators. Women make up two-thirds of the victims. Victims ages 60–63 make up 7.6% of cases, those ages 85 and older represent 23.1% (Tatara, 1993). According to the National Resource Center on Elder Abuse, in cases of domestic elder abuse 30% involved adult children, 15% involved spouses, and 17.8% involved other family members. Thirty-seven percent of the incidents were identified as neglect, 26% physical abuse, and 20% financial or material exploitation (Goldstein, 1995).

Data from the New Haven Established Population for Epidemiologic Studies in the Elderly pooled with records from the Connecticut adult protective services (APS) for the elderly characterized consequences of elder abuse, neglect, and self-neglect in 1988. Of 2,812 older community residents, 204 were seen by protective services over a 9-year period. In 38 cases, the allegations of abuse or self-neglect were refuted by an in-home visit. Of the 176 that were verified, 72.7% were cases of self-neglect, 17% neglect by caregivers, 5.7% cases of abuse, and 4.5% financial exploitation. After adjusting for other biomedical and sociodemographic risk factors, mortality was threefold greater among those who had been abused, neglected, or exploited compared to the remainder of the cohort. Mortality was 1.7 times higher among self-neglect cases compared to the remainder. Notably, causes of death did not differ among cases and the rest of the cohort. Deaths among abuse cases were not related to injury, leading the authors to speculate that interpersonal distress within the social network ("negative support") conveyed the additional mortality (Lachs et al., 1998). Although 19% of the allegations were refuted upon in-home examination, this additional mortality is likely to be more than a study of protective services cases would indicate.

Findings from the National Elder Abuse Incidence Study

A more rigorous estimate became available in 1998 from the National Elder Abuse Incidence Study mandated by Congress and carried out by the National Center on Elder Abuse at the American Public Human Services Association in collaboration with Westat Inc., a social science and survey research firm. Communities were selected to reflect a representative sample for the ethnic, socioeconomic, and geographic distribution of the population ages 60 and over. Definitions based on the various state and federal documents were operationalized by consensus. Incidence data were collected from (1) APS or the area agency on aging as well as (2) other community agencies and entities (senior centers, visiting nurses, banks) which might serve as sentinels for elder abuse without having formal reporting responsibility. The sentinel sampling, adapted from studies of child abuse, was conceived to estimate the number of cases observed by the standardized definitions but which, for whatever reason, did not appear on the APS case roster.

Findings largely confirmed earlier estimates based on less reliable methodologies. There were some 450,000 new cases of elder abuse or neglect detected in 1996 of which only one-quarter were ever reported to an APS. Adding the number of persons who seriously neglected themselves elevates the figure to 551,000. Thus by the most conservative yet scientifically reliable estimates, the number of new elder abuse victims represents more than 1% of the 44 million Americans ages 60 and older. This does not include ongoing cases that require the surveillance of APS and omits the number of abused persons in hospitals, nursing homes, board-and-care, and adult homes. Based on information from the community sentinels, for every case investigated by APS, four more meet criteria.

The characteristics of the victims and perpetrators were as follows. After controlling for their greater proportion in the aged population, women were victims of abuse or neglect at higher rates than males. Persons ages 80 or older were abused or neglected at two to three times their proportion of the population. When the perpetrator could be identified, in 90% of cases that individual was a family member. Two-thirds of the time the person was the victim's child or spouse. Males more frequently committed acts of abuse. African Americans were overrepresented in the ranks of the abused; Latinos were underrepresented. Persons who seriously neglected themselves tended to be either frail, confused, or depressed.

The Many Forms of Elder Mistreatment

Table 10.1 categorizes the three forms of elder mistreatment. They span the most easily detected physical abuse to the more subtle, difficult-to-uncover psychological and financial abuses. Physical abuse ranges from assault, which may be related to fits of rage or alcohol abuse, to premeditated isolation, starvation, and withholding of medication or medical care. However, in some instances physical assault may be self-defense against violence directed at the caregiver (Fulmer & Paveza, 1998). Here the underlying precipitant is disinhibition due to dementia rather than willful malice. Neglect is more often unintentional than

TABLE 10.1. Types of Elder Mistreatment

Physical	Psychological	Financial
Assault	Humiliation	Theft
Neglect	Harassment	Extortion
Restraint	Manipulation	Misuse of property
Isolation	Inattention	Misuse of funds
Starvation	Instilling fear	Blocked access to funds
Sleep deprivation	Intimidation	Blocked access to property
Withheld medication	Preemptive decision making	
Simple ←	EASE OF DETECTION →	Complex

Note. Adapted from Benton and Marshall (1991). Copyright 1991 by W. B. Saunders Co. Adapted by permission.

purposeful. Disadvantaged, socially isolated family members with little information and few resources may simply be overwhelmed, not knowing where to turn for help. With physical abuse, the malicious character of the behavior is easily inferred, whereas neglect may represent a call for help.

Psychological abuse obviously accompanies every episode of physical abuse. And it is important to recall that violence is usually preceded by verbal assault. Episodic outbursts are more often encountered than conscious manipulation, inattention, or intimidation. Some families exhibit a combative style of interaction which may seem abusive to outsiders but represents more a mode of expression. Yet when the older family member is intimidated, the content and intensity of the expression may be genuinely abusive. Similarly, threats to leave the elder unattended or abandoned to a nursing home may reach the threshold of psychological abuse (Lau & Kosberg, 1979). However, exhausted caregivers who need respite or alternative care arrangements may threaten a nursing home out of desperation rather than malice, particularly when the patient refuses a home health aide. Again, differentiating malicious intent from understandable frustration may not be easy.

Financial abuse is an exploitation of the older person's property or funds. It more often takes the form of surreptitiously cashing the pensioner's check, credit theft, and expropriation of checking accounts, bonds, or equities. Refusal to allow necessary care or services in the home in order to inherit more of the elder's financial legacy is also an abuse (Brenneman & Lucey, 1996). Certainly some senior citizens would rather bequeath their funds to family than expend their resources on care. And in impoverished areas, senior entitlements may be a valuable commodity which the elderly willingly contribute to the family's welfare. However, loss of entitlements such as Medicaid or Medicare Part B, which requires the senior to pay a premium, are cause for concern if not suspicion. More insidious are direct mail schemes which declare potential winnings in elder-friendly large print with the real probabilities after the initial investment in a microscopic font. Tampering with a competent senior's mail may be a federal offense, but some families find it less offensive to screen the postal materials for exploitive potential.

DETECTION

Clearly, when abuse or neglect is suspected the patient needs to be interviewed separately from family or caregiver. Mental status of the patient should be observed with and without the caregiver present. Vague, fearful responses regarding injury, illness, and care needs should alert the examiner to see the patient alone. Patients who avoid eye contact with family or who are reluctant to speak in their presence should be asked privately about concerns for their safety. Thoughts of suicide should be asked about directly, particularly when affect is depressed or constricted. Key to the detection of abuse is an awareness of the attributes of both victims and perpetrators as well as the situations in which abuse occurs (Table 10.2). This risk/vulnerability model guides efforts to detect abuse and preventive interventions (Fulmer &

TABLE 10.2. Elder Abuse and Neglect Risk Profile

High-risk elderly	High-risk caregiver
Female	Problem drinker
Advanced age	Abuses medications, drugs
Dependent	Cognitively impaired
Problem drinker	Mental illness, emotional lability
Intergenerational conflict	Caregiving inexperience
Internalizes blame	Economically troubled or dependent
Excess loyalty	Abused as a child
Past abuse	Stressed
Stoicism	Socially disengaged
Isolation	Blames others, lacks understanding
Impairment	Unsympathetic, hypercritical
Provocative	Unrealistic

Note. Adapted from Kosberg (1988). Copyright 1988 by the Gerontological Society of America. Adapted by permission

Paveza, 1998). Much of the clinical literature on detection is anecdotal but does provide clues and assessment tools for the practitioner. The Akron General Medical Center Geriatric Abuse Protocol (Costa, 1993) is one such effort to structure the assessment. Table 10.2 provides the commonly accepted risk profile. In brief, the person at high risk of abuse or neglect is more often a woman of advanced age who is isolated and dependent, has been victimized before, and may be cognitively impaired. The person at risk of being a perpetrator is an economically, socially disadvantaged family member who is mentally ill or abusing alcohol or another substance. Cognitive impairment, lack of caregiver skills, and a history of childhood abuse round out the brief profile (American Medical Association, 1992).

Because elder abusers are most often family members, the shame of being abused often impairs the victim's ability to divulge the information (Dolon & Blakely, 1989). Financial exploitation by the family is a particularly insidious form of abuse and may explain why home care services that might have prevented a medical emergency have been withheld. Detection of abuse, neglect, or exploitation begins with history taking. Dramatic inconsistencies regarding injury, a history of admissions to several different hospitals, clinics, or doctors involved in care, and claims that the patient is "accident prone" all should raise concerns. Problems with medication compliance or lost prescriptions leading to repeated hospitalizations in which the patient is easily stabilized should also raise suspicions. Isolation from formal and informal social support despite available entitlements through Medicare or Medicaid is another risk factor that should be considered. Caregiver pathology (substance abuse, mental illness) and exhaustion should also be noted. Queries regarding household composition, how many rooms, and how many occupants will provide concrete details of the adequacy of the environment and potential for mistreatment (Lachs et al., 1994).

The signs and symptoms of abuse and neglect characterize several kinds of maltreatment (Table 10.3). The most important of these are (1) frequent, unexplained crying and (2) persistent unexplained suspicion of or fear of one or more individuals in the home. Physical findings suggestive of abuse or neglect include poor hygiene, malnutrition, poor nail care, decubiti, and fresh or healing wounds about face, back, buttocks. Pattern bruises (belt buckle) and missing patches of hair are signs of abuse, whereas finger marks about the arms of legs may indicate nothing more that capillary fragility and the caregiver's well-meaning efforts to assist the dependent person's mobility. Genital, breast, or anal bruises or bleeding are obviously cause for more aggressive examination. Contractures are preventable and their presence indicates less than ideal care and at times frank neglect.

TABLE 10.3. Detection of Elder Abuse and Neglect

History	Dramatic inconsistencies regarding injury
	Several hospitals, clinics, or doctors involved
	"Accident prone"
	Medication compliance
	Isolation from formal and informal social support
	Caregiver pathology (substance abuse, mental illness)
	Household composition, loss of entitlements
Physical	Poor hygiene, malnutrition, poor nail care, decubiti
	Fresh or healing wounds about face, back, buttocks
	Pattern bruises (belt buckle), missing patches of hair
	Genital, breast, or anal bruises; bleeding
	Contractures
	Grey Turner's sign (flank bruising)
	Cullen's sign (periumbilical bruising)
Mental status	Observed with and without caregiver, unexplained crying
	Suicidality
Home visit	Absence of assistive devices, filth, vermin infestation

Note. Data from Benton and Marshall (1991).

The House Call

A home visit may be the single most effective measure for both detection and prevention. Referral to a visiting nurse agency for an in-home assessment is a key maneuver both to minimize risk and to assess the reliability of the caregiver. The majority of caregivers will welcome an in-home assessment to ensure the safety of the environment and provide coaching on care skills. Explanations as to why a house call is rejected will be informative and sensitize the next practitioner who encounters the problem. Caregivers who repeatedly cancel the appointment despite promising constant availability to their impaired relative should not inspire confidence. The in-home assessment will detect needs and recommend assistance of which the overwhelmed caregiver and patient may not be aware. Absence of assistive devices, an unhygienic environment, and lack of food and drink (empty refrigerator) should be noted.

The in-home assessment will enable the practitioner to recommend a plan of care to support the caregiver and the patient. That the cost of care will be an issue should come as no surprise. The practitioner should be frank and open and propose a modest trial care plan that can be renegotiated at a future date once the patient and caregiver have assessed the value of the services. A weekly visit from a nurse or 4 hours of service, once a week, from a home health aide will not provide absolute protection, but it will reduce risk. The plan need not be ideal to represent a distinct improvement but it does need to get started. Some older persons will neglect their needs or their spouse's despite substantial resources out of a misplaced concern to "save for a rainy day." This stance is understandable for the present older generation who lived though deprivations of the Great Depression, World War II, the Holocaust, and legalized racial segregation. Yet reluctance to purchase care that will clearly extend the person's autonomy and well-being may reach delusional proportions. A capacity assessment by the practitioner with referral for a guardianship proceeding via protective services may be necessary.

INTERVENTION

Interventions (Table 10.4) for elder abuse and neglect derive from the theories posited to explain the causes (Table 10.5). Theory also guides the initial interview with the suspected perpetrator. It is assumed that by addressing the problems of the caregivers, who make up the majority of perpetrators, the needs of the older victim can be met without coercion or nursing home admission. When abuse is suspected, the discussion with the patient and caregiver will require tact, sensitivity, persistence, and circumspection. Acknowledging the victim's dependency and the burden placed on the caregiver allows an opportunity to assess the presence of depression, substance abuse, and social isolation. Inquiries as to caregiver stress related to exhaustion and marital or financial difficulties should be attempted in order to identify needs for counseling or supportive services of home health aides or respite care. Detection of alcohol or substance abuse, depression, or other mental illness will identify the need for mental health treatment.

Outright ageism and sociopathy are less frequently encountered but will clarify the need for a more confrontational, coercive approach. Denials are to be expected, as is uncertainty on the part of the practitioner. Inability to reach a firm conclusion should not be cause for alarm. Documenting the signs and suspicions in the emergency room record

TABLE 10.4. Interventions When Elder Abuse Is Suspected

Discussion	Patient and caregiver
Consultation	Social services, psychiatry, rape team
Documentation	Signs and suspicions (tort liability is negligible)
Home visit	Safety assessment, evaluation of equivocal signs
Hospitalization	Primary, secondary, and tertiary prevention
Insuring follow-up	Visiting nurse service, Protective Services Administration

Note. Data from American Medical Association (1992).

TABLE 10.5. Theories Regarding the Causes of Elder Abuse

Theory	Rationale
Ageism	Denigration of the aged leads to abuse and neglect
Impairment	Mental and physical dependency makes the elderly vulnerable
Abuser pathology	Mentally ill, addicts, sociopathic persons
Family dynamics	Abuse is learned and normative, maintains enmeshment
Internal stress	Caregivers act abusively when depressed or depleted
External stress	Caregivers abusive due to life crises, finances, marriage

Note. Data from Fulmer et al. (1984).

will build the case for the next encounter and lower the threshold for a formal report or referral. Psychiatric consultation can be of assistance in evaluating the patient once abuse is suspected and the seemingly inappropriate disposition is discharge home. If sexual abuse is suspected the hospital rape team should be contacted. The social services department is more often the avenue specified by legislative mandate to follow through for cases in which abuse or neglect is suspected. Whether or not reporting is mandatory, the emergency room clinician should seek assistance if there is suspicion of abuse. If the level of suspicion is high and the person refuses an in-home assessment, a referral to protective services is indicated. Protective services agencies are empowered to provide emergency interventions both for care and financial security. Yet their case workers are often overburdened and telephone follow-up on the practitioner's part may be critical to ensure that aftercare is achieved. In rare cases hospitalization may be required to prevent abuse or confirm the extent of neglect and necessary treatment. However, it is often more realistic to minimize risk with community services than to temporarily eliminate risk with hospitalization. An array of supportive services from home care providers can supply a quite reasonable safety net. Nonetheless, nursing home placement is often the result when a seriously self-neglecting older person is reported to protective services (Lachs et al., 1998).

SUMMARY

As the number of older adults increases, so will reports of elder mistreatment and the need for effective interventions. Data on the scope of the problem, particularly self-neglect, are limited. Information on prevention is more anecdotal than systematic. However, it is clear that effective interventions require several elements (Goldstein, 1996): (1) the clinician's awareness of the signs, symptoms, and definitions of elder abuse; (2) the use of assessment protocols with proven validity and reliability

(Costa, 1993; Fulmer & Paveza, 1998); and (3) practitioners' awareness of the adult protective laws in their states and the community resources available in the region. Mandatory elder abuse reporting laws are based on child abuse legislation and, depending on locale and enforcement, may be less than ideal when applied to presumed competent adults (Sellers et al., 1992). Optimal intervention will also include protection of privacy rights, continuity of care to reduce recurrence, and appropriate attention to the needs of both the victim and perpetrator. As a result, the use of a multidisciplinary team approach is the fourth critical element. And because the profile of the abuser is so often characterized by mental illness or substance abuse, mental health specialists will more often than not be involved in the case. Finally, an in-home assessment is pivotal to primary, secondary, and tertiary prevention. One's initial reaction to an abused or neglected older person may be rage or demoralization. Yet a punitive attitude toward the perpetrator may interfere with meeting the patient's immediate needs. The availability of knowledgeable colleagues can buffer the anger as well as prevent despair. A less distressed associate may be able to identify interventions the primary assessor may be to too overwhelmed to consider. However, the capacity to recognize and reduce the risk of elder mistreatment is well within the reach of informed practitioners.

For further information contact the National Resource Center on Elder Abuse, American Public Welfare Association, 810 First Street, NE, Suite 50, Washington, DC 20002-4205; 202-682-2470.

APPENDIX

Definitions of Elder Abuse, Neglect, and Exploitation

The following definitions were developed for the National Elder Abuse Incidence Study of domestic elder abuse, neglect, and exploitation of elders living in noninstitutionalized settings (U.S. Department of Health and Human Services Administration in Aging and the Administration for Children and Families; *http://www.interinc.com/NCEA/Incidence Study/main.html: National Center on Elder Abuse*).

Physical abuse is the use of physical force that may result in bodily injury, physical pain, or impairment. Physical abuse may include but is not limited to such acts of violence as striking (with or without an object), hitting, beating, pushing, shoving, shaking, slapping, kicking, pinching, and burning. The unwarranted administration of drugs and physical restraints, force-feeding, and physical punishment of any kind also are examples of physical abuse.

Sexual abuse is nonconsensual sexual contact of any kind with an elderly person. Sexual contact with any person incapable of giving consent also is considered sexual abuse; it includes but is not limited to unwanted touching and all types of sexual assault or battery such as rape, sodomy, coerced nudity, and sexually explicit photographing.

Emotional or psychological abuse is the infliction of anguish, emotional pain, or distress. Emotional or psychological abuse includes but is not limited to verbal assaults, insults, threats, intimidation, humiliation, and harassment. In addition, treating an older person like an infant; isolating an elderly person from family, friends, or regular activities; giving an older person a "silent treatment"; and enforced social isolation also are examples of emotional or psychological abuse.

Neglect is the refusal or failure to fulfill any part of a person's obligations or duties to an elder. Neglect may also include a refusal or failure by a person who has fiduciary responsibilities to provide care for an elder (e.g., failure to pay for necessary home care service, or the failure on the part of an in-home service provider to provide necessary care). Neglect typically means the refusal or failure to provide an elderly person with such life necessities as food, water, clothing, shelter, personal hygiene, medicine, comfort, personal safety, and other essentials included as a responsibility or an agreement.

Abandonment is the desertion of an elderly person by an individual who has assumed responsibility for providing care or by a person with physical custody of an elder.

Financial or material exploitation is the illegal or improper use of an elder's funds, property, or assets. Examples include but are not limited to cashing checks without authorization or permission; forging an older person's signature; misusing or stealing an older person's money or possessions; coercing or deceiving an older person into signing a document (e.g., contracts or a will); and the improper use of guardianship, or power of attorney.

Self-neglect is characterized as the behaviors of an elderly person that threaten his/her own health or safety. Self-neglect generally manifests itself in an older person's refusal or failure to provide himself/herself with adequate food, water, clothing, shelter, safety, personal hygiene, and medication (when indicated). For the purpose of this study, the definition of self-neglect *excludes* a situation in which a mentally competent older person (who understands the consequences of his/her decisions) makes a conscious and voluntary decision to engage in acts that threaten his/her health or safety.

Signs of Abuse and Neglect

Physical Abuse

- Bruises, black eyes, welts, lacerations, and rope marks
- Bone fractures, broken bones, and skull fractures

- Open wounds, cuts, punctures, untreated injuries, and injuries in various stages of healing
- Stains, dislocations, and internal injuries/bleeding
- Broken eyeglasses/frames, physical signs of being subjected to punishment, and signs of being restrained
- Laboratory findings of medication overdose or under utilization of prescribed drugs
- An elder's report of being hit, slapped, kicked, or mistreated
- An elder's sudden change in behavior
- A caregiver's refusal to allow visitors to see an elder alone

Sexual Abuse

- Bruises around the breasts or genital area
- Unexplained sexually transmitted disease or genital infections
- Unexplained vaginal or anal bleeding
- Torn, stained, or bloody underclothing
- An elder's report of being sexually assaulted or raped

Emotional Abuse

- Emotional upset or agitation
- Extreme withdrawal and noncommunication or nonresponsiveness
- An elder's report of being verbally or emotionally mistreated

Neglect

- Dehydration, malnutrition, untreated bedsores, and poor personal hygiene
- Unattended or untreated health problems
- Hazardous or unsafe living conditions (e.g., improper wiring, no heat or no running water)
- Unsanitary or unclean living conditions (e.g., dirt, fleas, lice on person, soiled bedding, fecal/urine smell, inadequate clothing)
- An elder's report of being neglected

Abandonment

- The desertion of an elder at a hospital, nursing facility, or other similar institution
- The desertion of an elder at a shopping center or other public location
- An elder's own report of being abandoned

Financial or Material Exploitation

- Sudden changes in a bank account or banking practice, including an unexplained withdrawal of large sums of money by a person accompanying the elder
- The inclusion of additional names on an elder's bank signature card
- Unauthorized withdrawal of funds using an elder's ATM card
- Abrupt changes in a will or in other financial documents
- Unexplained disappearance of funds or valuable possessions
- Provisions of substandard care or bills unpaid despite the availability of adequate financial resources
- The provision of services that are not necessary
- Discovery of an elder's signature forged for financial transactions or for the titles of the elder's possessions
- Sudden appearance of previously uninvolved relatives claiming rights to an elder's affairs and possessions
- Unexplained sudden transfer of assets to a family member or someone outside the family
- An elder's report of financial exploitation

Self-Neglect

- Dehydration, malnutrition, untreated or improperly attended medical conditions, and poor personal hygiene
- Hazardous or unsafe living conditions (e.g., improper wiring, no indoor plumbing, no heat or no running water)
- Unsanitary or unclean living quarters (e.g., animal/insect infestation, no functioning toilet, fecal/urine smell)
- Inappropriate and/or inadequate clothing, lack of necessary medical aids (e.g., eyeglasses, hearing aid, dentures)
- Grossly inadequate housing or homelessness

REFERENCES

American Medical Association. (1992). *Diagnostic and treatment guidelines on elder abuse and neglect.* Chicago: Author.

Benton, D., Marshall, C. (1991). Elder abuse. *Clinics in Geriatric Medicine, 7,* 831–845.

Block, M. R., Sinnott, J. D. (Eds.). (1979). *The battered elder syndrome: An exploratory study.* College Park, MD: University of Maryland Center on Aging.

Brenneman, K. S., Lucey, C. R. (1996). Elder maltreatment. In D. B. Reuben, T. T. Yoshikawa, & R. W. Besdine (Eds.), *Geriatrics review syllabus* (pp. 59–61). New York: American Geriatrics Society.

Costa, A. J. (1993). Elder abuse. *Primary Care, 20,* 375–389.

Dolon, R., Blakely, B. (1989). Elder abuse and neglect: A study of adult protective service workers in the United States. *Journal of Elder Abuse and Neglect, 1,* 31–49.

Fulmer, T., McMahon, D., Bear-Hines, M., et al. (1992). Prevalence of abuse, neglect, abandonment, violence and exploitation: An analysis of all geriatric patients seen in one emergency department over a six month period. *Journal of Emergency Nursing, 12,* 505–510.

Fulmer, T., Paveza, G. (1998). Neglect in the elderly patient. *Nursing Clinics of North America, 33,* 457–466.

Fulmer, T., Street, S., Carr, K. (1984). Abuse of the elderly: Screening and detection. *Journal of Emergency Nursing, 10,* 131.

Goldstein, M. Z. (1995). Elder abuse. In I. Kaplan & B. J. Sadock (Eds.), *Comprehensive textbook of psychiatry* (6th ed., pp. 2652–2656). Baltimore, MD: Williams & Wilkins,

Goldstein, M. Z. (1996). Families of older adults. In J. Sadavoy, L. W. Lazarus, L. F. Jarvik, et al. (Eds.), *Comprehensive review of geriatric psychiatry—II* (2nd ed., pp. 881–906). Washington, DC: American Psychiatric Press.

Kosberg, J. I. (1988). Preventing elder abuse: Identification of high risk factors prior to placement decisions. *Gerontologist, 28,* 43–50.

Lachs, M. S., Berkman, L., Fulmer, T., et al. (1994). A prospective community-based pilot study of risk factors for the investigation of elder mistreatment. *Journal of the American Geriatrics Society, 42,* 169–173.

Lachs, M. S., Williams, C. S., O'Brien, S., et al. (1998). The mortality of elder mistreatment. *Journal of the American Medical Association, 280,* 428–432.

Lau, E., Kosberg, J. I. (1979, September/October). Abuse of the elderly by informal care providers. *Aging,* pp. 11–15.

Lehtonen, R., Pahkinen, E. J. (1996). *Practical methods for design and analysis of complex survey* (rev. ed.). Chichester: Wiley.

National Center on Elder Abuse. (1997, September 9). NCEA—The incidence study. *http://www.interinc.com/NCEA/Incidence Study/main.html: National Center on Elder Abuse.*

Pillemer, K. A., Finklehor, D. (1988). The prevalence of elder abuse: A random sample survey. *Gerontologist, 28,* 51–57.

Tatara, T. (1989). Toward development of estimates of the national incidence of elder abuse based on currently available data: An exploratory study. In T. Filison & D. Ingram (Eds.), *Elder abuse: Practice and policy* (pp. 153–165). New York: Human Services Press.

Tatara, T. (1993). Understanding the nature and scope of domestic elder abuse with the use of state aggregate data: Summaries of key findings of a national survey of state APS and aging agencies. *Journal of Elder Abuse and Neglect, 5,* 35–57.

Tatara, T. (1995). *An analysis of state laws addressing elder abuse, neglect, and exploitation.* Washington, DC: National Center on Elder Abuse.

Sellers, C. S., Folts, W. E., Logan, K. M. (1992). Elder maltreatment: A multidimensional problem. *Journal of Elder Abuse and Neglect, 4,* 5–23.

Sengstock, M. C., Liang, J. (1982). *Identifying and characterizing elder abuse.* Detroit, MI: Wayne State University Institute of Gerontology.

Steinmetz, S. K. (1981, January–February). Elder abuse. *Aging,* pp. 6–10.

U.S. House of Representatives, Subcommittee on Health and Long Term Care, Select Committee on Aging. (1981). *Elder abuse: An examination of a hidden problem* (Publication No. 97–277). Washington, DC: U.S. Government Printing Office.

11

Alcohol and Substance Abuse

Treatment of substance abuse among older adults will become increasingly important as the number of aged Americans increases. The abuse of psychoactive substances is a major contributor to excess morbidity and mortality among persons of all ages and socioeconomic strata regardless of race or ethnicity. Alcohol and tobacco account for the majority of substance abuse–related death and disability in the United States; the former through cerebrovascular and hepatic disease, accidents, and violence, the latter through chronic pulmonary disease and malignancy. Patterns of substance abuse in late life are substantially different from that observed among younger adults. However, treatment may be less challenging. Effective diagnosis and treatment requires a nonpunitive, supportive, but persistent approach. This means the capacity to collect a substance intake history and the ability to formulate a treatment plan or referral strategy to an addiction specialist or residential treatment setting. It is also important for the practitioner to manage negative feelings toward patients who decline treatment or who are chronic abusers.

PREVALENCE OF ALCOHOL PROBLEMS AMONG OLDER ADULTS

Alcohol abuse and dependence by far exceed the individual and social morbidity associated with abuse of illicit substances. Although depression and anxiety are the principal reversible mental disorders of women, men experience equivalent rates in alcohol and substance abuse. A large minority of alcoholics and substance abusers suffer a concurrent major mental disorder (Blow et al., 1992b; Speer & Bates,

208

1992). Among persons 60 years of age or older the prevalence of alcohol disorders varies by gender, ethnicity, and setting. In the NIMH Epidemiologic Catchment Area Community Survey, the lifetime prevalence of alcohol disorders for men ranged from 13% of whites to 22% of Hispanics to 24% among African Americans. Among women the rates varied from 1% of Hispanics, 2% of whites, and 3% of African Americans. The 6-month prevalence of alcohol disorder without specifying race was 1.7% for men, 0.1% for women (Helzer et al., 1991).

However, in clinically defined populations the prevalence is considerably higher, reflecting the morbidity associated with alcohol abuse (Carlen et al., 1994). Among nursing home patients, 20% will have a history of alcohol abuse or dependence. Seventeen to 30% of patients seen in psychiatric practice report alcohol as a complicating factor in their illness. From 15 to 25% of medical and surgical patients whether hospitalized or ambulatory also have alcohol-related problems (Kranzler et al., 1990). Alcohol is involved in 10% or more of emergency room admissions. And a significant minority of residents in alcoholic rehabilitation facilities are 60 years of age or older (Liberto & Oslin, 1995). More than one-third of elderly alcoholics experienced onset of the disorder after age 60. However, the prevalence of problem drinking declines after age 50 due to premature demise, underreporting, diagnostic criteria that may not be relevant to older adults, and unidentified comorbidity (Bucholz et al., 1995; Finlayson, 1995a).

PREVALENCE OF NONALCOHOL
SUBSTANCE ABUSE IN LATE LIFE

The incidence of addiction to illicit substances after the age of 65 approaches 0 with prevalent cases representing abusers who have aged into geriatric status. Middle-age opiate addicts more often "mellow out," die, transition to alcohol or prescription medications with abuse potential, or enter methadone programs (Barnas et al., 1992). More problematic among older persons is the misuse of prescribed medications. Individuals over 65 receive 30% of all prescriptions (Sheahan et al., 1989). They consume more prescribed and over-the-counter (OTC) medications than any other age group. Two-thirds take an OTC drug daily. Aging also makes the individual more vulnerable to drug effects and interactions (Finlayson, 1995b). Products containing alcohol or caffeine as well as cold and allergy remedies with anticholinergic antihistamines or sympathomimetics are problematic for seniors. The most frequently misused agents are sedative/hypnotics, narcotic analgesics, and the nonsteroidal anti-inflammatory agents. They impair cognition

(Foy et al., 1995), jeopardize the liver or kidneys, or erode the gut when used improperly (Katz et al., 1998).

PHARMACODYNAMICS OF ALCOHOL IN THE AGED

The vulnerability of older persons to even modest intake is due to the pharmacodynamics of alcohol in advanced age (see Table 11.1). The toxicity of alcohol is induced at lower concentrations as a result of (1) age-related diminished volume of distribution (total body water), (2) diminished hepatic clearance, (3) increased blood–brain barrier permeability, and (4) increased receptor sensitivity. Tolerance for alcohol declines with age while sensitivity increases. The acute intake of alcohol suppresses hepatic metabolism while the chronic use increases microenzymal metabolism (Beresford & Lucey, 1995). This leads to a number of interactions with commonly prescribed medications. The sedative effects of psychotropics and valproate are increased. Even low-risk psychotropics can be lethal in overdose with alcohol. Acute alcohol ingestion also increases the effects of anticoagulants, hypoglycemics, and phenytoin and can precipitate disulfiram-like reactions with β-lactams, cephalosporins, sulfonylurea, and the hypoglycemics. Chronic use decreases the effects of anticoagulants, hypoglycemics, and phenytoin (Forster et al., 1993).

TABLE 11.1. Pharmacodynamics of Alcohol in the Aged

Toxicity induced at lower concentrations
    Diminished volume of distribution (total body water)
    Diminished hepatic clearance
    Increased blood–brain barrier permeability
    Increased receptor sensitivity

Capacity to develop dependence and tolerance diminishes with age
Conventional diagnostic criteria may not be relevant in late life
    Amount consumed may be pathologic but below midlife threshold
    Mean corpuscular volume (MCV) not a reliable indicator of abuse
    Social and occupational impact less prominent due to retirement

Acute use suppresses hepatic metabolism

Chronic use increases microenzymal metabolism

Interactions with commonly prescribed medications
    Increased sedative effects with psychotropics and valproate
    Acutely increases effects of anticoagulants, hypoglycemics, phenytoin
    May induce disulfiram-like reactions with β-lactams, cephalosporins,
        sulfonylurea, hypoglycemics
    Chronically decreases effects of anticoagulants, hypoglycemics, phenytoin

UNCERTAIN DIAGNOSTIC CRITERIA

Conventional diagnostic criteria may not be relevant in late life due to both social and physiological factors. DSM-IV divides substance-related problems into abuse and dependence (see Table 11.2). The term "substance abuse" indicates episodic but patterned misuse of which the individual is aware and which poses a threat to well-being. Dependence entails abuse but is distinguished by the person's preoccupation with the substance, the development of tolerance, dose escalation, and signs of an abstinence syndrome. Unfortunately, the separation of abuse from dependence becomes more difficult with age. Older adults may be problem drinkers without consuming large quantities and without experiencing withdrawal (Korrapati & Vestal, 1995).

The social and occupational impact of alcohol, which is critical to the diagnosis of abuse, may be less salient in late life due to retirement. The retired, socially isolated older male may fill the void with alcohol yet genuinely not report loss of social or occupational activities associated

TABLE 11.2. DSM-IV Diagnostic Criteria for Substance Abuse and Dependence

Abuse

Any of the following:
- Recurrent use resulting in failure to fulfill roles and responsibilities
- Continued use despite awareness of directly related social, occupational, mental or physical problems, or failed obligations which are caused or made worse by substance abuse
- Recurrent use in hazardous situations
- Recurrent substance related legal problems (disorderly conduct, DWI)

Dependence

Three or more of the following:
- Continued use despite awareness of directly related social, occupational, mental, or physical problems
- Often taken in larger amounts or longer than intended
- Persistent desire or failure to control intake
- Preoccupation with procurement, intake, or recovery
- Frequent impairment at work, school, or the home
- Social, work, or recreational activities abandoned or reduced as a result of substance use
- Marked tolerance (dose escalated or effects diminished by 50%)
- Withdrawal symptoms or substance use to avoid or alleviate withdrawal

Note. Adapted from American Psychiatric Association (1994). Copyright 1994 by the American Psychiatric Association. Adapted by permission.

with drink. The older woman who continues to have a bedtime sherry despite the development of stroke, dementia, or use of hypoglycemics may not be aware of the danger that alcohol poses. In either case the practitioner may not be alert to signs of an incipient problem because the quantity consumed or the impact seems minimal. The Substance Abuse Among Older Adults Consensus Panel for the Treatment Improvement Protocol Series (TIPS) (1998) recommends the terms "at-risk" and "problem" drinkers. At-risk drinkers have functional, health, or social problems which may be complicated by alcohol intake in even modest amounts but have not encountered difficulties. Problem drinkers are those whose intake is clearly excessive, as well as those who meet DSM-IV (American Psychiatric Association, 1994) criteria for abuse and dependence.

SYMPTOM PRESENTATION
OF ALCOHOL ABUSE IN OLD AGE

The symptoms of late-life alcohol abuse are most commonly nonspecific (see Table 11.3) and may include self-neglect, falls, and other injuries. Confusion, irritability, or emotional lability, depression, and sleep disturbance may be reported by family or caregivers. Unexplained diarrhea, malnutrition, and hypothermia may be the result of chronic alcohol overconsumption. Comorbid psychiatric disorders, particularly depression, are not infrequent. Of older adults abusing alcohol, major health problems are present in 90%, with chronic obstructive pulmonary disease occurring in 25%. Dementia from any cause is seen in 25 to 60% (Gambert & Katsoyannis, 1995). Both static and circumscribed, as well as pervasive, progressive cognitive deficits can result

---

TABLE 11.3. Symptom Presentation of Alcohol Abuse in Older Adults

Symptom presentation is most commonly nonspecific and may include the following:
    Self-neglect, falls, injuries, automobile accidents
    Confusion, amnesia, lability, depression, sleep disturbance, irritability
    Diarrhea, malnutrition, hypothermia, drowsiness, slurred speech
    Social isolation, withdrawal from family

Symptoms of intoxication, dependence, withdrawal less frequent

Comorbid psychiatric disorder particularly depression, cognitive impairment, or substance abuse not infrequent

Major health problems in 90%, chronic obstructive pulmonary disease in 25%

Dementia from any cause seen in 25–60%

from prolonged dependence on alcohol. A relatively small ingestion of alcohol may be associated with extensive cognitive impairment that should be reversible (Tarter, 1995; Alterman et al., 1990). However, the symptoms of intoxication, dependence, and withdrawal are less frequently observed, suggesting that the alcohol abuse in the aged may be physiologically easier to treat than in younger persons.

DETECTION AND SCREENING

Detection rates of alcohol abuse or dependence range from 27 to 37% of affected individuals depending on the experience of the physician. Diagnostic recognition is lowest for whites, women, and those with at least a high school diploma (Adams et al., 1996). The frequency with which treatment is offered is even lower (McInnes & Powell, 1994). TIPS (1998) recommends that 60-year-olds be screened for alcohol and prescription drug abuse as part of their annual assessment. The panel recommends a "brown bag approach" in which older adults are asked to bring every pill or capsule they take, including OTC and prescription medications, vitamins, and botanicals. Screening is also appropriate when certain physical symptoms are present or if the older person is recently bereaved or experiencing other major life changes. Questions about alcohol or medication abuse are best linked to a medical condition when screening older people. Thus screening instruments are more effective when used as part of a medical history in either a patient interview or self-report format or as a semistructured interview with a concerned friend, spouse, or family member. Screening is best introduced with a transitional statement such as the following: "Alcohol can affect your health and may interfere with medications. It is important that I know how much you drink and whether you have experienced any problems with drinking" (Babor et al., 1992, p. 35). TIPS (1998) cites additional examples: "I'm wondering if alcohol may be the reason why your diabetes isn't responding as it should" (p. 27), or "Sometimes one prescription drug can affect how well another medication is working. Let's go over the drugs you're taking and see if we can figure this problem out" (p. 27).

A number of screening instruments are useful to detect alcohol-related problems (see Table 11.4). TIPS (1998) recommends the CAGE Questionnaire (Buchsbaum et al., 1992; Ewing, 1984) and the Michigan Alcohol Screening Test—Geriatric Version (MAST-G) to screen for alcohol use among older whites (Blow et al., 1992a) and the Alcohol Use Disorders Identification Test (AUDIT) for alcohol problems among older members of ethnic minority groups (Saunders et al., 1993;

TABLE 11.4. Alcohol Abuse Screening Instruments

TWEAK[a]

TWEAK (Tolerance, Worry about drinking, Eye opener, Amnesia, Can't cut down drinKing) plus:
- How many drinks does it take before you begin to feel the effects of alcohol?
- How many drinks does it take before alcohol makes you fall asleep or pass out?
- Are there times when you drink and afterward you can't remember what you said or did?

CAGE Questionnaire[b]

Have you ever felt you should Cut down on your drinking?
Have people Annoyed you by criticizing your drinking?
Have you ever felt bad or Guilty about your drinking?
Have you ever had a drink first thing in the morning to steady your nerves or to get rid of a hangover (Eye opener)?

Scoring: Item responses on the CAGE are scored 0 for "no" and 1 for "yes" answers, with a higher score an indication of alcohol problems. A total score of 2 or greater is considered clinically significant.

Michigan Alcoholism Screening Test—Geriatric Version (MAST-G)[c]

After drinking have you ever noticed an increase in your heart rate or beating in your chest?	Yes	No
When talking with others, do you ever underestimate how much you actually drink?	Yes	No
Does alcohol make you sleepy so that you often fall asleep in your chair?	Yes	No
After a few drinks, have you sometimes not eaten or been able to skip a meal because you didn't feel hungry?	Yes	No
Does having a few drinks help decrease your shakiness or tremors?	Yes	No
Does alcohol sometimes make it hard for you to remember parts of the day or night?	Yes	No
Do you have rules for yourself that you won't drink before a certain time of the day?	Yes	No
Have you lost interest in hobbies or activities you used to enjoy?	Yes	No
When you wake up in the morning, do you ever have trouble remembering part of the night before?	Yes	No
Does having a drink help you sleep?	Yes	No
Do you hide your alcohol bottles from family members?	Yes	No
After a social gathering, have you ever felt embarrassed because you drank too much?	Yes	No
Have you ever been concerned that drinking might be harmful to your health?	Yes	No
Do you like to end an evening with a nightcap?	Yes	No
Did you find your drinking increased after someone close to you died?	Yes	No
In general, would you prefer to have a few drinks at home rather than go out to social events?	Yes	No

Are you drinking more now than in the past?	Yes No
Do you usually take a drink to relax or calm your nerves?	Yes No
Do you drink to take your mind off your problems?	Yes No
Have you ever increased your drinking after experiencing a loss in your life?	Yes No
Do you sometimes drive when you have had too much to drink?	Yes No
Has a doctor or nurse ever said they were worried or concerned about your drinking?	Yes No
Have you ever made rules to manage your drinking?	Yes No
When you feel lonely, does having a drink help?	Yes No

Scoring: Five or more "yes" responses are indicative of an alcohol problem. For further information, contact Frederic C. Blow, PhD, at University of Michigan Alcohol Research Center, 400 E. Eisenhower Parkway, Suite A, Ann Arbor, MI 48108, (734) 998–7952.

Alcohol Use Disorders Identification Test Questionnaire (AUDIT)[d]

Circle the number that comes closest to the patient's answer.

1. How often do you have a drink containing alcohol?

(0) Never (1) Monthly (2) 2 to 4 (3) 2 to 3 times (4) 4 or more
               or less   times a month a week   times a week

2. How many drinks containing alcohol do you have on a typical day when you are drinking?

(0) 1 or 2 (1) 3 or 4 (2) 5 or 6 (3) 7 to 9 (4) 10 or more

3. How often do you have six or more drinks on one occasion?

(0) Never (1) Less than (2) Monthly (3) Weekly (4) Daily or
               monthly   almost daily

4. How often during the last year have you found that you were not able to stop drinking once you had started?

(0) Never (1) Less than (2) Monthly (3) Weekly (4) Daily or
               monthly   almost daily

5. How often during the last year have you failed to do what was normally expected from you because of drinking?

(0) Never (1) Less than (2) Monthly (3) Weekly (4) Daily or
               monthly   almost daily

6. How often during the last year have you needed a first drink in the morning to get yourself going after a heavy drinking session?

(0) Never (1) Less than (2) Monthly (3) Weekly (4) Daily or
               monthly   almost daily

7. How often during the last year have you had a feeling of guilt or remorse after drinking?

(0) Never (1) Less than (2) Monthly (3) Weekly (4) Daily or
               monthly   almost daily

(*continued on next page*)

TABLE 11.4 (*continued*)

8. How often during the last year have you been unable to remember what happened the night before because you had been drinking?

(0) Never   (1) Less than   (2) Monthly   (3) Weekly   (4) Daily or
             monthly   almost daily

9. Has you or someone else been injured as a result of your drinking?

(0) No   (2) Yes, but   (4) Yes, during the last year
             not in the
             last year

10. Has a relative or friend or a doctor or other health worker been concerned about your drinking or suggested you cut down?

(0) No   (2) Yes, but   (4) Yes, during the last year
             not in the last
             year

Record sum of individual item scores here.

Scoring: Questions 1–8 are scored 0, 1, 2, 3, or 4. Questions 9 and 10 are scored 0, 2, or 4 only. The response is as follows:

	0	1	2	3	4
Question 1	Never	Monthly or less	2 to 4 times per month	2 to 3 times per week	4 or more times per week
Question 2	1 or 2	3 or 4	5 or 6	7 to 9	10 or more
Questions 3–8	Never	Less than monthly	Monthly	Weekly	Daily or almost daily
Questions 9–10	No		Yes, but not in the last year		Yes, during the last year

Saunders et al. (1993) suggest two cutoff points depending on the purpose of the screening. A threshold score of 8 yields higher sensitivity, 10 or more produces higher specificity. Higher scores on the first three items only, suggest hazardous alcohol use. Higher scores on items 4 through 6 indicate alcohol dependence. Isolated elevations on the 7–10 items suggest harmful alcohol use.

[a]From Chan et al. (1993). Copyright 1993 by Lippincott Williams & Wilkins. Reprinted by permission.
[b]From Ewing (1984). Copyright 1984 by the American Medical Association. Reprinted by permission.
[c]From Blow et al. (1992). Copyright 1992 by Lippincott Williams & Wilkins. Reprinted by permission.
[d]From Schmidt et al. (1995). Copyright 1995 by the *Southern Medical Journal*. Reprinted by permission.

Schmidt et al., 1995). The MAST-G and AUDIT are somewhat lengthy but show good sensitivity and specificity. Shorter mnemonic screens, the CAGE and TWEAK (Chan et al., 1993), are easy to remember but may be insensitive with older populations. Thus, when history is suspect or unclear or denial is evident, a collateral informant should be sought out with the permission of the patient. Most older adults will allow the practitioner to share the care plan with family, which opens an opportunity to discuss concerns.

ASSESSMENT

Assessing the patient's motivation and surveying other sources of therapeutic leverage are critical. The American Society for Addiction Medicine (1996) describes six dimensions to the assessment of substance abuse problems adapted here to late-life presentations. The first dimension deals with acute intoxication and danger of withdrawal. If the person is presently intoxicated, how dangerous is the condition? Are signs of withdrawal present or escalating? Is there a risk of seizures? Is there sufficient community support to make home detoxification safe? Second, are there biomedical conditions or complications other than withdrawal that need to be addressed now or in the future to allow treatment of the substance abuse problem? Third, do comorbid mental illness or psychosocial problems complicate the treatment? Are the problems manageable through treament of substance abuse or are they severe enough to warrant separate treatment of referral to a specialist? The fourth dimension focuses on the patient's acceptance or rejection of treatment. What is the basis and depth of the patient's motivation? Is the patient protesting or feeling coerced? If treatment is accepted, how strongly does the patient agree with other's perception that there is a serious problem? Is compliance an affectation assumed only to avoid negative consequences, or does the patient genuinely "own the problem" and acknowledge the threat to health and autonomy?

Fifth, what factors exist that might promote relapse or continued abuse? Does the patient have countervailing skills, habits, or information? What problems are likely to emerge if the patient is not engaged in treatment? How aware is the patient of cues to drink or misuse medication? What will fill the void once drinking no longer occupies the patient's time? Is there family or staff at the senior center available to reinforce the patient's efforts at abstinence? Will the patient waive confidentiality and allow the practitioner to share the treatment plan?

The final dimension concerns the recovery environment. Among retirees, boredom and loneliness are ready cues to drink. Thus the practitioner's awareness of the patient's social fabric and leisure pursuits is critical to successful intervention. Are there family members, social contacts, recreational pursuits, or living situations that will undercut engagement or treatment follow through? Are there supportive relationships, financial or religious resources, or leisure interests that increase the chances of success? Are there medical or functional conditions (nursing home admission) that will serve as motivators? Each of these assessment dimensions leads to realistic appraisal for patient and practitioner alike.

TREATMENT

Outpatient treatment is acceptable in most instances in which alcohol intake has reached the point of impairing the individual's autonomy (see Table 11.5). In some cases a change from daily to episodic use may reduce the individual's risk sufficiently. In other cases (e.g., when harm is certain or after repeated serious threats) abstinence should be the goal. TIPS (1998) recommends a sequential approach to treatment. The initial approach functions as either a referral strategy or treatment itself depending on the patient's willingness to engage and the severity of the problem (Bien et al., 1993). Because seniors typically are ashamed of their drinking, effective interventions should be non-confrontational and supportive and assure confidentiality. The intervention should be individualized and include feedback regarding the assessment, counseling to enhance motivation, education about physiological risks, techniques for behavior modification, the use of written materials and self-help manuals (see "Books for Patients and Families"

TABLE 11.5. Treatment of Alcohol Problems among the Elderly

Outpatient
    Assessment of motivation and social sources of therapeutic leverage
    Change sought through support rather than confrontation
    Emphasize alcohol's effects on comorbid conditions (diabetes, hypertension, falls)
    Focus on contributing issues (bereavement, loneliness, boredom)
    Rebuild social ties and rhythms (clubs, church, synagogue)
    Withdrawal symptoms treated with short acting benzodiazepines may be prolonged
    Antidepressant if depression or sleep disturbance persists for 4 weeks
    Antipsychotic may be needed for hallucinations or paranoia
    Antabuse (disulfiram) hazardous, naltrexone better
    Age-appropriate Alcoholics Anonymous or peer support group
    Al-Anon for enabling members of the social network
    Individual, group, marital, and family therapy as indicated
    Management of practitioner vulnerabilities
        Failure to suspect the problem due to patient's age
        Therapeutic nihilism or ageism
        Intense feelings toward help-rejecting, self-destructive patients

Hospitalization may be necessary if . . .
    BAL > 100 mg/dl
    Life threatening withdrawal signs (dehydration, seizures, tachycardia, hypertension, confusion)
    Presence of unstable comorbid disorders
    Outpatient treatment failed, polydrug abuse
    Suicidal intent or suicidal ideas with previous attempts
    Social factors (lives alone, spouse or companion is an enabler or abuser)

above this chapter's Reference list), and mutually agreed-on goals (TIPS, 1998).

The older person will feel less stigmatized and defensive if recommendations are fit into an overall care plan (Kofoed et al., 1987). The primary emphasis falls on improved health, mental capacity, and independence rather than elimination of the abused substance. Reducing intake is the means to each end (Fleming et al., 1997). Patients will need information about how their drinking patterns fit into the population norms for older adults. Older men should consume no more than one drink per day (somewhat lower limits for women) and a maximum of two drinks on any drinking occasion (e.g., New Year's Eve or weddings) (TIPS, 1998). The reasons for and circumstances surrounding drinking ("why, when, where") need to be explored to understand the role of alcohol in the older adult's life. Social isolation, and family problems need to be identified as potential areas of intervention. Some older modest but at-risk drinkers may not be aware that problems in physical, psychological, or social functioning are alcohol related. The patient may need coaching on sensible drinking limits and how to cut down or quit. Such coaching includes pursuing leisure opportunities that do not involve alcohol, getting reacquainted with hobbies and early-life interests, educational venues, volunteer activities (Dobson, 1988).

A contract of agreed-on drinking limits or abstinence, signed by the patient and the practitioner, may be particularly effective (Meichenbaum & Turk, 1987). Psychotherapy should focus on teaching skills to rebuild the social support network and address depression, grief, or loneliness and general problem solving (Harris & Miller, 1990; Egan, 1994; Carstensen et al., 1985). See Chapter 7 for a more detailed description of psychotherapeutic methods. For the senior with genuine alcohol dependence, an age-appropriate peer support group (Alcoholics Anonymous and others) should be recommended. Support groups (Al-Anon and others) should be part of the treatment plan, not just for those who are enabling members of a social network but for others as well (Dunlop, 1990).

When First Efforts Fail

Although a purely supportive approach will not fit all cases, without a supportive rapport, confrontational interventions will be perceived as either accusatory or punitive. When the practitioner lacks sufficient evidence or leverage, persons close to the substance-abusing patient may be asked to share their firsthand experiences of the problem behavior. The process may require preparation of family or friends prior to the meeting and is contingent upon the consent of the patient. The format is a show of concern not of force and should be limited to one or two friends, care providers, or family. Grandchildren, nieces, and nephews should be included only if they are adults. Bringing in child relatives will only embarrasses the older patient and cause resentment (TIPS, 1998).

"Motivational counseling" may also be required of the older person who rejects the practitioner's or the family's concerns (Miller & Rollnick, 1991). In motivational counseling the practitioner accepts the older adult's perspective as a starting point in order to identify the negative consequences of drinking or prescription drug abuse as they emerge. Specific events are used to shift the patient's perceptions about the consequences of the behavior and to acquire insights about alternatives. The practitioner shows confidence in the patient's capacity for change. Motivational counseling avoids labeling, moralizing, and confrontation; accepts ambivalence about change as the norm; and places the responsibility for change on the patient.

Practitioner fantasies of rescuing the older patient may be as common and as ultimately frustrating as the patient's rejecting help or denying the seriousness of the problem. Managing the practitioner's negative reactions to their self-destructive patients is one of the more challenging and frequent dilemmas of working with substance abusers. Intense practitioner feelings are often engendered by hasty assessment, including failure to plumb the patient's motivation or the need for ongoing support and therapeutic attention. Threatening to sever the therapeutic relationship if the person does not abstain is rarely effective and places the practitioner in a futile contest of wills (National Institute on Alcohol Abuse and Alcoholism, 1995).

More often what appears to be an impasse can be mediated by focusing on shared and at times modest goals of treatment (Prochaska et al., 1992). Preferable is an informed consent model in which the practitioner openly acknowledges the patient's choice to reject therapeutic advice. Risks of continued intake are expressed and documented, as is the patient's refusal to accept treatment recommendations for the specific problem. Clearly there are instances in which continued use of alcohol is eminently dangerous and presents an insurmountable obstacle to continued treatment, but such instances are rare.

Pharmacological Interventions

A dramatic or life-threatening abstinence syndrome may be less common in advanced age. However, symptoms of withdrawal may be prolonged. As a result, treatment with short-acting benzodiazepines (lorazepam, oxazepam) may also be prolonged. The patient needs to be informed from the outset that the ultimate goal is to be benzodiazepine free due to associated risks (Pomara et al., 1985). Fears of becoming dependent can be allayed in that older patients rarely escalate the dose. Antipsychotics may be needed if hallucinations or paranoia appear. More frequently an antidepressant will be required if mood disorder persists beyond the fourth week of abstinence. Persistent sleep disturbance may require a sedative antidepressant rather than an increased dosage of a benzodiazepine. Antabuse (disulfiram) poses hazards to the elderly, particularly those with medical comorbidities. Naltrexone (ReVia) rarely causes difficulties for older persons and may reduce drinking relapses (Litten et al., 1996). Once lab tests indicate that the patient is not in renal failure and that transaminases are not more than four times normal, naltrexone may be started at 15 mg daily. It is increased to 50 mg within 48 hours. Transaminases and bilirubin should be evaluated every 3 months thereafter. Efforts to eliminate smoking should not be deferred (Gordon & Kannel, 1983; Hurt et al., 1993). Wellbutrin may be an adjunctive or alternative pharmacological intervention for older adults whose cardiovascular disease contraindicates the use of a nicotine patch.

Hospitalization is recommended when the blood alcohol level reaches 100 mg/dl or when the abstinence syndrome is potentially life threatening as indicated by the occurrence of seizures, tachycardia, hypertension, or confusion (National Institute on Drug Abuse and Alcoholism, 1995). Also the presence of complicating comorbid disorders or social factors may require that the patient be hospitalized. The highest risk of suicide among any age group is seen in socially isolated, depressed older white males who use alcohol. Hospital admission is not necessary for all patients with depression or suicidal ideas (see Chapter 12). But when alcohol or suicidal intent is present the consideration for hospital admission becomes more serious. Residential treatment should be recommended for cases in which relapse occurs following hospitalization, when outpatient treatment has failed, or when polydrug abuse (alcohol or sedative/hypnotics with analgesics) is a problem. Cognitive impairment may remit after detoxification but will take time to reach maximum recovery (Center for Substance Abuse Treatment, 1995). Thus, home care services are not necessarily permanent.

When the patient has accepted referral to a substance abuse specialist or inpatient setting, the practitioner should become an active member of the recovery network. Sixty to 80% of relapses occur within 3 to 4 months (Vaillant et al., 1983). The assessment of successful outcome should include not only abstinence or reduced consumption but also improved physical functioning, quality of life, and well-being (TIPS, 1998).

PRESENTATION OF A CASE

The following case taken from my records illustrates the principles of effective treatment of late-life substance abuse. Readers should note the early efforts to establish rapport, set realistic goals, leverage social reinforcement, close off avenues of abuse, and retain optimism. Opportunities to support self-esteem and mastery appeared in the mid-phase but were complicated by the patient's resistance. Techniques from cognitive-behavioral therapy including "homework" and a calendar to objectively document the baseline pattern of abuse and effect of treatment were critical to the success of the effort. The case also illustrates the use of substitute medication for target symptoms.

Mr. R, a 71-year-old retired silversmith, was referred to reduce his dependence on lorazepam 2 mg 4 times daily and phenobarbital 60 mg twice daily. There was a long history of sedative use. His one effort to reduce his dosing brought on "headaches and nerves." As a child he was diagnosed with a neurasthenic circulatory disturbance and was bothered by essential tremor. He did well in school and was drafted to serve in World War II at age 19. He was taking five amytal tablets daily upon discharge until he switched to phenobarbital in midlife. The tremor interfered with his work but he was able to maintain steady state until his freelance smithing played out and he started lorazepam. He subsequently found full-time work but escalated the dose to 8 mg daily at the time of retirement and under the stress of his daughter's financial difficulties. He takes butalbital "once or twice a week for headache." His marriage of 48 years yielded one son and one daughter. His wife lost both brothers to alcoholism, calls him "a junkie," but has never threatened to separate. A mental status exam revealed a man appearing younger than 71 who was eager to cooperate and open about his anger and disappointment at the less than supportive attitude he has found among "the other psychiatrists." There was no evidence of cognitive impairment, delusions, or hallucinations. His Mini-Mental Status Exam (MMSE) score was 29.

The initial plan sought to reduce phenobarbital by 25% and to eliminate it before reducing the lorazepam. He allowed the plan to be shared with his son, who supported the effort. Mr. R was informed that the therapeutic contract would not provide for lost pills or prescriptions. Supportive psychotherapy during dose reduction to augment his motivation and increase in his exercise routine were also suggested.

Second Session

Mr. R and his wife, who accompanied him to the interview at the practitioner's office, reported no ill effects from gradual reduction in phenobarbital. With the therapist, the couple reviewed the goals of gradually eliminating the phenobarbital and reducing if not eliminating lorazepam. Further review of symptoms revealed sleep disturbance, irritability, and Mr. R's "feeling like something's going to happen" when he skips a dose. Mr. R and his wife were cautioned that some discomfort would have to be tolerated. The exercise regimen was also discussed.

Third Session

Mr. R reported complaints from phenobarbital reduction but he took more butalbital than usual during the previous week. However, he is walking regularly. The therapist planned to stop phenobarbital, cut lorazepam to 2 mg t.i.d., 1 mg at hour of sleep (h.s.).

Fourth Session

The therapist received a telephone call from Mr. R, who "ran out of pocket change and had no way of keeping his appointment." He has been taking three butalbital a day of which the practitioner was not aware and has continued with half a tablet of phenobarbital despite being asked to reduce it to h.s. only. Mr. R complained of the tremors and has taken on a project he fears he may not be able to complete. The practitioner advised him to bring a calendar to the next visit so that they might track his pills more exactly.

Fifth Session

During this session Mr. R was complaining of difficulty with tremor. He forgot to bring in his pills and a calendar, but the practitioner complimented him on his success with phenobarbital reduction to h.s. only and holding the butalbital to one pill daily. The use of propranolol to reduce tremor was also introduced.

Sixth Session

Mr. R brought in his calendar which demonstrated one to two butalbital per day, four lorazepam tabs, but no phenobarbital. However, he worries that the tremor will ruin his silverwork. He also wonders whether the butalbital is merely a substitute for the phenobarbital. The therapist and patient agreed on the following: He will minimize if not eliminate the butalbital in preparation for reducing lorazepam. He will also try 20 mg propranolol each morning before beginning silver smithing. He also brought in his sculpture of Will Rogers from 1983, which was quite good.

Seventh Session

Mr. R has been keeping his calendar nicely. He was able to eliminate butalbital and is using 20 mg propranolol to good effect. He will cut lorazepam to 3 mg in the morning and 4 mg h.s. He and the therapist made another appointment in 3 weeks and planned to try another cut.

Eighth Session

Mr. R was in good spirits, has been to the indoor swimming pool twice, and continues to find the propranolol effective in combating his tremor. Having used 3 mg in the morning and 4 mg h.s. of lorazepam for a month he is eager to reduce to 2 mg and 4 mg.

Ninth Session

Mr. R presented more silverwork at this session and a lively discussion of Mr. R's museum pieces ensued. He has tolerated last month's lorazepam reduction and is willing to reduce further to 1 mg once a day in the morning and 4 mg h.s. He feels further reductions may be difficult and the therapist renewed his intent not to rush the process.

Tenth Session

Mr. R enjoyed the summer's increased physical activity, finished his most recent commission, and is planning another. He has done well with the 1 mg once a day in the morning and 4 mg h.s. He seems eager to reduce.

Eleventh Session

Mr. R preferred to continue at 4 mg of lorazepam at night to ensure good sleep. The therapist will see him in 1 month and suggest that a reduction would be benign as well as reminding him that elimination is not the therapist's goal.

36 Months Later

Mr. R. preferred to continue with 4 mg lorazepam each night. He has never escalated the dose or augmented it with other psychoactive agents. He weathered the death of his brother without excess grief. He continues his silversmithing and swimming.

SUMMARY

Substance abuse is a prevalent public health problem which often goes undetected in older adults. The practitioner's willingness to educate the patient without being punitive coupled with a realistic optimism regarding treatment offers the best hope of reducing the personal and social costs of substance abuse. Generalists working with older substance abusers should acquire knowledge of (1) simple screening techniques, (2) signs and symptoms of late-life drug and alcohol problems, (3) pharmacological, behavioral, and psychosocial interventions including peer support programs and residential treatment, and (4) empathic care of persons not yet ready for substance abuse treament.

BOOKS FOR PATIENTS AND FAMILIES

Falvo, D. (1994). *Effective Patient Education: A Guide to Increased Compliance* (2nd ed.). Gaithersburg, MD: Aspen.

Hazelden Foundation. (1991). *How to Talk to an Older Person Who Has a Problem with Alcohol or Medications.* Center City, MN: Author.

Miller, W. R., Munoz, R. F. (1976). *How to Control Your Drinking.* Englewood Cliffs, NJ: Prentice-Hall.

Myers, J. E. (1989). *Adult Children and Aging Parents.* Alexandria, VA: American Counseling Association.

Wolfe, S. M., Fugate, L., Hulstrand, E. P., et al. (1988). *Worst Pills, Best Pills: The Older Adult's Guide to Avoiding Drug-Induced Death or Illness.* Washington, DC: Public Citizen Health Research Group.

REFERENCES

Adams, W. L., Barry, K. L., Fleming, M. F. (1996). Screening for problem drinking in older primary care patients. *Journal of the American Medical Association, 276*(24), 1964–1967.

Alterman, A. I., Kushner, H., Holahan, J. M. (1990). Cognitive functioning and treatment outcome in alcoholics. *Journal of Nervous and Mental Disease, 178*(8), 494–499.

American Psychiatric Association. (1994). *Diagnostic and statistical manual of mental disorders* (4th ed.). Washington, DC: Author.

American Society of Addiction Medicine. (1996). *Patient placement criteria for the treatment of substance-related disorders* (2nd ed.). Washington, DC: Author.

Babor, T. F., de la Fuente, J. R., Saunders, J., et al. (1992). *AUDIT: The Alcohol Use Disorders Identification Test: Guidelines for use in primary health care.* Geneva, Switzerland: World Health Organization.

Barnas, C., Rossmann, M., Roessler, H., et al. (1992). Benzodiazepine and other psychotropic drug abuse by patients in a methadone maintenance program: Familiarity and preference. *Journal of Clinical Psychopharmacology*, 12(6), 397–402.

Beresford, T. P., Lucey, M. R. (1995). Ethanol metabolism and intoxication in the elderly. In T. P. Beresford & E. S. Gomberg (Eds.), *Alcohol and aging* (pp. 117–127). New York: Oxford University Press.

Bien, T. H., Miller, W. R., Tonigan, J. S. (1993). Brief interventions for alcohol problems: A review. *Addiction, 88*, 315–335.

Blow, F. C., Brower, K. J., Schulenberg, J. E., et al. (1992a). The Michigan Alcoholism Screening Test—Geriatric Version (MAST-G): A new elderly-specific screening instrument. *Alcoholism: Clinical and Experimental Research, 16*, 372.

Blow, F. C., Cook, C. A., Booth, B. M., et al. (1992b). Age-related psychiatric comorbidities and level of functioning in alcoholic veterans seeking outpatient treatment. *Hospital and Community Psychiatry, 43*, 990–995.

Bucholz, K. K., Sheline, Y., Helzer, J. E. (1995). The epidemiology of alcohol use, problems, and dependence in elders: A review. In T. P. Beresford & E. Gomberg (Eds.), *Alcohol and aging* (pp. 19–41). New York: Oxford University Press.

Buchsbaum, D. G., Buchanan, R. G., Welsh, J., et al. (1992). Screening for drinking disorders in the elderly using the CAGE questionnaire. *Journal of the American Geriatrics Society, 40*, 662–665.

Carlen, P. L., McAndrews, M. P., Weiss, R. T., et al. (1994). Alcohol-related dementia in the institutionalized elderly. *Alcoholism: Clinical and Experimental Research, 18*, 1330–1334.

Carstensen, L. L., Rychtarik, R. G., Prue, D. M. (1985). Behavioral treatment of the geriatric alcohol abuser: A long-term follow-up study. *Addictive Behaviors, 10*(3), 307–311.

Center for Substance Abuse Treatment. (1995). *Detoxification from alcohol and other drugs* (DHHS Publication No. SMA 95–3046). Washington, DC: U.S. Government Printing Office.

Chan, A. W. K., Pristach, E., Welte, J. W., et al. (1993). Use of the TWEAK Test in screening for alcoholism/heavy drinking in three populations. *Alcoholism: Clinical and Experimental Research, 17*, 1188–1192.

Dobson, K. S. (Ed.). (1988). *Handbook of cognitive-behavioral therapies*. New York: Guilford Press.

Dunlop, J. (1990). Peer groups support seniors fighting alcohol and drugs. *Aging, 361*, 28–32.

Dunlop, J., Skorney, B., Hamilton, J. (1982). Group treatment for elderly alcoholics and their families. *Social Work in Groups, 5*, 87–92.

Egan, G. (1994). *The skilled helper: A problem-management approach to helping* (5th ed.) Pacific Grove, CA: Brooks/Cole.

Ewing, J. A. (1984). Detecting alcoholism: The CAGE Questionnaire. *Journal of the American Medical Association, 252*, 1905–1907.

Finlayson, R. E. (1995a). Comorbidity in elderly alcoholics. In T. P. Beresford & E. Gomberg (Eds.), *Alcohol and aging* (pp. 56–69). New York: Oxford University Press.

Finlayson, R. E. (1995b). Misuse of prescription drugs. *International Journal of the Addictions, 30,* 1871–1901.

Fleming, M. F., Barry, K. L., Manwell, L. B., et al. (1997). Brief physician advice for problem alcohol drinkers: A randomized controlled trial in community based primary care practices. *Journal of the American Medical Association, 277,* 1039–1045.

Forster, L. E., Pollow, R., Stoller, E. P. (1993). Alcohol use and potential risk for alcohol related adverse drug reactions among community-based elderly. *Journal of Community Health, 18,* 225–239.

Foy, A., O'Connell, D., Henry, D., et al. (1995). Benzodiazepine use as a cause of cognitive impairment in elderly hospital inpatients. *Journal of Gerontology: Biological Sciences and Medical Sciences, 50*(2), 99–106.

Gambert, S. R., Katsoyannis, K. K. (1995). Alcohol-related medical disorders of older heavy drinkers. In T. P. Beresford & E. Gomberg (Eds.), *Alcohol and aging* (pp. 70–81). New York: Oxford University Press.

Gordon, T., Kannel, W. B. (1983). Drinking and its relation to smoking, blood pressure, blood lipids, and uric acid: The Framingham Study. *Archives of Internal Medicine, 143,* 1366–1374.

Harris, K. B., Miller, W. R. (1990). Behavioural self-control training for problem drinkers: Components of efficacy. *Psychology of Addictive Behaviour, 4*(2), 90–92.

Helzer, J. E., Bucholz, K., Robins, L. N. (1991). Five communities in the United States: Results of the Epidemiologic Catchment Area Survey. In J. E. Helzer & G. J. Canino (Eds.), *Alcoholism in North America, Europe, and Asia* (pp. 71–95). New York: Oxford University Press.

Hurt, R. D., Eberman, K. A., Slade, J., et al. (1993). Treating nicotine addiction in patients with other addictive disorders. In C. T. Orleans & J. Slade (Eds.), *Nicotine addiction: Principles and management* (pp. 310–326). New York: Oxford University Press.

Katz, I. R., Sands, L. P., Bilker, W., et al. (1998). Identification of medications that cause cognitive impairment in older people: The case of oxybutynin chloride. *Journal of the American Geriatrics Society, 46,* 8–13.

Kofoed, L. L., Tolson, R. L., Atkinson, R. M., et al. (1987). Treatment compliance of older alcoholics: An elder-specific approach is superior to "mainstreaming." *Journal of Studies on Alcohol, 48,* 47–51.

Korrapati, M. R., Vestal, R. E. (1995). Alcohol and medications in the elderly: Complex interactions. In T. P. Beresford & E. Gomberg (Eds.), *Alcohol and aging* (pp. 42–69). New York: Oxford University Press.

Kranzler, H. R., Babor, T. F., Lauerman, R. J. (1990). Problems associated with average alcohol consumption and frequency of intoxication in a medical population. *Alcoholism: Clinical and Experimental Research, 14,* 119–126.

Liberto, J. G., Oslin, D. W. (1995). Early versus late onset of alcoholism in the elderly. *International Journal of the Addictions, 30,* 1799–1818.

Litten, R. Z., Allen, J., Fertig, J. (1996). Pharmacotherapies for alcohol problems: A review of research with focus on developments since 1991. *Alcoholism: Clinical and Experimental Research, 20,* 859–876.

McInnes, E., Powell, J. (1994). Drug and alcohol referrals: Are elderly substance abuse diagnoses and referrals being missed? *British Journal of Medicine, 308,* 444–446.

Meichenbaum, D., Turk, D. (1987). *Facilitating treatment adherence: A practitioner's guidebook.* New York: Plenum Press.

Miller, W. R., Rollnick, S. (1991). *Motivational interviewing.* New York: Guilford Press.

National Institute on Alcohol Abuse and Alcoholism. (1995). *The physicians' guide to helping patients with alcohol problems* (NIH Publication No. 95–3769). Rockville, MD: Author.

Pomara, N., Stanley, B., Block R., et al. (1985). Increased sensitivity of the elderly to the central depressant effects of diazepam. *Journal of Clinical Psychiatry, 46,* 185–187.

Prochaska, J. O., DiClemente, C. C., Norcross, J. C. (1992). In search of how people change: Applications to addictive behaviors. *American Psychologist, 47*(9), 1102–1114.

Saunders, J. B., Aasland, O. G., Babor, T. F., et al. (1993). WHO collaborative project on early detection of persons with harmful alcohol consumption: II. Development of the screening instrument "AUDIT." *Addiction, 88,* 791–804.

Schmidt, A., Barry, K., Fleming, M. (1995). A new screening test for the detection of problem drinkers: The Alcohol Use Disorders Identification Test (AUDIT). *Southern Medical Journal, 88,* 52–59.

Sheahan, S. L., Hendricks, J., Coons, S. J. (1989). Drug misuse among the elderly: A covert problem. *Health Values, 13*(3), 22–29.

Speer, D. C., Bates, K. (1992). Comorbid mental and substance disorders among older psychiatric patients. *Journal of the American Geriatrics Society, 40,* 886–890.

Substance Abuse Among Older Adults Consensus Panel for the Treatment Improvement Protocol Series (TIPS) 26. (1998). Frederic C. Blow, PhD, Consensus Panel Chair, U.S. Department of Health and Human Services, Public Health Service, Substance Abuse and Mental Health Services Administration, Center for Substance Abuse Treatment, Rockwall II, 5600 Fishers Lane, Rockville, MD 20857 (DHHS Publication No. SMA 98–3179).

Tarter, R. E. (1995). Cognition, aging, and alcohol. In T. P. Beresford & E. Gomberg (Eds.), *Alcohol and aging* (pp. 82–97). New York: Oxford University Press.

Vaillant, G. E., Clark, W., Cyrus, C., et al. (1983). Prospective study of alcoholism treatment: Eight-year follow-up. *American Journal of Medicine, 75,* 455–460.

12

Recognition and Reduction of Suicide Risk

The highest rates of suicide are found in the elderly, ranging from less than 3/100,000 among African American women to more than 60/100,000 among white males entering their ninth decade (Vital Statistics, 1996). At present rates, which have remained stable for more than 10 years, the number of deaths due to suicide among older persons will double over the next 40 years. Both social (Durkheim, 1891/1951) and psychopathological (Conwell et al., 1990b, 2000) factors contribute to suicidal vulnerability. Precisely how biomedical and sociodemographic factors interact to increase the risk of late-life suicide is unclear. Addressing the sociodemographic risk factors requires a broad-based public health campaign beyond the individual's practitioner's capacity. Nonetheless, the informed practitioner's awareness of risk factors, countervailing forces, and interventions offers the opportunity to reduce the morbidity and mortality of late-life suicidality.

Sociologists and journalists assert that the increase in late-life suicides reflects elder fears of dependency, nursing homes, and unwanted invasive care (Angell, 1990; Tolchin, 1989). In contrast, clinical scientists argue that depression and serotonergic disturbances are the driving force behind late-life suicide (Mann & Stoff, 1997). Chronic illness, alcoholism (Murphy et al., 1992), and the availability of firearms (Kaplan et al., 1998; Marzuk et al., 1992) have also been cited, as well as a greater social acceptance of suicide among the elderly (Grabbe et al., 1997). However, this apparent antagonism between biomedical and sociological causes indicates much about desirable interventions. An appreciation of the biomedical and sociodemographic suicide risk profile will allow mental health and primary care practitioners to focus on the individual's vulnerability. Table 12.1 displays the commonly ac-

TABLE 12.1. Risk Profile for Late-Life Suicide

Clinical

Expressed intent
Depression or other nondementing mental disorder
Alcohol use, moderate to heavy
Cancer, heart disease, lung disease
Chronic pain
Poor self-assessed health
Smoking

Sociodemographic

White male
Age 85 years or older
Firearms purchase, possession
Divorced, widowed
Recent life change event

Historical

Previous attempt
Lethality of attempt (firearms, jumping from height)
Family history of attempted or completed suicide
Low probability of rescue
Recent visit to primary care physician or mental health specialist
Anniversary of loss

cepted risk profile of suicidality among older Americans, including the social and psychopathological components.

TRENDS IN THE PREVALENCE
OF LATE-LIFE SUICIDE

By 1987 the rate of 21.6 suicides per 100,000 older adults exceeded that at the 1965 inception of Medicare, reversing the downward trend in elderly suicide that began in 1933 (Kennedy et al., 1996). The rate of late-life suicides increased despite advances in the economic and health status of older adults. Suicide is the tenth leading cause of death among older adults and the third most common cause of death from injury following falls and automobile accidents (Grabbe et al., 1997). Close to 7,000 seniors kill themselves each year, accounting for one-third of all suicides (Dyer, 1992). Present rates, based on death certificates and family reports, are an underestimate (Miller, 1978). Survivors' guilt over missing the warning signs biases reports toward calling them accidents rather than suicides. For every completed late-life suicide, there are at least four attempts. The number of physically ill isolated older adults who suicide through self-neglect is unknown (Osgood, 1992). Public opinion polls suggest that as many as 600,000 adults ages 60 or older have considered suicide over a 6-month period (Gallup, 1992a). If the percentage of older suicides increases no further, the number of late-life suicides will double over the next 40 years (Whanger, 1989).

International Prevalence Data

In 1996 the World Health Organization called upon member nations to address the growing problem of suicide. Kennedy and Tannenbaum's (in press) summary of the international data highlights the social character of suicide. First, men commit suicide at all ages, at rates from two to four times that of women, culminating in twelve to one by age 85. Second, rates for both men and women increase with age, rising precipitously at 75 years. Third, variations by nation and geography are as substantial as those observed by age and gender. Suicide in Spanish-speaking and Catholic nations are slightly lower, with the exception of Cuba and France. Nations from the former commonwealth (England and Wales, Scotland, Northern Ireland, Canada) are among the lowest. The highest rates appear in the geographically contiguous states of Austria, Hungary, and Bulgaria, exceeding the elevated prevalence of the Russian Federation. Because the patterns are so consistent across the nations they are unlikely to be artifacts of different reporting methods.

GENDER, RACE, AND SOCIAL FACTORS

Male gender is a risk factor regardless of age. Above age 65, 80% of suicides are male (U.S. Public Health Service, 1999). The preponderance of white males among elderly suicides has been the case since the turn of the century (McIntosh, 1985), but suicide rates in African American men have also increased since 1968. Explanations for the high rates of elderly suicide particularly in older white males include divorce and loss of status related to retirement (McIntosh & Santos, 1981). The rate for divorced men is 3.2 times that for married men and 18.9 that for married women (Meehan et al., 1991).

The contributions of retirement and social disengagement to suicidal risk are difficult to assess (Atchley, 1980). The conditions surrounding retirement rather than the event itself often determine the psychological impact of giving up work. Differences in life retirement satisfaction are based on whether leaving the workplace was mandatory or voluntary, the occupational level of the position surrendered, opportunities for future employment, volunteer work or leisure pursuits, and financial status. Disengaged (Cummings & Henry, 1961) older adults may have given up social roles and responsibilities for a more self-centered, satisfying life. On the other hand, social isolation is an accepted risk factor for suicide. Living alone and loneliness may be the most highly correlated social variable in late-life suicide (Barraclough et al., 1974; Batchelor & Napier, 1953). However, among older adults who live alone, few consider themselves isolated and fewer still attempt suicide.

HISTORICAL AND GENERATIONAL EFFECTS

Woodbury et al. (1988) suggested that the suicide rate among elderly white males would stabilize, not increasing until the cohorts born after 1947 reach 65. They find little evidence to suggest that physical disability and mental disorders, which are higher among older women than among men, explain the stable rate of suicides among women. The low rates for women and the high rates for men over the 20-year period beginning in 1962 were more consistent with social rather than psychobiological etiology. However, it remains to be seen whether older adult cohorts passing into their seventh to ninth decades in the new millennium will experience the same flattening of the suicide rate curve observed in previous cohorts.

McCall (1991) also suggests that relative societal affluence has been associated with suicide trends among elderly white males in previous decades. The increased prevalence of depression and suicide attempts among younger persons threatens a substantial increase in late life suicide into the 21st century as post-baby boomers age. The present cohort of younger adults shows a higher rate of suicide than that among their grandparents at the younger ages (Haas & Hendin, 1983). Thus the psychopathology of younger adults and the coming socioeconomic–demographic shifts in the next century suggest that historical and generational effects will make late-life suicide a more pressing public health problem.

METHODS OF DEATH

It is the greater lethality of methods and the lesser likelihood of rescue which distinguishes suicide attempts between the young and old. Firearms are the most common method of suicide among older men and women and more common than among persons less than 65. Sixty-five percent of suicides among older persons are firearm related (Osgood, 1992). A firearm in the home increases the risk of suicide more than fourfold (Kellerman et al., 1992). The usual household methods of suicide, death by hanging, suffocation, knifing, and poisoning with nonprescription medications vary by locale. Varying rates for falling from heights and carbon monoxide poisoning reflect differences in high-rise housing and automobile ownership (Marzuk et al., 1992). Among nursing home residents, self-starvation may be suicidal, although most self-starving persons typically deny that their behavior is suicidal ("just helping God along") (Osgood, 1992). Advanced age offers less likelihood of survival after an attempted suicide. Thus the cathartic effect of a suicide attempt sometimes observed among younger adults who mobilize themselves and their family for genuine change is unlikely in the older person (van Praag & Plutchik, 1985).

Efforts to reduce the lethality of suicide attempts yield modest benefits. Suicide rates from firearms have fallen since the institution of handgun control measures in New York (Marzuk et al., 1992). The detoxification (reduction of carbon monoxide) of coal gas was followed by a reduction in suicides in England and the Netherlands. However, there appeared to be a compensatory rise in medication overdoses suggesting a substitution of methods in response to a change in the availability of lethal means. Rates of self-poisoning remained stable despite a significant decline in the use of barbiturates during the period of study. The decrease in barbiturates was made up for with the use of nonopiate analgesics and other prescription drugs (Lindsey, 1986). Reducing the accessibility of suicidal methods may reduce suicidal attempts among ambivalent, impulsive ambivalent persons but not among those determined to kill themselves. However, risk factors such as access to firearms and unnecessarily dangerous prescription drugs are alterable. Reduced availability of more lethal methods might result in substitution of less deadly methods, with the net effect on mortality beneficial nonetheless (Brown, 1979).

PHYSICAL ILLNESS

Among individuals 60 years of age and older as many as 70% may have had a physical illness directly contributing to the completion of suicide (Mackenzie & Popkin, 1987). Diseases of the heart, lung, and central nervous system are frequently cited (Horton-Deustch et al., 1992). Clark (1992) found that 20% of older persons committing suicide had visited their physician within 1 day of death. Their physicians recalled patient presentations of vague physical complaints and denial of mental symptoms when specifically questioned. In contrast, their families reported depression, problems with alcohol, and prescription medications. Some late-life suicides result from a perception of terminal illness that cannot be verified by medical examination (Conwell et al., 1990a; Murphy, 1977). However, it is unclear that these distorted perceptions are delusions or simply an expression of hopelessness which has often been linked to suicidality (Beck et al., 1985; Green, 1981; Uncapher et al., 1998).

EXCESSES OF MODERN MEDICINE

Some (Angell, 1990) argue that medical advances have extended life beyond meaning, that older suicides "fear living more than dying because they dread becoming prisoners of technology" (Tolchin, 1989). There is also a significant relationship between suicide and anticipation of nursing home admission (Loebel et al., 1991). The "Kervorkian cure" of physician assisted suicide is perhaps the most troubling example of anticipatory suicide ("Kervorkian cure," 1990). Quill's (1991) report of assisted suicide, "Death with Dignity," describes a lengthy, deeply informed patient–physician relationship and as such represents the opposite end of the spectrum from Kervorkian's cases where neither the patient's suffering nor the physician's knowledge of his patient's condition seems compelling.

Miller (1978) identified the threshold of suicide as a "level of unbearability" reflecting the accumulation of life experiences, resources and coping mechanisms. However, the distinction between a rational preference for death over unbearable disability and a suicidal impulse due to mental illness in late life is not easily determined. "Subintentioned death" (Shneidman, 1963), "hidden suicide" (Merloo, 1968), and "indirect self-destructive behavior" (Nelson & Farberow, 1982) are used to describe masked or passive suicide, but the range of behaviors considered indirectly threatening is difficult to specify for practical purposes (Linehan, 1997). Conwell et al.'s (1990a) report on six of eight elderly suicides who had delusional concerns over cancer further questions the validity of "rational suicide." There is little evidence that physically ill older adults suicide in the absence of a depressive or other mental disorder (Shaffer, 1993).

ATTITUDES OF OLDER ADULTS
REGARDING SUICIDE

Although depression and physical illness are common antecedents of late-life suicide, the elderly more often cite loneliness as the major reason to consider suicide. They also cite financial problems, poor health, depression, alcohol problems, "not taking prescription drugs properly," feelings of worthlessness, and isolation. When asked where a suicidal friend could go for help, only 13% identify physicians or clergy. Close to 25% could not identify any source of help. Of those who admitted having attempted suicide, only 13% had sought any form of help prior to the attempt. More than three-quarters had not talked to anyone about their intentions beforehand. When asked about attitudes toward late-life suicide, 42% agreed that physicians should assist in suicide when there is incurable illness or intractable suffering. More than one-third agreed that late-life suicide should be viewed differently from teenage suicide. More than a quarter of the sample agreed that late-life suicide was a personal decision in which others should not be involved (Gallup Organization, 1992b). In summary, older adults do not see suicidal ideas as a health care problem, which makes recognition of suicidal patients all the more difficult.

THE NEUROBIOLOGY OF SUICIDALITY

The decrease in brain serotonergic function thought to result from an age-related increase in monoamine oxidase activity has been implicated in suicide. Serotonergic dysfunction is also associated with depressive disorders, panic disorder, and suicidal behavior in younger adults. If serotonin acts as a "break" against suicidal impulses, alcohol is surely the "accelerator" (Holden, 1992). This suggests an age-related risk of suicide which may be dissociated from conventional categories of mental disorders (Mann & Stoff,1997). The Hemenway et al. (1993) study showing a marked relationship between smoking and suicide demonstrated an increased relative risk for women ages 60 and above. The authors suggest that smoking, as a self-medicating behavior to counter depression, is an indirect risk factor for suicide.

MENTAL DISORDERS AND SUICIDE

Studies of psychiatric patients indicate that a depressive episode is present in from two-thirds (Gurland & Cross, 1983) to nine-tenths (Conwell et al., 1990b) of older adults who commit suicide. Severity of depressive symptoms rather than the presence of psychosis correlates with completed suicide (Clayton, 1985). However, information from community samples suggests that depressive disorders may play a less prominent role in late-life suicide. Wiessman et al. (1989) reported the frequency of suicidal thoughts and a history of suicide attempts among participants of the Epidemiologic Catchment Area studies (Weissman et al., 1989). Surprisingly, no relationship between depressive disorder and suicide attempts or suicidal thoughts was observed. Panic attacks and panic disorders but not advanced age were related to suicidal ideas and attempts. Although not all older adults who express suicidal ideas attempt suicide, it is thought that most elderly suicides have verbalized the thought (Osgood, 1992). Based on mortality statistics and survey data, at least 5% of older persons have thought of suicide in the last year but only 1% of that number will have died of suicide. Thus some measure of suicidal thinking, like that found in such instruments as the Zung Self-Rating Depression Scale (1985) or the Hamilton Depression Rating Scale (1960), is worth incorporating when the risk profile or clinical suspicions run high.

PERSONALITY AND NEUROPSYCHOLOGY

The personality profile of older suicide attempters remains elusive (Weissman, 1974). Studies of younger adults find hostility and impulsiveness. Older suicide attempters are more often described as hypochondriacal, with restricted social interests. Pathological jealousy and suspiciousness are observed in some instances but overall individuals seem psychologically frail and constricted (Batchelor & Napier, 1953). Neuroticism may also be characteristic of suicidal persons (Costa, 1991). Chronic suicidal ideas may be expressed by persons with dramatic, impulsive personality disorders and persons with posttraumatic syndromes (Jamison & Baldessarini, 1999). Neuropsychological investigations of suicide attempters describe a constriction in executive cognitive function (i.e., planning and problem solving) leaving suicide more likely given the lack of perceived alternatives (Weishaar & Beck, 1990). Similarly, being closed to novelty or new experience has also been associated with suicide attempts in late life (Duberstein et al., 1999).

THE CLINICAL ASSESSMENT OF SUICIDAL
THOUGHT AND BEHAVIOR

Model intervention programs are few but offer examples of service linkage across communities for effective intervention (National Institute of Mental Health, 1997). However, for the individual practitioner, intervention begins with the suspicion of suicidal ideas and follows with an individual risk assessment detailed in Table 12.2. Risk assessment is of no value if the clinician is unwilling to ask about suicidal thought. Few patients ever volunteer their thoughts of suicide unless asked to do so. Assessment of risk entails an awareness of characteristics that elevate vulnerability as well as those countervailing factors that make the impulse to suicide less likely (Plutchik et al., 1996) as shown in Table 12.3. The imminence of risk will dictate the clinician's response. Obviously, those at the highest risk are persons who have expressed suicidal intent with a plan to do so (Hirschfeld & Russell, 1997). Suicidal intent is different from the wish for death expressed by the very old and terminally ill who are not depressed and when asked deny any thought of self-harm.

When the patient answers yes to "Have you had thoughts of suicide recently?" the follow-up question should be, "Have you thought about how you would do it?" or "Do you plan to harm yourself or think you can't resist the impulse to do so?" The details of the plan are important. Are the means lethal; is there no chance for rescue? Is there a firearm in the home? Affirmative responses to these questions indicate imminent risk. Alcoholic intake, psychosis, delirium, and delu-

TABLE 12.2. Practitioner-Based Interventions to Reduce the Risk of Late-Life Suicide

When few risk factors are present
    Annual screening for depression
    Advanced directives (Patient Self-Determination Act)
    Encourage abstinence or moderation in alcohol intake
    Encourage active social network

When several risk factors are present but suicidal ideas are denied
    All the above and . . .
    Optimize treatment of depression, anxiety, insomnia, pain, alcohol abuse

When risk factors and thoughts of suicide are present but without intent or a plan
    All of the above and . . .
    Make family aware of elevated risk and ensure physician availability
    Family or third party to remove lethal means and alcohol
    Identify countervailing forces (concern for family, religion, life event goals)
    Fix an appointment (not as needed), ask that family attend

When lethal means are at hand, a plan is expressed, or intent is evident
    Refer for emergency psychiatric evaluation (involuntary if needed)
    Consider hospitalization, electroconvulsive therapy

When suicide has been attempted with lethal means, or countervailing forces are not available to prevent recurrent attempts
    Emergency psychiatric evaluation (involuntary if need be)
    Hospitalize if intent not convincingly recanted or attempt is a recurrence

TABLE 12.3. Countervailing Forces That Might Lessen the Older Adult's Likelihood of Acting on a Suicidal Impulse

Supportive, involved family
Presence of spouse
Social network
Financial security
Physically independent
Alcohol abstinence
Dementia (inability to sequence steps toward death)
Positively anticipated life events in family members (e.g., graduation, bar or bat mitzvah, confirmation, marriage, childbirth)
Religious beliefs and values (optimistic rather than fatalistic)
Advanced directives, health care proxy
Practitioner's optimism and concern, regular appointments for ongoing care
Treatment of depression, anxiety, insomnia, pain

Note. Data from Plutchik et al. (1996).

sions of guilt or desperation ("It's the only way out") make the impulse more difficult to resist and further suggest the need for immediate protective action. Persons who acknowledge suicidal ideas but deny intent should also be asked about prior attempts, again with emphasis on lethality and family history of suicidal behavior. Such persons may exhibit long-term risk of suicide but do not require immediate action. Although suicidal ideas may arise in numerous contexts, suicidal intent is a result of depression until proven otherwise. Older adults do not suicide on impulse or as imitation but as a calculated maneuver. Fears that the practitioner will precipitate suicidal ideas or acts are unfounded (Zimmerman et al., 1995).

MANAGEMENT OF ACUTE SUICIDAL RISK

If the risk is imminent, an emergency psychiatric examination and continuous supervision are necessary. Staff should remain with the patient until transportation can be arranged by ambulance to the emergency room. Police should be called if the patient refuses (Hirschfeld & Russell, 1997). When death is imminent, concern for confidentiality is inappropriate. Family who refuse to allow the evaluation of an immanently suicidal relative may need to be confronted by police as well and reminded that the gravity of the situation requires immediate action, at the least the opinion of a psychiatrist.

When the risk of suicide is less acute, the options are less extreme. First, staff should seek permission from the patient to put an informed social safety net in place. This may include family, senior center staff, close friends, or clergy. Here the approach is open collaboration in which patient and clinician are not asking that others take on the burden of preventing suicide but rather that they be aware that the risk is being managed aggressively. Enlisting the increased support of others is accompanied by added attention of the clinician through a scheduled phone call and office appointment. Getting the patient to agree to such steps is evidence of a willingness to resist the suicidal impulse.

Practitioners should ensure that lethal means (fire arms, medications with narrow safety range) and alcohol are removed by family or friends from the patient's area. This is again done with the patient's consent with the express purpose of restoring a sense of control over the suicidal impulses. It is also important to ask what has kept the person from suicide—concern for family, religious, or philosophical beliefs? Do they endure for some future event, a graduation, confirmation, bar or bat mitzvah of a young family member? Each of these countervailing forces can be reinforced. Finally, if depression, anxiety disorder, or alcohol abuse is present it should be treated aggressively with close follow-up. Patients who refuse the steps listed previously are obviously cause for concern and may require hospitalization if the level of risk cannot be reduced. Alternatively, a second opinion or psychiatric evaluation is indicated. Chapter 2 provides greater detail on the treatment of anxiety and depression; Chapter 11 discusses alcohol and substance abuse.

Electroconvulsive therapy (ECT) is the most rapidly effective treament for suicidal intent associated with severe or delusional depression. Persons who have made a near lethal attempt (gunshot wound, hanging, jumping) and continue to express suicidal intention and those who remain at high risk despite medication are better treated immediately with ECT. Depending on the locale and patient's physical status, ECT may be available on an outpatient basis. More often ECT requires hospitalization, and most patients and families will prefer a trial of medication before accepting ECT.

Psychotropic medications with proarrhythmic or hypotensive effects should be avoided because of lethal risk in overdose. Sertraline, paroxetine, nefazodone, venlafaxine, mirtazapine and citalopram are preferred over, nortriptyline, desipramine, trazodone, phenelzine, and Wellbutrin (seizure threshold). Patient and family need to be counseled that depression, apathy, and despair do not remit with the initial administration of any of these agents. However, agitation and sleep disturbance may respond more rapidly to paroxetine, nefazodone, or mirtazapine which have sedative properties at the proper dose. Some persons, particularly those begun on a nonsedating antidepressant,

will benefit from the addition of a benzodiazepine (lorazepam) to reduce anxiety and insomnia. However, medication is no substitute for
close follow-up. Phone checks in addition to the scheduled appointment will help to manage side effects, sustain hope, and increase compliance. The clinician's interest will also give the patient something to
live for and sustain the family during the crisis. Equally important, apathy may remit before despair allowing the suicidal impulse to overwhelm the person in the early days of treament despite apparent improvement. Close attention should continue until improved mood is
sustained (Hircshfeld & Russell, 1997).

MANAGEMENT OF CHRONIC SUICIDAL RISK

The management of chronic suicidality focuses on the reduction of risk
factors, augmentation of countervailing forces, and psychotherapy.
The risk factors include suicidal ideation, social isolation, and untreated illness, most notably hypothyroidism, congestive heart failure,
lung disease, agoraphobia, depression, alcohol, or sedative abuse. The
literature on behavioral and psychosocial interventions for suicidal
persons randomized to routine or specialized care is not extensive but
suggests that persons benefiting the most are those at higher risk (van
der Sande et al., 1997; Linehan, 1997, Weishaar & Beck, 1990). Here the
emphasis should be placed on the benefits of routine care rather than
on the lack of superior outcomes with specialized efforts. Richman
suggests two forms of psychotherapy for older adults with suicidal
tendencies. Family therapy allows the tensions and anxieties that contributed to suicidal thoughts or behaviors to be examined without
fears of destroying the family's integrity. The goal is to advance the
function of the individual as well as the protective influence of the
family. Richman (1996) is convinced that covert messages encouraging
the death of the older member are frequent. Group therapy with depressed, suicidal older adults focuses on reducing alienation, loneliness, and the sense of abandonment that accompanies the losses of late
life. A homogeneous rather than mixed group is preferred.

WHEN PREVENTION FAILS

With late-life suicide, risk reduction may be more realistic than risk
elimination. Some persons are determined to take their lives and will
not abandon or divulge their intentions despite family and the practitioner's best efforts. When suicide occurs it frequently provokes

rage and despair in family and caregivers alike. A postmortem meeting to support the family's bereavement and lessen self-blame is helpful. Inevitably, questions will arise about what could have been done to prevent the act. Yet it is important that the clinician avoid assigning or accepting responsibility for the death. Some will feel that suicide was the best choice or was understandable but others will not. The goal of the postsuicide meeting is expression and exploration rather than consensus. Differences of opinion are encouraged. The clinician should accept these reactions as part of the process of grieving. (Chapter 7 provides a fuller discussion of treament of the bereaved.) Rosenberg et al. (1989) discuss the portrayal of adolescent suicide in the media. They emphasize the importance of not dramatizing the suicide so as not to foster imitation. Labeling suicidal thought as normative may increase rather than decrease the prevalence of suicidal ideas. Rather, the distress which leads to suicide should be acknowledged and portrayed as a missed opportunity for help. This avoids painting the deceased as a heroic victim with no escape who ultimately gains control of death.

Finally, because suicide may provoke a record review by the local health authority, it is important that documentation reflect steps taken to reduce suicidal risk and the patient's and family's responses. The options presented and duties assigned should be stated in outline form. When family or patient demand outpatient treatment over the practitioner's preference for hospitalization, the interchange should be noted as well as responses to recommendations such as removal of firearms and alcohol, not leaving the patient alone, institution of antidepressant medication, and willingness to accept follow-up phone calls and appointments. Criteria for treatment failure should be explicit so that a rejected hospitalization recommendation may be revisited. Telephone contacts should be noted with intention to follow through on preventive measures. Was the patient or family able to carry out the recommended steps? If preventive steps or supportive supervision have not been carried out, the recommendation for hospitalization should be restated.

PUBLIC POLICY AND PREVENTION

The benefits of programs to reduce late-life suicide are few and their impact has been questioned (Mercer, 1989). Educational offerings for the professions and public at large, case finding, and legislative action are minimal. Model programs recognize the interrelations of the social, medical, and mental health determinants of late-life suicide. Aggressive case finding, integration of programs across social agencies and health care entities, education and training of practitioners, and appropriate interventions including peer support and follow-through are essential elements. The Seattle "gatekeepers" program is one such model effort which claims a reduction in suicides (Goldstein et al., 1993).

The development of suicide counseling centers has not been accompanied by a reduction in elderly suicide rates (Brown, 1979). No more than 4% of calls to suicide hotlines are from the elderly (Osgood, 1992). The development of profiles describing high-risk populations has also had little effect on suicide rates. The problem of suicide across the lifespan is in part responsible for the development of the National Center for Injury Prevention and Control at the Centers for Disease Control (Shaffer, 1993). Although intervention programs for late-life suicide are few, there is considerable evidence for the reduction in suicides across all age ranges through efforts that have little to do with mental health providers. These include the reduction of carbon monoxide from coal gas, the reduction in prescriptions of barbiturates, the introduction of antidepressants with less toxicity in the event of overdose, and efforts to reduce the possession of handguns. Two studies indicate a connection between the prominence of press coverage and both the overall rates and choice of lethal methods. The Austrian Association for Suicide Prevention promulgated guidelines for the press that resulted in reductions of space given to the reports and the frequency with which suicide appeared on the front page (Etzersdorfer et al., 1992). A reduction in front-page reportage was associated with both a reduction in total suicides by year and in subway suicides.

Companion pieces from the *New England Journal of Medicine* illustrate the importance of seemingly superficial semantic options. Quill et al. (1992) use the phrase "physician assisted suicide" for individuals who are hopelessly, and soon to be terminally ill, whereas Brody (1992) in contrast uses "assisted death." Labeling the assisted death of a terminally ill individual as a suicide risks influencing public opinion to be more accepting of genuine suicides of depressed or misguided individuals who are neither hopelessly nor terminally ill. Just as the schools have become the base for programs to counter teenage suicide, religious institutions seem a reasonable choice for senior citizens. Efforts to reduce late-life suicides will have an impact on the suicidal risk of future generations by preventing suicide from becoming a bitter family legacy.

The Patient Self-Determination Act (Omnibus Budget Reconciliation Act of 1990) should be a more prominent standard of clinical practice, as routine as the annual assessment. A discussion of these sensitive, difficult decisions could well reduce fears that loss of control will result in unwanted care. Reduction in the availability of lethal means (handgun control) should also be attempted. Reducing the lethality of suicidal methods may not decrease the morbidity but should reduce the mortality of suicide attempts. Even if other methods are substituted so that the attempt rate does not fall, the net effect would still be beneficial.

Concerns over health costs threaten to displace the need for changes in public policy discussion that might lead to reduced late-life suicide rates (Emanuel & Battin, 1998). Clearer terminology regarding suicide, palliative care, assisted death, and euthanasia is needed. Is the right to die in the context of intractable pain or shortness of breath the same as the right to suicide in less compelling circumstances? Can we avoid legitimizing suicide if we continue to ignore the duality of social and psychopathological causation in less than desperate situations? Ultimately, effective policy will incorporate social, psychopathological, legal, and ethical dimensions of the problem.

SUMMARY

Late-life suicide is premeditated, characterized by male gender, untreated depression, social isolation, physical illness, disability, and fewer attempts with more lethal methods and outcomes. The most recent estimates indicate that present mental health and social services which should reduce the associated morbidity and mortality are not doing so. The lack of specialized intervention programs and the scarcity of outcome studies reflect the antagonism between the social and psychopathological theories of etiology. However, this antagonism may indicate as much about desirable interventions as it does about the lack of agreement. Any effective understanding about the causes and prevention of elderly suicide must address both social pathology and psychopathology. The Surgeon General's call to action (U.S. Public Health Service, 1999) to reduce suicide rates reinforces this perspective. Public acceptance of physician-assisted suicide (Altman, 1997) makes the problem all the more urgent.

REFERENCES

Altman, L. K. (1991, July 27). Jury declines to indict a doctor who said he aided in a suicide. *The New York Times*, p. 1.
Angell, M. (1990). Prisoners of technology: The case of Nancy Cruzan. *New England Journal of Medicine, 322*, 1226–1228.

Atchley, R. C. (1980). *Social forces in later life.* San Francisco, CA: Wadsworth.

Barraclough, B. M., Bunch, J., Nelson, B., et al. (1974). A hundred cases of suicide: Clinical aspects. *British Journal of Psychiatry, 125,* 355–373.

Batchelor, I. R. C., Napier, M. B. (1953). Attempted suicide in old age. *British Medical Journal, 2,* 1186–1190.

Beck, A. T., Steer, R. A., Kovacs, M., et al. (1985). Hopelessness and eventual suicide: A 10-year prospective study of patients hospitalized with suicidal ideation. *American Journal of Psychiatry, 142,* 559–563.

Brody, H. (1992). Assisted death: A compassionate response to a medical failure. *New England Journal of Medicine, 327,* 1384–1388.

Brown, J. H. (1979). Suicide in Britain: More attempts, fewer deaths, lessons for public policy. *Archives of General Psychiatry, 36,* 1119–1124.

Clark, D. C. (1992, December 10). Remarks at the "Too Young to Die" conference on the National Suicide Survey, conducted by Empire Blue Cross and Blue Shield and the Gallup Organization, Inc., New York.

Clayton, P. J. (1985). Suicide. *Psychiatric Clinics of North America, 8,* 203–214.

Conwell, Y., Caine, E. D., Olsen, K. (1990a). Suicide and cancer in late life. *Hospital and Community Psychiatry, 41,* 1334–1339.

Conwell, Y., Lyness, J. M., Duberstein, P., et al. (2000). Completed suicide among older patients in primary care practices: A controlled study. *Journal of the American Geriatrics Society, 48,* 23–29.

Conwell, Y., Melanie, R., Caine, E. D. (1990b). Completed suicide at age 50 and over. *Journal of the American Geriatrics Society, 38,* 640–644.

Costa, P. T. (1991). *Depression as an enduring disposition.* Paper presented at NIMH Consensus Development Conference on the diagnosis and treatment of depression in late life, Bethesda, MD *(Program and Abstracts,* p. 45).

Cummings, E., Henry, N. E. (1961). *Growing old: The process of disengagement.* New York: Basic Books.

Duberstein, P. R., Conwell, Y., Seidlitz, L., et al. (1999). Age and suicidal ideation in older depressed inpatients. *American Journal of Geriatric Psychiatry, 7,* 289–296.

Durkheim, E. (1951). *Suicide.* New York: Free Press. (Original work published 1891)

Dyer, E. R. (1992, December 10). Comments at the "Too Young to Die" Conference on the National Suicide Survey, conducted by Empire Blue Cross and Blue Shield and the Gallup Organization, Inc., New York.

Emanuel, E. J., Battin, M. P. (1998). What are the potential cost savings from legalizing physician assisted suicide? *New England Journal of Medicine, 339,* 157–172.

Etzersdorfer, E., Sonneck, G., Nagel-Kuess, S. (1992). Newspaper reports and suicide [Letter to the Editor]. *New England Journal of Medicine, 327,* 502–503.

Gallup, G. H. (1992a, December 10). Remarks at the "Too Young to Die" Conference on the National Suicide Survey, conducted by Empire Blue Cross and Blue Shield and the Gallup Organization, Inc., New York.

Gallup Organization. (1992b). *Executive summary: Attitude and incidence of suicide among the elderly.* Princeton, NJ: Author.

Goldstein, M., Colenda, C. C., Kennedy, G. J., et al. (1993). *Models of geropsychiatric practice*. Washington, DC: American Psychiatric Press.

Grabbe, L., Demi, A., Camann, M. A., et al. (1997). The health status of elderly persons in the last year of life: A comparison of deaths by suicide, injury, and natural causes. *American Journal of Public Health, 87,* 434–437.

Green, S. M. (1981). Levels of hopelessness in the general population. *British Journal of Clinical Psychology, 20,* 11–14.

Gurland, B. J., Cross, P. J. (1983). Suicide among the elderly. In M. K. Aronson, R. Bennet, & B. J. Gurland (Eds.), *The acting-out elderly* (pp. 205–215). New York: Hawthorn Press.

Haas, A. P., Hendin, G. E. (1983). Suicide among older people: Projections for the future. *Suicide and Life-Threatening Behavior, 13,* 147–154.

Hamilton, M. (1960). A rating scale for depression. *Journal of Neurology, Neurosurgery and Psychiatry, 23,* 56–62.

Hemenway, D., Solnick, S. J., Colditz, G. A. (1993). Smoking and suicide among nurses. *American Journal of Public Health, 83,* 249–251.

Hirschfeld, R. M., Russell, J. M. (1997). Assessment and treatment of suicidal patients. *New England Journal of Medicine, 337,* 910–915.

Holden, C. (1992). A new discipline probes suicide's multiple causes. *Science, 256,* 1761–1762.

Horton-Deutsch, S. L., Clark, D. C., Farran, C. J. (1992). Chronic dyspnea and suicide in elderly men. *Hospital and Community Psychiatry, 43,* 1198–1203.

Jamison, K., Baldessarini, R. J. (1999). Effects of medical interventions on suicidal behavior. *Journal of Clinical Psychiatry, 60*(Suppl. 2), 117–122.

Kaplan, M. S., Adamek, M. E., Rohades, J. A. (1998). Prevention of elderly suicide: Physicians' assessment of firearm availability. *American Journal of Preventive Medicine, 15,* 60–64.

Kellerman, A. L., Rivara, F. P., Somes, G., et al. (1992). Suicide in the home in relation to gun ownership. *New England Journal of Medicine, 327,* 467–472.

Kennedy, G. J., Metz, H., Lowinger, R. (1996). Epidemiology and inferences regarding the etiology of late-life suicide. In G. J. Kennedy (Ed.), *Suicide and depression in late life* (pp. 3–22). New York: Wiley.

Kennedy, G. J., Tannenbaum, S. (in press). Suicide in late life: International perspectives. *Psychiatric Quarterly.*

Kevorkian cure: Death [Editorial]. (1990, December 12). *The New York Times,* p. E17.

Lindsey, J. (1986). Trends in self-poisoning in the elderly 1974–1983. *International Journal of Geriatric Psychiatry, 1,* 37–43.

Linehan, M. M. (1997). Behavioral treatments of suicidal behaviors: Definitional obfuscation and treament outcomes. *Annals of the New York Academy of Science, 836,* 302–328.

Loebel, J. P., Loebel, J. S., Dager, S. R., et al. (1991). Anticipation of nursing home placement may be a precipitant of suicide among the elderly. *Journal of the American Geriatrics Society, 39,* 407–408.

Mackenzie, T. B., Popkin, M. K. (1987). Suicide in the medical patient. *International Journal of Psychiatry in Medicine, 17,* 3–22.

Mann, J. J., Stoff, D. M. (1997). A synthesis of current findings regarding neurobiological correlates and treatment of suicidal behavior. *New York Academy of Science, 836,* 352–363.

Marzuk, P. M., Leon, A. C., Tardiff, K., et al. (1992). The effect of access to lethal methods of injury on suicide rates. *Archives of General Psychiatry, 49,* 451–458.

McCall, P. L. (1991). Adolescent and elderly white male suicide trends: Evidence of changing well-being? *Journals of Gerontology: Social Sciences, 46,* S43–S51.

McIntosh, J. L. (1985). Suicide among the elderly: Levels and trends. *American Journal of Orthopsychiatry, 55,* 288–293.

McIntosh, J. L., Santos, J. F. (1981). Suicide among minority elderly: A preliminary investigation. *Suicide and Life-Threatening Behavior, 11,* 151–166.

Meehan, P. J., Saltzberg, L. E., Sattin, R. W. (1991). Suicides among older United States residents: Epidemiologic characteristics and trends. *American Journal of Public Health, 81,* 1198–1200.

Mercer, S. O. (1989). *Elder suicide: A national survey of prevention and intervention programs.* Washington, DC: American Association of Retired Persons.

Merloo, J. (1968). Hidden suicide. In H. L. P. Resnick (Ed.), *Suicidal behaviors: Diagnosis and management* (pp. 256–272). Boston: Little, Brown.

Miller, M. (1978). Geriatric suicide: The Arizona study. *Gerontologist, 18,* 488–495.

Murphy, G. E., Wetzel, R. D., Robins, E., et al. (1992). Multiple risk actors predict suicide in alcoholism. *Archives of General Psychiatry, 49,* 459–463.

Murphy, G. K. (1977). Cancer and the coroner. *Journal of the American Medical Association, 237,* 786–788.

National Institute of Mental Health. (1997). Prevention of suicidal behavior in older primary care patients. *NIH Guide, 26.*

Nelson, F. L., Farberow, N. L. (1982). The development of an Indirect Self-Destructive Behavior Scale for use with chronically ill medical patients. *International Journal of Social Psychiatry, 28,* 5–14.

Osgood, N. J. (1992, December 10). Remarks at the "Too Young to Die" conference on the National Suicide Survey, conducted by Empire Blue Cross and Blue Shield and the Gallup Organization, Inc., New York.

Plutchik, R., Botsis, A. J., Weiner, M. B., et al. (1996). Clinical measurement of suicidality and coping in late life: A theory of countervailing forces. In G. Kennedy (Ed.), *Suicide and depression in late life* (pp. 83–102). New York: Wiley.

Quill, T. E. (1991). Death and dignity: A case of individualized decision making. *New England Journal of Medicine, 324,* 691–694.

Quill, T. E., Cassel, C. K., Meier, D. E. (1992). Care of the hopelessly ill: Proposed criteria for physician assisted suicide. *New England Journal of Medicine, 327,* 1380–1384.

Richman, J. (1996). Psychotherapeutic approaches to the depressed suicidal older person and family. In G. Kennedy (Ed.), *Suicide and depression in late life* (pp. 103–119). New York: Wiley.

Rosenberg, M. L., Eddy, D. M., Wolpert, R. C., et al. (1989). Developing strategies to prevent youth suicide. In C. R. Pfeffer (Ed.), *Suicide among youth: Perspectives on risk and prevention* (pp. 203–225). Washington, DC: American Psychiatric Press.

Shaffer, D. (1993). Suicide: Risk factors and the public health. *American Journal of Public Health, 83,* 171–172.

Shneidman, E. S. (1963). Orientation towards death: A vital aspect of the study of lives. In R. White (Ed.), *The study of lives* (pp. 146–185). New York: Prentice-Hall.

Tolchin, M. (1989, July 19). When long life is too much: Suicide rates among the elderly. *The New York Times,* p. A1.

Uncapher, H., Gallagher-Thompson, D., Osgood, N. J., et al. (1998). Hopelessness and suicidal ideation in older adults. *Gerontologist, 38,* 62–70.

U.S. Public Health Service. (1999). *The Surgeon General's call to action to prevent suicide.* Washington, DC: U.S. Department of Health and Human Services.

van der Sande, R., van Rooijen, L., Buskens, E., et al. (1997). Intensive in-patient and community intervention versus routine care after attempted suicide. A randomized controlled intervention study. *British Journal of Psychiatry, 171,* 35–41.

van Praag, H. M., Plutchik, R. (1985). An empirical study on the "cathartic effect" of attempted suicide. *Psychiatry Press, 16,* 123–130.

Vital Statistics of the United States. (1996). Mortality, Part A, 1992. Hyattsville, MD: National Center for Health Statistics (U.S. Department of Health and Human Services Publication 367).

Weishaar, M. E., Beck, A. T. (1990). Cognitive approaches to understanding and treating suicidal behavior. In S. J. Blumnethal & D. J. Kupfer (Eds.), *Suicide over the life cycle: Risk factor assessment, and treatment of suicidal patients* (pp. 469–498). Washington, DC: American Psychiatric Press.

Weissman, M. M. (1974). The epidemiology of suicide attempts, 1960 to 1971. *Archives of General Psychiatry, 30,* 737–746.

Weissman, M. R., Klerman, G. L., Markowitz, J. S., et al. (1989). Suicidal ideation and suicide attempts in panic disorder and attacks. *New England Journal of Medicine, 321,* 1209–1214.

Whanger, A. D. (1989). Inpatient treatment of the older psychiatric patient. In E. Busse & D. G. Blazer (Eds.), *Geriatric psychiatry* (pp. 234–246). Washington, DC: American Psychiatric Press.

Woodbury, M. A., Manton, K. G., Blazer, D. G. (1988). Trends in US suicide mortality rates 1968 to 1982: Race and sex differences in age, period and cohort components. *International Journal of Epidemiology, 17,* 356–362.

World Health Organization. (1996). *Prevention of suicide: Guidelines for the formulation and implementation of national strategies.* Geneva: World Health Organization.

Zimmerman, M., Lish, J. D., Lush, D. T., et al. (1995). Suicidal ideation among urban medical outpatients. *Journal of General Internal Medicine, 10,* 573–576.

Zung, W. W. K. (1985). A self-rating depression scale. *Archives of General Psychiatry, 12,* 63–70.

13

Mental Health Consultation in the General Hospital, Home, or Nursing Facility

Traditional mental health care settings are inadequate to meet the needs of older adults (Gurland et al., 1988). Mental health specialists must adapt their expectations and approach to be effective in alternative venues and to diversify their portfolio of practice sites to ensure financial viability. These sites include general hospitals, nursing homes, senior citizen centers, retirement communities, and certified home health agencies. The material that follows is meant to inform the primary provider of what to expect from the mental health consultant and to teach the mental health consultant an effective, efficient orientation. See related topics in chapters dealing with specific diagnoses, elder abuse, and legal and ethical issues (competency assessment, conflict mediation).

PATTERNS OF MENTAL HEALTH CONSULTATION

Caplan (1970) provides the basic orientation for mental health consultation by defining the consultant relationships in four patterns. First, the consultant's attention may be directed at the patient's problem as defined by the provider who requested the consultation. Second, the consultant may focus more on the person requesting the service with the patient being a relatively secondary or indirect concern. Third, the focus may be the program or setting of the patient's care. Fourth, the consultation may be directed more to the administration rather than to the patient, consultee, or program. Added to the traditional models are two others. These include (1) consultations for family members who may be struggling with the patient, staff, or administration and (2) the consultation to meet regulatory requirements or address deficiencies noted by agency surveyors (Jackson, 1997). Obviously the field of care demands a fluid rather than rigidly patterned relationship from the consultant. Throughout the examples that follow, the models expand and contract to accommodate the consultant's role from participant observer to advocate. And once established, the consultant can move freely from one model to the next depending on the need.

MODELS AND METHODS

Greenhill proposed a number of models and methods through which mental health services (Greenhill, 1979) and training (Greenhill & Kilgore, 1950) might be delivered in the setting of medical and surgical units. The consultation model in which the primary physician refers the patient for psychiatric evaluation is the bedrock but not the sole support for all other models. These include the liaison model in which a consulting psychiatric service is assigned to work with patients and physicians from specific hospital units designated by the parent department, usually medicine. The milieu model extends the liaison model to encompass the cultural anthropology and social psychology of patient care. A greater collaboration with social work and nursing staff results, but the primary physician remains responsible for identification and triage of cases (Small & Fawzy, 1988). The psychiatrist is identified by milieu staff as an "insider" in the ward culture (Mohl, 1979).

The critical-care model is a subdivision of the milieu model in which the liaison is forged with an intensive care unit rather than a parent department. The biological psychiatry model is an analogous subdivision of the consultation model in which the psychiatrist relies more on expertise in neuroscience and psychopharmacology and less on psychodynamics and social psychology. However, Greenhill's ideal is an integral model in which any member of the health care team may request psychiatric consultation.

The distinguishing characteristic of the integral model is a focus on primary prevention by early identification of populations at high risk for episodes of mental illness or difficulty collaborating with treatment. These populations are characterized by certain conditions and medical procedures (e.g., substance abuse and hemodialysis) which are frequently accompanied by psychological sequelae and by characteristics such as advanced age or disadvantaged ethnic minority status. The final component of the integral model is a quality assurance auditing procedure that ensures the appropriateness of psychiatric care.

Empirical Models

Strain et al. (1985) identified empirical models of mental health training for primary care physicians in which consultation/liaison psychiatrists participate. Similarly, McKegney and Schwartz (1986) described the organizational and treatment issues that arise between consultation/liaison psychiatry and behavioral medicine. Both reviews emphasize diversity and the limitations that arise out of the "local politics" under which the programs evolved. However, the effectiveness of the programs, whether the focus is patient care, clinical training, or research, depends on strong leadership, mutually perceived needs, and realistically defined goals (Perez et al., 1985; Popkin et al., 1984; Rosse et al., 1986; Ruskin, 1985). As with any collaborative effort, the smaller, more specialized component of the program (i.e., mental health) is vulnerable to the preferences and personalities of the larger. Gallagher et al. (1990) describe both the promise and problems in the development of a behavioral medicine service at the University of Vermont College of Medicine. Although the biopsychosocial diagnostic net espoused by Gallagher is conceptually well suited to the problems of the elderly, few individuals referred to his service were found to have cognitive disorders. Thus despite conceptual readiness, not all consultation/liaison and behavioral medicine services will be psychogeriatric as well.

Mental Health Consultation in the General Hospital

Older adults make up 12% of the population of the United States, but they account for more than 35% of the admissions to acute care beds. Their hospital stays average 30% longer than those of younger individuals (Beland et al., 1991) and from 40 to 50% experience some form of psychiatric disorder before discharge (Goldstein et al., 1993). Lipowski (1983) was among the first to argue that consultation/liaison experience with older patients from the medical and surgical units makes psychiatrists effective psychogeriatricians.

Studies that followed Lipowski's call to integrate consultation/liaison and geriatric psychiatry identified aspects of consultant knowledge and practice that were particularly relevant to the elderly (Unützer & Small, 1996). Goldberg (1989) identified a number of areas in which the consultation/liaison psychiatrist must show geriatrics expertise. First, the stress of hospitalization with its unfamiliar environments, complex evaluations, and uncertainties of treatment are more threatening for the elderly. Forced dependency, although temporary, may be overwhelming to a frail but previously independent older adult. Second, the presence of multiple medical conditions and age-related increases in physiological heterogeneity makes it more difficult to minimize the risk of adverse reactions to medications. Diagnosis is similarly made more difficult by the multiplicity of ongoing treatments and conditions. The result is a more frequent finding of dementia, delirium, and affective disorders with anxiety and somatoform and personality disorders seen less often.

Third, the density and persistence of cognitive impairment as well as negative social stereotypes and age-related biases (Butler, 1975; Kiloh, 1961) may mislead well-intentioned primary care physicians and consultants as to the efficacy of psychiatric intervention in late life. Fourth, interview techniques require modification to attend to sensory impairments and social expectations of older persons. Auditory acuity in the higher frequencies is frequently degraded in old age. To compensate, the consultant should speak in lower tones, remain in full sight, and conduct the interview in as quiet an environment as possible. The social approach should be more deferential than familiar or casual. A collateral source of information, usually a family member, is crucial both to give an objective view of the older patient's prior level of function and support and to minimize the burden of detail placed on the older primary informant. Family engagement is also important to reinforce whatever therapeutic recommendations the consultant might offer (Small & Fawzy, 1988). Fifth, a thorough grounding in the biological determinants of mental impairment and age-related changes in physiology, as well as expertise in psychopharmacology, is essential. Finally, the consultant must be knowledgeable in the assessment of the person's capacity to make health care decisions.

Limitations of Consultation in the General Hospital

Acute inpatient services do not allow for longer-term relationships needed to adequately care for the dementia patient, nor do they prepare the psychiatrist for community outreach or practice in long-term-care facilities. Observing a dementia patient's family develop nursing skills and stratagems to manage difficult behavior is not possible in a setting in which hospital staff are expected to complete such assignments. Similarly, serial trials of medications for refractory late-life depressive episodes may not be compatible with the treatment of more acute medical or surgical conditions. However, in relying on referrals from third parties, geriatric psychiatry is more similar to consultation/liaison than to general psychiatry. Older adults are more likely to be referred by family, social service agencies, or their primary physicians than are younger individuals who find mental health services more acceptable. The financial incentives of caring for a population with federal entitlements for mental health care (Medicare part B) cannot be overlooked in an era in which even the most altruistic service must be economically viable. The incomplete penetration of the Medicare enrollees by managed care entities offers a window of opportunity (profitability).

However, despite significant reform of Medicare payments for psychiatric care, patients receiving domiciliary and outpatient services remain at a considerable disadvantage compared to those served in the hospital. Although there is no longer a per-year cap on outpatient psychiatric reimbursement, the copayment (i.e., the out-of-pocket expense to the patient) is 50% compared to 20% of the Medicare-approved charge for inpatient procedures. In states (unlike New York) in which the majority of nursing home residents are not Medicaid recipients, this policy means that substantially less than the 50% copayment for a nursing home visit may be recoverable. Of note, consultation and follow-up codes, evaluation and management (E&M) codes requiring limited physical exam and systems review (routine when medicating older persons), and home care codes incur a 20% copayment. Clearly the financial incentives weigh heavily in favor of a practice diversified between consultations to nursing homes and general hospitals, with office visits and house calls making up the balance.

Consultation in the Emergency Room

Although the number of older adult admissions to emergency rooms is proportionate to their representation in the community, their use of resources once admitted to the emergency room is disproportionately large. And although there may be fewer psychiatric patients among elderly emergency room admissions, there is a much greater percentage of individuals with dementia (Gottlieb et al., 1982). The frequency with which dementia or acute confusion complicates the emergency room stay of older patients indicates the need for mental health specialists to be an integral part of the emergency room team. Models in which mental health services are provided in a separate psychiatric emergency room seem not ideal for the elderly (Goldstein et al., 1993).

Older adults are particularly vulnerable to the disorienting effect of a busy emergency room. Putting the senior patient at ease is the first priority. Family members are a valuable source of history as well as a reassuring presence for any patient in the emergency room. Anxiety, suspiciousness, evasiveness, or confusion that are not reduced by the family's presence should alert the clinician that behavioral disturbance will have to be managed at the same time that investigative procedures are undertaken. Because family members are the most frequent perpetrators of elder abuse, it is also important to observe their interactions with the patient (see Chapter 10).

Emergency pharmacological interventions should be considered when agitation impairs the person's capacity to collaborate in diagnostic or therapeutic procedures. When the underlying cause of agitation can be rapidly addressed (e.g., the relief of pain or correction of a metabolic disturbance), psychotropics should be deferred. When agitation is the result of simple anxiety or sleep deprivation due to the emergency room or intensive care unit (ICU) ambiance, a low dose of a benzodiazepine without active metabolites may be useful (lorazepam 0.5 mg orally or i.m.). The advantages of lorazepam are short duration of action and freedom from anticholinergic and extrapyramidal side effects. Adverse reactions are rare but include respiratory depression, confusion, and paradoxical disinhibition. When delirium, delusions, or hallucinations are present haloperidol (0.5 mg i.m. or orally) is preferred. It is less sedative and more likely to induce parkinsonian signs, but generally preferred when respiratory or cardiovascular collapse is a threat. Whichever psychotropic is chosen, follow-up to monitor efficacy may be required at frequent intervals. Older adults vary tremendously in their capacity to metabolize medications and may ultimately require doses outside the practitioner's range of experience or comfort. Psychiatric consultation should be sought when agitation does not respond to routine measures.

Avoiding Assault by Estimating the Hierarchy of Threat

The effective management of patient violence depends on one's ability to predict imminent assault and to approach the hierarchy of threat in an objective, systematic manner. Interventions to reduce the threat of an assault start with an assessment of the patient, the setting, and the clinician's feelings. When the practitioner's initial reaction is terror (Adler & Shapiro, 1973), to unconsciously label the patient a drunk, criminal, or sociopath (Lion & Pasternak, 1973), or to expect the worst, it will prove difficult to put the threat in an accurate perspective. Conversely, a false sense of personal security may blind the clinician to genuine warning signs. As a result, putting the patient at ease, gaining cooperation, and structuring a preventive environment may be delayed.

Rapidly determining whether the patient is a high, medium, or low risk for assault allows a rational path through a period of under-standable fear and uncertainty. History and diagnosis are used to define longer-term or medium- and low-risk status, but it is motor behavior that is the best clue to a high risk of violence within the ensu-ing 30–60 minutes (Dubin, 1981). Table 13.1 presents a hierarchy of characteristics recommended to predict assaultiveness (Kennedy et al., 1999). It is important to recognize that assaults rarely arise "out of the blue" and early intervention can prevent the escalation of threat into the realm of physical aggression (Dibella, 1979). Obviously, the psy-chotic, agitated, enraged older person who is menacing in both posture and speech requires immediate help to regain control. However, the demented, aphasic, visually impaired older resident of a nursing facil-ity who is verbally threatening during bath time also requires care to prevent a self-protective response from becoming an assault. In the former case, a calm, careful interview focused on the patient's feelings and desperate need for control can secure permission for tranquilizing medication and/or diagnostic procedures. In the latter case, alerting

TABLE 13.1. Hierarchy for Predictors of Assault

History	Diagnosis	Behavior
High risk: Imminent danger, requires immediate action		
Recent assault	Psychosis	Verbal threats
Severe injury	Mania	Hyperactivity
Several episodes	Delirium	Autonomic arousal
	Intoxication	Clinched fists, jaws
		Coiled spring stance
		Weapons possession
Medium risk: Long-term risk, clearly requires precautions		
Past assault	Personality disorder	Verbal abuse
Minor injury	Paranoid	Agitation, panic
No precipitant	Antisocial	
Arrests	Borderline	
Threats	Alcohol abuse	
Low risk: Uncertain but may require precautions		
Threats only	Dementia	
Poor insight	Seizure disorder	
	Sensory deficits	
	Aphasia	
	Head injury	

Note. Adapted from Kennedy et al. (1999). Copyright 1999 by Advanstar Com-munications Inc. Adapted by permission.

staff that this particular nursing home resident requires more time and more sensory cues in order not to be frightened by the simple act of bathing may eliminate the aggressive outbursts.

Effective treatment of violence in clinical settings is based on understanding that an assault arises out of the patient's sense of vulnerability. And that threatening behavior is a last chance defense against overwhelming loss of security and control. The best approach to assaultiveness is talk—not confrontation or correction of false perceptions but empathic interaction designed to verbally elicit desperate feelings in place of violent acts. The practitioner should assure the disturbed individual that loss of control will not be allowed and that what is to follow in the exchange is meant to restore a sense of safety. The panicky, psychotic person terrified by the disintegration of personality needs to gain control over feelings in order to regain control of aggressive impulses. The patient may not be aware of the extent to which the threatening behavior frightens others. Therefore the clinician should first reflect in a calm manner that the patient's threats are taken seriously. "You look very upset, and people are scared, can we talk about it? Tell me what's wrong; it will help. You don't have to hurt yourself or anyone else. If you lose control I can call for security, but first let's make sure you stay in control." In short, the clinician must help the patient defend against intolerable feelings and ensure that limits are set.

Patients at high risk for assault should not be interviewed alone. The interviewer may wish to have family or hospital security nearby during the interview, but it is rarely necessary for security personnel to remain in the room. Again, body language rather than content of speech is the best indicator of imminent violence. If the patient cannot sit down and cannot relinquish a menacing posture or threatening gestures in response to verbal interventions, security personnel or other staff should be called to demonstrate a show of force. The presence of security is generally sufficient to reassure staff and patient alike that aggression is under control so that verbal interventions may resume.

Restraints

When verbal approaches and a show of force are not enough to reduce assaultiveness, physical restraints will be required. Restraints should never be used as a threat. They should not be attempted without sufficient staff. They should be applied calmly, quietly, in a nonpunitive manner. Dubin (1981) suggest the following protocol for the use of restraints:

1. No less than four and preferably five persons (one for each limb and the head) should restrain the person. Leather restraints are the most reliable and least dangerous.
2. A staff member should explain why the person is to be restrained and remain with the person at all times to alleviate the fear of helplessness, impotence, and loss of control.
3. Limbs should be restrained with legs spread-eagled, one arm above the head the other at the patient's side.
4. Access for intravenous fluids should be insured.
5. Raise the head of the bed to reduce the risk of aspiration and the patient's feeling of vulnerability.
6. Restraints should be checked periodically for safety and comfort.
7. With restraints in place the physician reinstitutes verbal interventions and begins medication therapy. Most restrained patients will accept oral medication that should be administered in the most readily absorbed liquid form.
8. After the person regains control, one restraint at a time may be released at 5-minute intervals until only two restraints remain. It is inadvisable to keep a patient in one restraint so that the last two restraints should be removed together.
9. Always document the behavior that necessitated the use of restraints and alternative treatments that failed, the intervening verbal and pharmacological interventions, the course of treatment, and response during the period of restraint.

Weapons

Although restraints are an unpleasant reality of emergency care, nothing is more frightening than a patient threatening the use of a weapon in the clinic or emergency room or on a home visit. As emphasized previously, all threats emanate from fear, helplessness, and passivity. A weapon is the most dramatic symbol of these emotions (Salamon, 1976) and a remarkably effective means of engendering similar feelings in others. Again talk, time, and mastery of one's own sense of vulnerability are essential to relieve the person's need for desperate measures. Interviewers should never ask immediately for the weapon to be surrendered. First, they should give patients a chance to describe the fears that led them to arm themselves. This provides the opportunity to put verbal defenses in place. When the person feels less vulnerable, interviewers should ask that the weapon be placed on the floor so that security personnel can take possession after the interview. A clinician should never accept the weapon directly. If the patient refuses to relinquish the weapon, the interviewer should immediately call security. If the patient threatens the interviewer, it is best that he or she respond in a way that does not provoke the person to action or infect the person with his or her own sense of panic. The interviewer should calmly look the person in the eye, move slowly and deliberately, speak in a natural tone of voice, and keep speaking in a comforting, reassuring way, ask others to leave the room, and assure the patient that he or she is in control (Walker, 1983).

Consultation for End-of-Life Treatment Decisions and Palliative Care

The ideals of palliative care are rarely achieved. The major barriers to incorporating both the scientific basis and the practical methods of palliative care reside in prevailing physician practices (Hamel et al., 1995). The imperatives of cost containment will ultimately result in the adoption of aspects of palliative care. Ultimately, economic forces will shape physician behaviors without necessarily leading to the improved consumer satisfaction associated with genuine palliative care. Less coercive means exist to hasten the transition to comfort care when cure is not an option without sacrificing staff morale or the trust of patients and their families. What follows is meant to identify those less coercive means in order to improve end-of-life care.

Areas of particular interest include but are not limited to (1) management of pain, depression, sleep disturbance, anxiety, and agitation; (2) use of invasive diagnostic procedures; (3) use of more invasive treatments (dialysis, tube feeding, ventilators, chemotherapy, surgery), as well as less (antibiotics, psychotropics); (4) methods of obtaining health care proxy and advanced directives; (5) patterns of consultation with other specialties; (6) interactions with staff and family; (7) attention to religious preferences and values; (8) adaptation to patients and families of ethnic and racial origins different from those of the practitioner; (9) presentation of hospice and long-term-care options; (10) physician frustrations and satisfactions; and (11) physiologically futile treatment (see Chapter 14 for detailed discussion of futility).

Sloane (1998) describes the basic elements of palliative care. They include (1) companionship for the patients until death, (2) someone for the family to speak with during the end stage and after the patient's death, (3) periodic, passive range of motion exercises provided they can be performed without pain, (4) freedom from restraint, (5) limiting medications to those likely to have near-term benefits, (6) liberal treatment of pain, (7) skin care including frequent change of soiled linens and repositioning to prevent breakdown, (8) regular bowel care to prevent constipation and to facilitate elimination, (9) oral care for cleansing and to prevent dry mouth, (10) feeding appropriate to the goals of care and tailored to the patient's preferences and capacities, and (11) simple pleasures that the patient will enjoy, including massage, music, favorite foods, family photos, prayer, gentle bathing, comfortable clothes, and pets. In summary, recognizing the patient's end-stage condition, formulating new goals of care, and providing the basic elements of the care plan promise genuine satisfaction for the practitioner and considerable comfort for the patient and family.

Sloane (1998) has summarized the palliative or comfort-care approach to dementia patients and those with end-stage disease. First, the family and other caregivers should be informed that although the exact prognosis (survival time) is uncertain, the goals of care have changed now that the patient has reached the end stage. End-stage dementia is characterized by severe confusion (Mini-Mental Status Exam score of less than 3): inability to dress, go to the toilet, walk, little if any meaningful speech (five words or less), and, most important, specific medical complications within the last 90 days, including dehydration, pneumonia, urosepsis, and refusal or inability to consume adequate nutrition despite staff encouragement. These patients are bed-bound and no longer recognize family, friends, or their surroundings.

Some practitioners have intuitively developed a stance that allows them to cross discipline boundaries and barriers to palliative care. They anticipate and tolerate the ambivalence and uncertainty involved in the dying patient's care from family and staff. They routinely mediate conflict, delegate tasks, and define boundaries and end points (i.e., the limits of care). However, their naturally acquired approach and their more individual, perhaps charismatic qualities may not generalize to the average practitioner. Some practitioners will incorporate the elements of palliative care once exposed to them in conventional education venues of grand rounds, case conferences, and consultations. Others, because of orientation or interests, will prefer a consultant team to assist with palliative care techniques rather than to carry them out independently.

There are a number of mental health components to the provision of palliative care. These include the pharmacological relief of anxiety, depression, and sleep disturbance, as well as psychotherapeutic approaches to lessen the distress of the patient, family, and primary care staff. The purpose of psychosocial assessment and mental status exam is to determine treatable problems (anxiety, depression, psychosis, sleep disturbance) as well as to assess cognitive impairment which may contribute to the patient's difficulty in participating in the decision-making process (dementia) or which might require additional measures to resolve (delirium). Are there obvious personality traits that complicate the therapeutic relationship? For example, is the patient particularly needy, contentious, mistrustful, aloof, or withdrawn? Conversely, does the patient seem passive, indifferent, or impervious to the implications of the condition? Is there frank denial?

The social and family data collection should include work history, family configuration, and domicile. Is there evidence of marital discord, family enmeshment, and conflict? Has the person lived a more solitary life or always been part of an active social unit? What kind of work and responsibilities did the person perform? What is the religious affiliation? When were religious services or acts of private devotion last attended? An approach to a palliative care consultation follows.

General and Specific Tasks of the Palliative Care Consultation

General tasks

- Provide information, support, and tangible assistance (procedures and doctor's orders) for palliative care to patients, families, their health care providers, and the institution.
- Enhance the primary care provider's relationship with the patient, family, and institution.

Specific tasks

- Coordinate the activities of the team as it expands or contracts in the process of performing the consultation or providing direct care including respiratory and nutritional supports.
- Recommend, and if requested perform, procedures for the relief of dyspnea, pain, anxiety, depression, psychosis, and sleep disturbance.
- Engage in conflict mediation when end-of-life treatment preferences of the involved parties seem mutually exclusive; acquire advanced directives or appointment of health care proxy.
- Manage institutional risk and clarify individual responsibilities.
- Provide an emotionally, intellectually, and spiritually supportive microenvironment for palliative care to be carried out.
- Clarify the ethically acceptable options and imperatives as well as the decision-making process by which preferences for care are expressed.

A Model Palliative Care Team:
Composition and Responsibilities

- Nurse clinician (initial evaluation, triage to other team members, nursing liaison, acquire health care proxy)
- Critical care specialist (intensivist), pain management team member (relief of pain and dyspnea, respiratory support)
- Geriatrician, oncologist (focus on prognosis for function, survival, quality of life, nutrition, syndromal approach, acquire advance directives)
- Bioethicist, risk managers (clarify decision-making processes, ethical and legal options and imperatives, conflict mediation)
- Psychiatry, social service (relief of sleep disturbance, anxiety, depression, psychosis, provision of family counseling, and home care services)
- Clergy (spiritual support and clarification of religious values in health care decisions)

Presentation of a Case

A 96-year-old woman was admitted to the geriatric medicine unit from home with a change in mental status. Her evaluation revealed severe cognitive impairment, marked cortical atrophy, dehydration, pressure ulcers about the ankles and buttocks, and urinary tract infection. Intravenous fluids, nasogastric tube, and broad-spectrum antibiotics were begun, but the patient remained uncommunicative. Her widowed daughter was her sole companion and care provider in the home. The daughter initially portrayed her mother's decline as relatively abrupt, which staff found hard to accept. The mother's attending physician had not seen her in over a year, had not procured a heath care proxy or advanced directives, and had not discussed a do-not-resuscitate (DNR) order with staff or family. He had consulted gastroenterology for the placement of a gastrostomy feeding tube.

House staff were disturbed by the proposed invasive procedure, the patient's debilitated state, and prognosis in light of their suspicions that the patient's diagnosis was end-stage dementia rather than one of sudden unexplained decline. Nursing staff were concerned that the patient had been neglected and that the daughter was both an abuser and not capable of advocating in her mother's best interests. The attending physician showed little interest in a discussion about comfort care for the patient or the daughter's role in subsequent health care decisions.

He agreed that the patient's case could be presented in the weekly teaching conference to senior physicians in geriatric medicine and geriatric psychiatry. He chose not to attend despite being on the floor at the time.

In the conference, the daughter, who was a retired computer programmer, was neither evasive nor defensive. She was open about her inability to care for her mother at home during the last year leading up to this admission. The mother had previously been admitted to another acute care hospital because of a fractured hip. At that time her daughter had arranged for the services of a visiting nurse and physical therapist. However, the mother's cognitive status and gait both declined to the point where her daughter was providing for all activities of daily living. When the mother became incapable of going to her garden to sit in the sun, she told her daughter, "Don't make this [suffering] go on any longer than it has to." Her intake of food and fluids diminished, as did her spontaneous speech. When she became unresponsive, her daughter called 911. In the conference, the daughter did not think that she could ever care for her mother at home again. She knew her mother was gravely ill and was uncertain of "how much you [physicians] can really do for her. I know she would not have wanted all these tubes or to end up on a machine. I don't even know what I want you to do. I just think her clock has run out, guess it's been running down for the last year." She impressed the staff who attended the meeting as exceptionally concerned and capable, and they felt that she was pleading for the physicians to offer a prognosis and recommendations regarding care options.

After she left the conference, it was the team's consensus that the daughter did indeed have a sufficient directive from her mother to refuse artificial food and fluids, that she had functioned as her mother's *de facto* health care proxy for some time, and that she was presently operating in her mother's best interests. The physicians suggested that the daughter be presented with the recommendations that a DNR order should be written, that the gastrostomy not be placed, and that the nasogastric tube and intravenous lines not be replaced if they should become dislodged. The geriatric medicine attending and intern shared these recommendations with the daughter who agreed to the DNR order and to provide written instructions based on a subsequent discussion with risk management personnel to pursue comfort care only. The attending of record consented as well and wrote the DNR order. The mother died before the paperwork could be completed and the tubes pulled, but she was spared the gastrostomy and efforts at resuscitation.

MENTAL HEALTH CARE IN NURSING HOMES

Residential health care facilities (nursing homes) are not well served by mental health specialists. Borson et al. (1989) estimate that less than 1% of elderly nursing home residents who might benefit from psychiatric intervention receive it. Data from empirical studies indicate that models of practice described in the earliest consultation/liaison literature may guide the later development of psychogeriatric services in nursing homes. However, these models need to be adapted to the culture of the facilities. Jackson (1997) describes several aspects of the nursing home environment that the consultant should keep in mind. First, nursing homes are hierarchical and teamwork is not the norm. The hierarchy begins with a small upper echelon of administrators who have little contact with residents but have most of the authority. At the bottom are the certified nursing assistants who have the most contact with residents and their families but little apparent control on the rhythm of care (Smyer et al., 1988). However, Kayser-Jones (1995) suggests that the certified nursing assistants by virtue of their responsibilities have the greatest decision-making latitude over the daily lives of the most impaired residents.

Clearly, to gain entry the consultant must forge a relationship with administration. Yet to be clinically effective, an alliance with the nursing staff is critical. The request for consultation is more often initiated by nursing than by physician staff, not surprising when one considers who most often interacts with the resident or family. Nursing homes operate on a medical rather than psychosocial model despite the primary care physician's general absence from the site of care. The pace of decision making and care is slow compared to the hospital. Staff have had little training in mental health, frequently feel overburdened, and find it difficult to address negative reactions to troubling residents and families.

Nursing home care is stigmatized and heavily regulated, leaving staff with low morale and relatively high rates of turnover. Because of fears that they will be criticized or be assigned more work, staff often resist calling the primary care physician. Once called, the mental health consultant will need to work actively with both the primary care physician and the staff. The physician with rare exception will ask that the consultant carry out all aspects of the mental health care, but ongoing feedback is essential for effective intervention.

Jackson (1997) notes several goals of the mental health consultation. The most important are (1) to "treat the resident, not the psychiatric illness" and (2) to help the staff do their jobs. This means reducing problem behaviors, optimizing medications, reducing the use of restraints, and avoiding unnecessary procedures. Reducing survey deficiencies and ensuring compliance with the Omnibus Budget Reconciliation Act and Medicare regulations are also critical for the consultant and the facility (Health Care Financing Administration, 1991, 1992a, 1992b, 1992c).

There are several elements to staff assistance. Although some staff intuitively adapt their approach to modify problem behaviors, most need bedside teaching and in-service training. These activities will require time away from resident care but promise to increase efficiency and reduce stress. It is critical that the consultant acknowledges the stress of care and reinforces positive staff behaviors and self-esteem. Staff cannot examine how they contribute to the problem without first being given credit for their efforts and the genuine difficulty they encounter. The consultant cannot offer helpful suggestions without first having ascertained what interventions staff have exhausted. Communication and support between individual staff members and between shifts is emphasized to increase the consistency of the approach and to engender an adaptive rather than defensive posture. Because nursing home personnel have had little instruction in neurology, it is important to explain the reflexive nature of some residents' protective responses, which may seem willful and meant to harm (Rovner et al., 1990). Symptoms and motivation both of the resident and the family may need to be explained to staff.

Lippert et al. (1990) compared characteristics of psychiatric consultations for elderly patients in a Toronto general hospital to consultations in an affiliated nursing home. Several differences emerged. General hospital consultations were more frequently emergent, required contact with physicians as opposed to other health care personnel, required a greater number of visits in the 2 weeks immediately following the initial patient contact, and were less likely to employ psychotherapy as an intervention. Nursing home consultations in contrast were more frequently requested for management than diagnosis and entailed greater contact with allied health professionals than with physicians. Dementia was diagnosed in 70% of the nursing home consultations and 27% of the general hospital consultations.

Bienenfeld and Wheeler (1989) echo the need for a liaison model. Nursing home residents referred to their offices were often not accompanied by nursing staff who could serve as collateral informants for the presenting problem as well as therapeutic agents in their own right. Moreover, the identified patient generally represented only an isolated part of a more systemic clinical problem. Bienenfeld and Wheeler (1989) switched to an on-site evaluation followed by a case conference scheduled to bridge the nursing staff's change of shift. They also emphasized the need for ongoing contact with administrative staff to ensure that the program meets administrative as well as clinical interests. Medicare part B provided the bulk of reimbursement augmented by fees to the nursing home, which through careful documentation of services were then used to justify an increased Medicaid allotment to the facility.

Zarit and Zarit (1998) add several components to the consultation. First, the consultant needs an understanding of the setting and staffing. Despite the prevalence of dementia in nursing facilities, staff have had little training in the recognition and treatment of mental disorders and little familiarity with psychiatric terms. Second, the consultant should find the person (often the nurse or social worker) who initiated the request and also determine what the certified nursing assistant most familiar with the patient thinks. There is usually an explicit request written in the medical record such as "evaluate for depression." But the implicit problem may be more informative; for example, the certified nursing assistant finds her favorite resident no longer responds to family or engages in activities. Third, the consultant should read the record. Medical comorbidity and polypharmacy are the rule, not the exception, in nursing facilities.

Fourth, if the resident has involved family, the consultant should give them a call. They will provide both recent history and social background that will make the consult much more efficient and thorough. Staff will tell the consultant if the resident prefers family not to be contacted. Lacking a family member, there may be other staff who know the resident and can be counted on for diagnostic details and ultimately assisting with interventions. Fifth, the consultant should respond promptly and make the response relevant to the concerned staff. The note in the medical record should be concise and specific; lengthier communications should be passed on to the staff who initiated requested help and will implement your recommendations. Finally, the consultant should follow up to ensure the desired outcome or conversely to reassure staff that their efforts have not been in vain even if the resident cannot improve.

Parmalee and Lawton (1990) characterize nursing home care as a dialectic of autonomy and security. The residents deserve privacy and individual rights but require security and protection from one another as well as medical events. The dialectical balance shifts from time to time. The widespread use of restraints in the 1970s prevented falls and litigation. Yet in the 1990s these same restraints were seen as akin to the chains placed on the lunatics of Paris liberated by Pinel in the late 18th century (Streim et al., 1996). The regulatory environment under which nursing homes operate is extensive, with specific applications to mental health consultations, psychotropic medication, and psycho-therapy. Regulations promulgated first under the Omnibus Budget Reconciliation Act of 1987 (OBRA 87) defined antipsychotic medication as a restraint until proven otherwise. Subsequent regulatory language required that the specific reason for an antipsychotic be written in the record and at times in the order. A defined behavior and related diagnosis of psychosis should be identified. An effort to manage the problem behavior with environmental or interpersonal approaches should be documented. Attempts to reduce if not discontinue the antipsychotic should also be documented. Antidepressants do not fall under these procedures. Psychotherapy, particularly group sessions with dementia patients, may not be billed to Medicare if they appear to be substituted for activities therapy which should be provided through the nursing home's daily rate of reimbursement. The Office of the Inspector General's Project Operation Restore Trust published in 1996 (DHHS OEI-02-91-00861) focused on the five states with the highest number of Medicare and Medicaid beneficiaries. The Inspector General's report found that close to one-third of Medicare billed procedures, most often psychological testing and group therapy, were either not medically necessary or questionable. To guard against unfavorable audits, psychotherapy may be provided for major mental disorders, but the request for the service, as with all other mental health services, must come from the primary care provider in writing both on the consultation form and in the order sheet.

Presentation of a Case

On the eve of retirement, a 70-year-old corporate executive suffered a massive stroke. Heroic neurosurgical procedures saved his life but left him severely disabled. Upon admission to the nursing home, staff found his wife to be clinging and depressed and his children angry and demanding. Based on the patient's history and present condition there seemed little hope of significant recovery, and staff interpreted the family turmoil as resistance to mourning and separation. The oldest son in particular was frustrated that a more aggressive plan of rehabilitation had not been put in place. The family wasted no time in carrying their concerns to administration and a cascade of meetings followed. However, the relationship between staff and family became increasingly tense. There was a fundamental difference of opinion about the patient's prognosis best captured by one staff member's comment: "This family means well but they're just not being realistic—he'll never go home again." Staff felt that the family's request that the patient be evaluated by psychiatry for depression was little more than denial of the poor prognosis. Nonetheless, they were eager for a meeting with the family and the psychiatric consultant to decompress the situation. They also hoped to move the family to adjust to the patient's poor prognosis and to accept a less intensive level of care.

The consultant found the patient to be nearly somnolent but insightful when provided sufficient stimulation. Although the patient could not recall the date, he knew he was in a nursing home and that he needed help "with almost everything." He denied feeling depressed or hopeless. He was accurate about who in the family visited and how often and added, "They mean everything to me." There was an engaging quality to his rapport despite occasional lapses in attention. However, during physical therapy he seemed inattentive, drifting into sleep when not actively engaged. The goals of the physical care plan were indeed modest and included self-feeding but little else in the way of independence or ambulation. In an individual interview, his wife was tearful and admitted to being overwhelmed. The family interview included the resident's wife; son and his wife; staff from administration, medicine, nursing, social service, and rehabilitation; and the pastoral counselor.

The consultant framed the conference as a means to gain a clearer picture of the family's expectations as well as an avenue of support for both the patient and his wife. Any differences of opinion or perceptions could also be examined. The consultant asked not only for a recounting of medical events leading up to the nursing home admission but also for material about the patient's professional, social, and family life prior to his catastrophic illness. The wife, son, and daughter-in-law portrayed the patient as an exceptionally productive and sociable man who was an esteemed patriarch—the origin of much of the family's emotional and economic well being.

Immediately following the stroke, an emergency craniotomy had been required and was complicated by the need for a second surgical procedure within hours of the first. The man who had a week ago been chief executive of both his family and his corporation was poorly responsive and had been placed on combined phenytoin/phenobarbital therapy after surgery for seizure prophylaxis. The family was given an uncertain prognosis by a surgical staff whom they had barely met and who seemed pessimistic about any gains the patient might make in physical therapy. The psychiatry consultant recommended against transfer to a rehabilitation facility and showed little enthusiasm for bedside physical therapy.

At the nursing home the family was experiencing the same resistance previously encountered on the neurosurgery ward. They were aware of the poor prognosis, but they pointed out rightly that no one had attempted an aggressive rehabilitation approach. If it failed they could accept the result but would not accept the absence of a therapeutic trial. Moreover, this family catastrophe had occurred within less than 60 days. How could they accept the poor progress as definitive over so short a period given the fact that physical therapy had not been attempted with any degree of effort.

The psychiatric consultant responded, "It must be hard to maintain hope given all these obstacles, all the frustration," to which the daughter replied in tears, "That's why we keep pushing—to make sure Daddy has every chance. Nobody was prepared for this—we need him back home, not just for Mom but for all of us." Social work staff added, "Sometimes we need a push—you must have thought we didn't care." The consultant acknowledged that there was a genuine difference of opinion about prognosis but that there need not be any differences about testing the validity of the prognosis through a mutually agreed upon plan to push physical therapy, and that although he did not find that depression significantly contributed to the patient's disability, the somnolence might be related to the phenobarbital. Because the incidence of postsurgical seizures declines during the 6 months following craniotomy, it seemed reasonable to slowly taper the phenobarbital while continuing the phenytoin. Although the likelihood of full recovery seemed remote, a partial improvement might mean that round-the-clock nursing care would not be necessary. And with assistance, the patient just might return home with part-time help, which was well within the family's means.

As a result, a trial of increasingly aggressive physical therapy accompanied by a gradual reduction in the dose of phenobarbital was begun. The wife was seen in individual therapy by the social worker and was instructed by both nursing and physical therapy staff in ways to assist her husband's efforts to regain his strength and independence. With time the phenobarbital was eliminated and the patient became more accessible although with obvious deficits in cognition. The psychiatric consultant revisited and found no need for antidepressant medication or psychotherapy. Eight months after the stroke the former executive walked out of the nursing facility to return home with the help of his wife and the part-time home health aide.

CONSULTATION TO CERTIFIED HOME HEALTH AGENCIES: HOW TO MAKE A HOUSE CALL

Less than 5% of older community residents in need of mental health services receive care (Burns & Taube, 1990). Because of the stigma of mental illness and biases about the efficacy of mental health services in old age, older adults are less likely to be offered and to accept a referral for psychiatric care (Colenda et al., 1997). For frail elders the difficulty of travel compounds the problem. Older adults are reluctant to seek services for fear that disclosing their impairments would sacrifice their liberty. Case finding by social service agencies is also inadequate in that area agencies on aging and the mental health delivery systems lack systematic linkage (Lebowitz et al., 1987). Senior centers, service agencies, and nutrition programs may provide supportive services and counseling yet few seniors accept psychiatric consultation when agency staff recognize the need. As a result, few of these persons receive treatment and fewer still optimal treatment (Lasoski, 1986). The problem is all the more unfortunate because early intervention will prolong the older person's independence (Kennedy et al., 1996). Depression is a genuine risk factor for the development of dementia (Devanand et al., 1996). And the relationship between depression and disability is intimate and reciprocal (Kennedy et al., 1990, 1991). In addition, few seniors are aware of how advanced health directives (living will, health care proxy) can reduce their risk of unwanted end-of-life care. The result is an excess of avoidable disability (Kennedy, 1995). When coupled with the fact that treatment exists for depression and that treatments for the cognitive impairment of dementia are emerging, the implications for mental health practitioners are considerable (Kelman et al., 1994). Not surprisingly, Medicare-certified home health agencies are likely to encounter substantial unmet mental health needs among their older clients. Naturally occurring retirement communities (NORCs) also offer a unique opportunity to reduce the fragmentation of care.

Considerable information is available on specialized outreach programs for the mentally ill elderly (Cohen, 1996; Goldstein et al., 1993; Levy, 1985; Maddox & Glass,1989; Philipps & Liberman, 1988; Reifler et al., 1982) but not in the context of Medicare-certified home health agencies which have traditionally limited their services to nursing, social work, and physical or occupational therapy (Koren, 1986). Existing studies of outreach to the mentally ill elderly are descriptive with few controlled comparisons of interventions, personnel, or outcomes that might be used to establish the indications, benefits, cost offsets, or critical aspects of team composition. Nonetheless, they demonstrate a compelling need and document a variety of practical interventions and viable team configurations.

Among nonpsychiatric home care studies, measures of cost offsets, mortality, functional status, cognition, and rates of nursing home admission yield equivocal results. Failure to target appropriate patients and to manage the care and the care team may account for the observation that more home care means more cost without much improvement in the older person's function (Cummings & Weaver, 1991).

Between 1980 and 1990, the number of Medicare-certified home health agencies almost doubled, reaching an estimated annual cost of $4 billion. However, since 1987 more agency providers have left the Medicare market than entered due to tighter controls on eligibility criteria for the medical necessity of their services and the resultant uncertain profitability (Scalzi et al., 1994). In the present cost-containment environment, home care advocates will likely turn to other arguments, such as unmet needs (Ramsdell et al., 1989; Steele et al., 1987), consumer satisfaction (Kennedy et al., 1995), and the increase in late-life suicides (Mercer, 1989) to champion their cause.

Generalizations from Urban to Other Areas

I have previously reported my experience with two home care agencies in the Bronx (Kennedy et al., 1995). What follows is an abbreviated version emphasizing how the consultation principles apply to other areas as well. The Bronx Visiting Nurse Service outreach teams are composed of a full-time psychiatric nurse, social worker, and social work assistant as well as a part-time psychiatric consultant. Referrals come from clinics, community-based agencies, and the much larger non–mental health components of the parent agency. In-home care is envisioned as crisis intervention, evaluation, and referral with services terminated most often within 1 to 2 months.

The Montefiore Home Health Agency is the first hospital-based home health agency in the United States. Most referrals come from Montefiore Medical Center, an acute care hospital which is a major affiliate of the Albert Einstein College of Medicine. The agency's clientele are mainly isolated, physically disabled older persons.

At the Montefiore agency the new psychiatrist took a more active role, including direct treatment of a limited number of patients, educational conferences with staff, and introduction of a team approach to difficult cases. The consultant also coordinated psychiatric hospitalization and emergency room assessments. Initially this approach encountered resistance. First the agency retained a false dichotomy between mental and physical disorders and identified its mission as attention to the latter and an avoidance of the former. Efforts to screen out the mentally ill prior to admission reinforced the illusion that mental health problems were beyond the staff's responsibilities. Second, staff had received little training in mental health care. Because they did not expect to provide mental health services they did not always appreciate the need for mental health care skills. Finally, staff harbored unrealistic expectations regarding the psychiatrist, expecting to be magically relieved of problems once the psychiatrist "took over."

Case conferences were used to teach staff early signs of depression and dementia as well as effective responses to suicidality. Teaching in the field with referring staff generalized concepts introduced in the conferences to the home visits. The conferences imparted information and allowed staff to acquire a sense of mastery. Staff became less likely to act out uncertainty by denying the problem or shifting it to the psychiatrist.

When a new psychogeriatric consultant joined the Visiting Nurse Service, she entered an established team of mental health specialists but encountered similar problems. Differences in perspectives and priorities among the various disciplines were not uncommon. Referrals to the psychiatrist were most often focused on questions of impaired judgment, suicide risk and need for hospitalization, or institution of pharmacotherapy prior to linkage to clinic. The decision whether or not to hospitalize determined the immediacy of action. As a result, other treatment options were deemed less important because the team rarely provided other than brief, supportive psychotherapy. In addition, referral sites were expected to perform any procedures necessary for diagnosis and treatment so that the psychiatrist's interest in the diagnosis was viewed as a peripheral concern when the central question was whether or not to refer. Nonetheless, efforts to clarify the diagnosis, particularly when physical and mental disorders coexisted, remained essential to a more nuanced referral or to steps that might facilitate the acceptance of services.

At the outset, both staff and patients resisted an in-home visit from the psychiatrist. The former because their work became the subject of review by an as yet unincorporated team member; the latter because the nurses and social workers were seen as less of a threat than the psychiatrist. In response, the new psychiatrist used ongoing team meetings to invest herself in the group, to develop a collaborative educational expectation from colleagues, and to avoid overly rigid role definitions. It became clear that each clinical discipline brought a unique perspective to patient care but that much of their techniques and goals were overlapping. By acknowledging the shared character of clinical authority in the field, the psychiatrist's expertise was enhanced rather than devalued. The psychiatrist also began to meet periodically with chiefs of the various psychiatry and medicine clinics, which served as reception sites for referrals as well as a source of requests for in-home evaluations. These meetings reinforced cross-agency collaboration by clarifying referral procedures and admissions criteria, personalizing the bureaucracy of care and resolving disputes about the appropriateness of patient referrals.

In summary, at both agencies the incoming psychiatric consultants needed to form alliances and adapt their personal styles to the needs of the team and the administrative structure of the organization. Opportunities for leadership and teaching expanded once the dynamics of team interactions and the socialization of new members were in hand.

Survey of Referrals

Both the Montefiore Home Health Agency and the Visiting Nurse Service's Community Mental Health Outreach are certified home health agencies and serve the Bronx, where 150,000 persons ages 65 or older reside. Despite their contrasting missions, the survey of referrals found more similarities than differences. In both programs one-third of referrals were for persons 80 years of age or older and more than two-thirds were women. The most frequent diagnoses were disorders of mood or cognition, with anxiety and adjustment disorders amounting to less than one-fifth of all referrals. Suicidality was a problem of similar proportions, although the percentage of persons hospitalized by the Visiting Nurse Service Mental Health team was twice that of the Montefiore Home Health Agency. Also, more psychotic community residents were seen by the Visiting Nurse Service. Neither program was particularly successful in referring patients to outpatient clinics, which was not surprising given the nature of the referrals.

For the Visiting Nurse Service Mental Health Outreach team, 427 cases from referrals ages 55 and older were opened. Slightly less than one-third were referred for mental health consultation from within the parent home health agency. Close to one-quarter of cases were triaged to other agencies before consultation or not contacted because hospitalization or death intervened. Most of this group were persons requiring emergency medical care, the guardianship procedures of the Protective Services for Adults agency, or home health aide services for uncomplicated cases of dementia. More than one-third of patients either refused further services or resolved their presenting problems with one intervention. A number of these patients consented only to follow-up treatment by their primary care physician.

Case 1. A recently widowed woman with crippling cardiac valve disease had neglected her nutrition, hydration, and medication and admitted, "I would jump out the window but I haven't the courage." Her daughter in Virginia was contacted and informed that hospitalization seemed the only safe treatment plan given her deteriorating car-

diac status and suicidal expressions. She accepted psychiatric hospitalization only to reject it the next day. Because of uncertainty as to her
safety, both from cardiac collapse as well as from suicide, the Visiting
Nurse Service determined that continued in-home service was not reasonable, which precipitated a crisis. An order for an involuntary emergency room evaluation was obtained and the patient was admitted
over her objection to a psychiatric facility. Her daughter arrived threatening suit if her mother was not discharged to her care. The mother re-
canted her suicidal intent and accepted a home health aide and case
management services, which her daughter arranged before returning
south. She did not pursue psychiatric follow-up but developed an effective reliance on the home health aide and remained well.

This case illustrates several ethical dilemmas. Civil procedures
available to coerce the vulnerable person into a safe care plan are bureaucratic and time-consuming and may be traumatic. The power to
coerce care inevitably means that some parties will be unhappy with
the process even when the results seem ideal. The imperatives of respect for patient autonomy and the physician's responsibility not to
abandon an imperiled person pose a dilemma which can be managed
but not always resolved. Risk management that merely avoids malpractice actions is neither satisfying for the clinicians nor adequate for
agency policy. Consultants in ethics affiliated with an academic medical center offer added perspectives on rights, responsibilities, risk/
benefit analyses, and the decision making process that so often determines the outcome of perplexing situations (Hamerman et al., 1991).

Case 2. A retired pharmacist, discharged from the hospital after
hip fracture repair, found his disability unacceptable and his wife un-
sympathetic. He threatened suicide with pills. The home health agency
psychiatrist found the patient to have a major depression and arranged
for his wife to monitor sedatives. The patient responded positively to a
"no-suicide" contract with the psychiatrist. However, following several episodes of diarrhea, which required his wife's assistance, he felt
humiliated and threatened suicide when she was about to leave the
house, a threat she brushed off with characteristic sarcasm. He took 15
pills and was discovered by the home health aide and taken to the hospital by the Emergency Medical Service ambulance. At the end of a
short stay on the psychiatric unit, the home care team attended discharge planning and welcomed him back to their service, the first time
the agency had reinstituted care for a psychiatric admission.

Case 3. A man with end-stage renal disease and coronary atherosclerosis, who was apathetic, irritable, and slept poorly, denied depres-

sion and the need for treatment. After six sessions of in-home psychotherapy he accepted antidepressant medication. His mood improved and his internist agreed to monitor the medication. A short course of psychotherapy from the consulting psychiatrist had been necessary to gain acceptance of antidepressant medication.

Case 4. A person with severe pulmonary disease and history of stroke left her nursing home after securing the services of the home health agency. However, she was condescending and intolerant of home health aides who were not of her race, so much so that she ultimately refused all assistance, leading the agency to consider discharging her. The consulting psychiatrist was asked to prescribe medication to make her more tractable. The psychiatrist and director of social services made a joint visit but medication was not prescribed and the request to discharge the patient was challenged. Instead, the approach was shifted to an explanation of the patient's narcissistic personality disorder, her propensity to split staff into rescuers or persecutors, and her overblown sense of entitlement—all of which undercut her ability to gain the care she so clearly needed. A team approach was adopted, with the focus shifted to management of her personality disorder rather than indignation over her bigotry.

Four points emerge from the cases. First, socially isolated older persons with medical and psychiatric vulnerability are unsettling to serve in a context in which the providers have little control over the circumstances of care. Often a party other than the patient is requesting the service. As a result, patient trust and motivation may be less than desired. The mental health practitioner may feel pulled between two masters: the patient and the agency. Decisions to initiate or withhold treatment may be challenging. The agency may not be able to continue treatment indefinitely. Moreover, without the capacity to monitor compliance and adverse reactions, medication may not be safe. Ultimately the patient and physician may find themselves working at cross-purposes.

Second, home health agencies encounter pathology similar to that seen by specialized mental health outreach teams. However, they are unlikely to be overwhelmed by a seriously and persistently mentally ill and demented clientele. Arguing from experience with rural populations, Abraham et al. (1993) found that despite differing demographic, economic, cultural, and ethnic characteristics between two model outreach programs, one in Iowa the other in Virginia, the diagnostic mix was similar. Mood disorders were more prevalent than dementias but "coping/adjustment" disorders were the most frequently encountered diagnoses with anxiety, thought disorders, and substance abuse each accounting for 5% or less. The "coping/adjust-ment" category consisted of persons struggling with physical illness and disability themselves or with the care of a demented or disabled relative. My experience with a decidedly urban sample demonstrates similar proportions of the major diagnostic categories. Most important, persons with mood disturbances and coping/adjustment disorders should be relatively responsive to recognized, perhaps even modest interventions. They represent the group most likely to demonstrate cost offsets and the greatest gains in well being as a result of mental health home care.

Third, for effective referrals, the linkage across clinical disciplines and provider agencies requires foresight and incentives to be effective. Physicians are not well prepared for fieldwork in the community. Less than half of all U.S. medical schools require a home-care experience of their students (Steel et al., 1994). Fellowship-trained physicians from geriatric medicine or geriatric psychiatry programs have been required to work with a health care team and to make house calls, but their numbers will never be adequate to meet the need. Providing a contin-uum of care for home-bound isolated older community residents may require physicians to take on more of a case manager role. The burden of setting aside time for liaison activities both within the team and out-side the agency is considerable and represents a sizable challenge to funding sources.

Fourth, a substantial minority of frail seniors will need cardiovas-cular, orthopedic, or neurological procedures only available in a hospi-tal. These procedures remain more remunerative than routine, preven-tive, or outpatient care. As a result, services that capture patient needs for these more remunerative procedures offer an obvious incentive to the hospital. This is critical to the acute care technology available to re-verse stroke and heart attack, provided the patient receives the treat-ment within hours of symptom onset. In theory, then, the costs of home-based care may be offset by the increase in highly reimbursed procedures. From the public health point of view, these procedures are designed to prevent dependency as well as to save lives. The preven-tion of dependency translates into reduced caregiver burden, reduced nursing home admissions, and reduced costs of long-term institutional care, a health and economic goal shared by young and old alike.

Fifth, the relations between the home care team and the psychiat-ric consultant require skillful management. The Montefiore Home Health Agency, with a mission of care for physical disorders, tended to refer more patients than necessary for psychiatric evaluation and follow-up. In contrast, the Visiting Nurse Service's Geriatric Mental Health team needed encouragement to seek the psychiatric consultant's input beyond evaluations for admission, impaired decisional capacity, or involuntary care.

Whatever the future of Medicare, it is doubtful that the number of older adults in need of in-home psychiatric care will decrease or that the interdisciplinary, interagency problems we identified will disappear. To the extent that home care services survive in a cost-contained environment, recommendations for mental health consultants follow.

Recommendations for Mental Health Consultants to Home Care Agencies

- Consultants have little control over events in the community without the patient or a third party authorizing their actions or acting on their behalf. By behaving as an invited guest and team player, the consultant will less often be seen as a meddling intruder.
- Even when fully integrated into an existing team, the consultant's role in the agency remains that of consultant. Given the fluidity of clinical authority in home care, consultants may lead but more often they follow.
- Referrals of persons with persistent psychotic disorders and dementia may require considerable resources but they represent the minority of the case load and should not justify an agency's reluctance to provide mental health services.
- Consultants should review cases carefully before the home visit to identify critical issues and to make their colleague's latent agenda manifest. Biomedical and psychological dynamics may be of little use without an awareness of the social and financial situation.
- In-home treatment is not risk free. The consultant may minimize the chances of an adverse outcome, but risk cannot be eliminated. The informed-consent model in which risks, benefits, and alternatives are prioritized for the patient and family to accept or reject is most useful.
- Precipitating a crisis may be the only way to resolve an unsafe or intolerable situation. Altering the household equilibrium may threaten an enmeshed family for economic as well as psychodynamic reasons.
- Respect for patient autonomy and the physician's responsibility not to abandon imperiled persons pose an ethical dilemma that may be managed but not always resolved.
- Access to a consultant in law and ethics from an academic med-

ical center should be sought out to clarify the ethical dilemmas. Avoidance of tort liability is not a sufficiently high standard of excellence in care.

- Liaison with entities that give and receive the home care agency's referrals is an essential aspect of the consultant's job. Management of emergencies and admissions will be greatly facilitated.

- With support from the agency or family, the consultant will be able to administer a wide range of treatments from brief psychotherapy to the in-home management of suicidality.

SUMMARY

Effective geriatric mental health consultation requires a similar approach to the older patient no matter where the consultation is carried out. The consultant must compensate for the patient's sensory and cognitive deficits. Fears of abandonment, helplessness, isolation, and loss must be recognized. The needs of the staff and family caregivers must also be addressed. And to have genuine authority, the consultant must be aligned with the administrative and organizational culture of the care setting. However, the service delivery model will differ markedly by site. Consultants to residential health care facilities (nursing homes) and certified home health agencies (home care) should adopt a more psychosocial or liaison mode with a broader field for intervention and a longer-term orientation. The regulatory environment and staffing patterns make the consultation focus on the caregiving group as well as on the patient. Despite the prevalence of dementia, longer-term psychotherapy may be feasible due to the patient's accessibility. And a more complex, longitudinal approach to psychopharmacology is possible because the patients remain in place.

In contrast, the more medically modeled, patient-centered, or pure consultation approach may be best in the general hospital ward and emergency room. Here the pace is fast, the request is more often emergent, and access to the patient limited. However, the administrative hierarchy and regulatory environment of acute care is less of a burden. Disorders of cognition, more often delirium, may be the most frequent diagnoses so that facility with the evaluation of capacity and participation in end-of-life care are critical for the consultant. Skill with short-term psychotherapy and the emergency use of psychotropics are equally important.

Fellowship-trained geriatric psychiatrists will have worked in nursing homes and hospitals and have made house calls as part of their mandatory rotations. However, most practicing mental health specialists in geriatrics will have acquired these skills through clinical experience. The material presented here is meant to enhance the practices of that latter group. It is also offered to the primary care providers to expand their expectations of mental health consultants.

REFERENCES

Abraham, I. L., Buckwalter, K. C., Snustad, D. G., et al. (1993). Psychogeriatric outreach to rural families: The Iowa and Virginia Models. *International Psychogeriatrics, 5,* 203–211.

Adler, G., Shapiro, L.N. (1973). Some difficulties in the treatment of the aggressive acting out patient. *America Journal of Psychotherapy, 27,* 548.

Bienenfeld, D., Wheeler, B. G. (1989). Psychiatric services to nursing homes: A liaison model. *Hospital and Community Psychiatry, 40,* 793–794.

Borson, S., Lipzin, B., Nininger, J., et al. (1989). Psychiatry and the nursing home. *American Journal of Psychiatry, 144,* 1412–1418.

Burns, B. J., Taube, C. A. (1990). Mental health services in general medical care and nursing homes. In B. Fogel, A. Furino, & G. Gottlieb (Eds.), *Mental health policy for older Americans* (pp. 63–84). Washington, DC: American Psychiatric Press.

Butler, R. N. (1975). *Why survive: Growing old in America.* New York: Harper & Row.

Caplan, G. (1970). *The theory and practice of mental health consultation.* New York: Basic Books.

Cohen, C. I. (1996). Integrated community services. In J. Sadavoy, L. W. Lazarus, L. F. Jarvik, et al. (Eds.), *Comprehensive review of geriatric psychiatry—II* (pp. 1003–1034). Washington, DC: American Psychiatric Press.

Colenda, C. C., Greenwald, B. S., Crosset, J. H. W., et al. (1997). Barriers to effective psychiatric emergency services for elderly persons. *Psychiatric Services, 48,* 321–325.

Cummings, J. E., Weaver, F. M. (1991). Cost-effectiveness of home care. *Clinics in Geriatric Medicine, 7,* 865–873.

Devanand, D. P., Sano, M., Tang, M., et al. (1996). Depressed mood and the incidence of Alzheimer's disease in the elderly living in the community. *Archives of General Psychiatry, 53,* 175–182.

DiBella, G. A. W. (1979). Educating staff to manage threatening paranoid patients. *American Journal of Psychiatry, 130,* 207.

Dubin, W. R. (1981). Evaluating and managing the violent patient. *Annals of Emergency Medicine, 10,* 481–484.

Florio, E. A., Jensen, J. E., Hendryx, M., et al. (1998). One year outcomes of older adults referred for aging and mental health services by community gatekeepers. *Journal of Case Management, 7,* 74–83.

Gallagher, R. M., McCann, W. J., Jerman A., et al. (1990). The behavioral medicine service: An administrative model for biopsychosocial medical care, teaching, and research. *General Hospital Psychiatry, 12,* 283–295.

Goldberg, R. L. (1989). Geriatric consultation/liaison psychiatry. In N. Billig, P. V. Rabins, S. Krager, et al. (Ed.), *Issues in geriatric psychiatry, advances in psychosomatic medicine* (pp. 138–150). Basel: Krager.

Goldstein, M. Z., Colenda, C. C., Kennedy, G. J., et al. (1993). *Models of geropsychiatric practice.* Washington, DC: American Psychiatric Press.

Gottlieb, E., Waxman, H. M., Carner, E. D., et al. (1982). Geriatric psychiatry in the emergency department: Characteristics of geriatric and non-geriatric admissions. *Journal of the American Geriatric Society, 30,* 427.

Greenhill, M. H. (1979). Models of liaison programs that address age and cultural differences in reaction to illness. *Bibliotecha Psychiatrica, 159,* 77–81.

Greenhill, M. H., Kilgore, S. R. (1950). Principles of methodology in teaching the psychiatric approach to medical house officers. *Psychosomatic Medicine, 12,* 38–48.

Gurland, B., Toner, J., Mustille, A., et al. (1988). The organization of mental health services for the elderly. In L. Lazarus et al. (Eds.), *Essentials of geriatric psychiatry* (pp. 189–213). New York: Springer.

Hamel, M. B., Goldman, L., Teno, J., et al. (1995). Identification of comatose patients at high risk for death or severe disability: Support investigators. Study to understand prognoses and preferences for outcomes and risks of treatment. *Journal of the American Medical Association, 273,* 1842–1848.

Hamerman, D., Kennedy, R. D., Schulmerich, S., et al. (1991). The academic medical center and the community: Health care for the elderly. *Pride Institute Journal of Long Term Home Health Care, 10,* 42–52.

Health Care Financing Administration. (1991, September 26). Medicare and Medicaid: Requirements for long term care facilities, final regulations. *Federal Register, 56,* 48,865–48,921.

Health Care Financing Administration. (1992a, April). *State operations manual: Provider certification* (Transmittal No. 250). Washington, DC: U.S. Government Printing Office.

Health Care Financing Administration. (1992b, November 30). Medicare and Medicaid programs: Readmission screening and annual resident review. *Federal Register, 57,* 56,450–56,504.

Health Care Financing Administration. (1992c, December 28). Medicare and Medicaid: Resident assessment in long term care facilities. *Federal Register, 57,* 61,614–61,733.

Jackson, J. M. (1997). Nursing home practice. In A. P. Siegal, J. M. Jackson, G. Moak (Eds.), *Geriatric psychiatry practice management handbook* (pp. 5-1–5-77). Washington, DC: American Association for Geriatric Psychiatry.

Kayser-Jones, J. (1995). Decision making in the treatment of acute illness in nursing homes: Framing the decision problem, treatment plan, and outcome. *Medical Anthropology Quarterly, 9,* 236–256.

Kelman, H. R., Thomas, C., Kennedy, G. J., et al. (1994). Cognitive impairment and mortality in older community residents. *American Journal of Public Health, 84,* 914–919.

Kennedy, G. J. (1995). The geriatric syndrome of late-life depression. *Psychiatric Services, 46,* 43–48.

Kennedy, G. J., Inuogu, E., Lowinger, R. (1999). Psychogeriatric emergencies: Rapid response and life-saving therapies. *Geriatrics, 54,* 38–46.

Kennedy, G. J., Katsnelson, N., Laitman, L., et al. (1995). Psychogeriatric services at certified home health agencies. *American Journal of Geriatric Psychiatry, 3,* 339–347.

Kennedy, G. J., Kelman, H. R., Thomas, C. (1990). The emergence of depressive symptoms in late life: The importance of declining health and increasing disability. *Journal of Community Health, 15,* 93–104.

Kennedy, G. J., Kelman, H. R., Thomas, C. (1991). Persistence and remission of depressive symptoms in late life. *American Journal of Psychiatry, 148,* 174–178.

Kennedy, G. J., Lowinger, R., Metz, H. (1996). Epidemiology and inferences regarding the etiology of late life suicide. In G. J. Kennedy (Ed.), *Suicide and depression in late life: Critical issues in treatment, research and public policy* (pp. 3–22). New York: Wiley.

Kiloh, L. G. (1961). Pseudo-dementia. *Acta Psychiatrica Scandinavica, 37,* 336–351.

Koren, M. J. (1986). Home care—Who cares? *New England Journal of Medicine, 314,* 917–920.

Lasoski, M. C. (1986). Reasons for low utilization of mental health services by the elderly. In T. L. Brink (Ed.), *Clinical gerontology: A guide to assessment and intervention* (pp. 1–18). Binghamton, NY: Haworth Press.

Lebowitz, D. B., Light, E., Bailkey, F. (1987). Mental health center services for the elderly: The impact of coordination with area agencies on aging. *Gerontologist, 27,* 699–702.

Levy, M. T. (1985). Psychiatric assessment of elderly patients in the home. *Journal of the American Geriatrics Society, 33,* 9–12.

Lion, J. R., Pasternak, S. A. (1973). Countertransference reaction to violent patients. *American Journal of Psychiatry, 130,* 207.

Lipowski, Z. (1983). The need to integrate liaison psychiatry and geropsychiatry. *American Journal of Psychiatry, 140,* 1003–1005.

Lippert, G. P., Conn, D., Schogt, B., et al. (1990). Psychogeriatric consultation: General hospital versus home for the aged. *General Hospital Psychiatry, 12,* 313–318.

Maddox, G. L., Glass, T. A. (1989). The continuum of care: Movement toward the community. In E. W. Busse & D. G. Blazer (Eds.), *Geriatric psychiatry* (pp. 635–667). Washington, DC: American Psychiatric Press.

McKegney, F. P., Schwartz, C. E. (1986). Behavioral medicine: Treatment and organizational issues. *General Hospital Psychiatry, 8,* 330–339.

Mercer, S. O. (1989). *Elder suicide: A national survey of prevention and intervention programs.* Washington, DC: American Association of Retired Persons.

Mohl, P. C. (1979). The liaison psychiatrist: Social role and status. *Psychosomatics, 20,* 19–23.

Omnibus Reconciliation Act of 1987. Public Law No. 100–203, Subtitle C, Nursing Home Reform. Washington, DC: U.S. Government Printing Office.

Perez, E., Silverman, M., Blouin, B. (1985). Psychiatric consultation to elderly medical and surgical inpatients in a general hospital. *Psychiatric Quarterly, 57*, 18–22.

Philipps, C., Liberman, R. P. (1988). Community support. In R. P. Liberman (Ed.), *Psychiatric rehabilitation of chronic mental patients* (pp. 285–311). Washington, DC: American Psychiatric Press.

Popkin, M., Mackensie, T., Callies, A. (1984). Psychiatric consultation to geriatric medically ill inpatients in a university hospital. *Archives of General Psychiatry, 41*, 703–707.

Ramsdell, J. W., Swart, J. A., Jackson, J. E., et al. (1989). The yield of a home visit in the assessment of geriatric patients. *Journal of the American Geriatrics Society, 37*, 17–24.

Reifler, B. V., Kethley, A., O'Neill, P., et al. (1982). Five-year experience of a community outreach program for the elderly. *American Journal of Psychiatry, 139*, 220–223.

Rosse, R., Ciolino, C., Gural, L. (1986). Utilization of psychiatric consultation with an elderly medically ill inpatient population in a VA hospital. *Military Medicine, 151*, 583–586.

Rovner, B. W., German, P. S., Broadhead, J., et al. (1990). The prevalence and management of dementia and other psychiatric disorders in nursing homes. *International Psychogeriatrics, 2*, 13–24.

Ruskin, P. (1985). Geropsychiatric consultation in a university hospital: A report on 67 referrals. *American Journal of Psychiatry, 142*, 333–336.

Salamon, I. (1976). Violent and aggressive behavior. In R. A. Glick, A. T. Myerson (Eds.), *Psychiatric emergencies* (p. 109). New York: Grune & Stratton.

Scalzi, C. C., Zinn, J. S., Guilfoyle, M. J., et al. (1994). Medicare-certified home heath services: National and regional supply in the 1980's. *American Journal of Public Health, 84*, 1646–1648.

Sloane, P. D. (1998). Advances in the treatment of Alzheimer's disease. *American Family Physician, 58*, 1577–1586, 1589–1590.

Small, G., Fawzy, F. (1988). Psychiatric consultation for the medically ill elderly in the general hospital. Need for a collaborative model of care. *Psychosomatics, 29*, 94–103.

Smyer, M. A., Cohn, M. D., Brannon, D. (1988). *Mental health consultation in nursing homes.* New York: New York University Press.

Steel, R. K., Muslinger, M., Boling, P. A. (1994). Medical schools and home care [Letter to the Editor]. *New England Journal of Medicine, 331*, 1098–1099.

Steele, K. S., Bissonette, A., et al. (1987, October). *The home as a model setting for geriatric assessment.* NIH Consensus Development Conference.

Strain, J. J., Pincus, H. A., Houpt, J. L., et al. (1985). Models of mental health training for primary care physicians. *Psychosomatic Medicine, 47*, 95–110.

Streim, J. E., Rovner, B. W., Katz, I. R. (1996). Psychiatric aspects of nursing home care. In J. Sadavoy, L. W. Lazarus, L. F. Jarvik, et al. (Eds.), *Comprehensive review of geriatric psychiatry—II* (pp. 907–936). Washington, DC: American Psychiatric Press.

Unützer, J., Small, G. W. (1996). Geriatric consultation-liaison psychiatry. In J. Sadavoy, L. W. Lazarus, L. F. Jarvik, et al. (Eds.), *Comprehensive review of ge-*

riatric psychiatry—II (pp. 937–1002). Washington, DC: American Psychiatric Press.

Walker, J. I. (1983). *Psychiatric emergencies: Intervention and resolution.* Philadelphia: Lippincott.

Zarit, S. H., Zarit, J. M. (1998). Consultation in institutional settings. In *Mental disorders in older adults* (pp. 320–346). New York: Guilford Press.

14

Legal and Ethical Issues

The power of modern medicine threatens to outdistance public and professional notions of appropriate ethical behavior. The expansion of life-saving treatments has led to an expansion of both choice and conflict. Since the end of World War II, the balance of power has shifted from physician to patient to managed care organization; from paternalism to bureaucratic parsimony (Siegler, 1985). And the mercantilism of managed care has intensified inherent conflicts between patient and provider and added an entirely new set of disputes (Dubler, 1998; La Puma & Scheidermayer, 1996; Sorum, 1996). It will take time to evolve the rituals and relationships necessary for a new consensus. To cope with the growing ethical dilemmas faced by their patients and colleagues, practitioners need an awareness of the history of patient autonomy, decisional capacity assessment, bioethics consultation, and mediation techniques. These include the dynamic use of moral debate and principled positions to clarify if not balance the interests of those in conflict (Dubler & Nimmons, 1992). Common to all are the ideals of patient self-determination and well-being. What follows are history, principles, and procedures to approach both.

MODERN HISTORY OF THE DOCTOR–PATIENT RELATIONSHIP

The Nuremberg Code was developed in 1947 by American judges during the Doctors' Trial, which examined Nazi physicians accused of carrying out inhumane experiments with concentration camp prisoners (Shuster, 1997). Although the document focused on research with human subjects, it signaled a fundamental change in the doctor–patient balance of power. In the Hippocratic tradition, greater weight was given for the paternalistic authority of the physician to affect the patient's best interests (Sachs & Cassel, 1994). Physicians adhered to a set of principles that governed practice. The physician's assumed pledge of beneficence and nonmalfeasance (do no harm) added integrity to that authority. With the Nuremberg Code the balance shifted to a more patient-centered approach in which the physician's preferences or autonomy were given less weight. But there are other attributes of the relationship beyond its balance of power.

Although contractual on the surface, the relationship at depth is more fiduciary and covenantal (Finns, 1999). In the fee-for-service treatment setting, practitioners operate in the interests of their patients. In clinical research and in managed care, practitioners serve other interests as well. Yet clinical practice will progress slowly if at all without wider patient participation in research. The development of generalizable knowledge is critical in situations where the best treatment may be unknown. And given a finite level of resources, cost control will continue to be a legitimate concern for the patient, practitioner, and the public at large. Past inequities and unjust practices ensure that what ideally is a collaborative relationship runs the risk of becoming adversarial. This is especially true in the United States now that universal access to care has all but disappeared from partisan debate. The times demand greater openness and clarity in decision making. Practitioners need to develop the ability to identify genuine choices for the patient, to support the process of choosing, and to mediate the inevitable conflict. Because the avoidance of malpractice liability is the lowest ethical standard of care, practitioners, whether in managed care or otherwise, should ascribe to a higher set of principles.

AUTONOMY, ABANDONMENT, AND THE SANCTITY OF LIFE

At the heart of these principles are three elements. First is individual autonomy, the competent person's right to self-determination including the right to refuse necessary care. Respect for autonomy includes accepting the patient's preferences even when they represent bad or ill-considered judgment (Brock & Wartman, 1990). However, the second element, the professional's duty not to abandon, argues that the practitioner should not arbitrarily sever the relationship with a patient. The practitioner should also act in the patient's best medical interest when the person is endangered by impaired judgment (Kapp, 1992). In practical terms, if the patient refuses a necessary treatment as a direct result of cognitive impairment, it is abandonment for the physician to simply acquiesce. Similarly, if a patient sought treatment out of misinformation or delusional beliefs, it would be abandonment to provide unnecessary or inappropriate care. Finally respect for autonomy is entirely compatible with giving advice and arguing for what the practitioner thinks is best

Although respect for personal autonomy and the duty not to abandon imperiled persons are separate in the abstract, they are intimately linked in practice. Their linkage depends on the person's decisional capacity, the seriousness of the threat that the medical condition or situation poses, and the practitioner's capacity to reduce that threat. When the threat is equivocal, the prognosis uncertain, and the options for intervention ambiguous, capacity is less of a concern when a patient refuses. Any preference may seem reasonable. However, when the prognosis is dire and the intervention is likely to be highly beneficial, the patient's refusal will raise concerns about judgment, capacity, and possibly mental illness. Finally, the concept of the sanctity or dignity of life adds a metaphysical and to some a compelling aspect to the more individualistic concepts of autonomy and abandonment. Suicide and euthanasia may be seen to violate the dignity of life and trump concerns for individual autonomy.

Informed Consent and the Limits to Autonomy

Key to respect for autonomy and the duty not to abandon are the doctrine of informed consent and the ethic of truthfulness. Stated simply, patients have the right to know their diagnosis and prognosis as well as the risks, benefits, burdens, and alternatives of any proposed treatment or diagnostic procedure. However, the extent of information that should be conveyed for consent to be truly informed depends on the patient and the procedure. The goal is to inform rather than overburden. Many older persons rely on the beneficence and judgment of the physician when considering a procedure. Indeed, some will purposefully delegate their moral agency to the physician or family members. They may wish to minimize anxiety or irrational concerns that hearing about complications may make them more likely to occur. In some cultures important individual decisions are by tradition delegated to the family authority. No decision is considered valid until a family consensus has been reached (Alpers & Lo, 1999). Respect for the patients' wishes that others play a part, even take the lead, in decision making does not violate their autonomy as long as it is their choice and they appreciate the consequences. Their physical assent remains essential even if they delegate the responsibility for consent to others. One cannot force a person to act autonomously or to consider options with care and circumspection. Impaired persons may be coerced into receiving care by court order but the process is hardly one of informed consent.

For procedures in which it is assumed that the average person is readily familiar and the risk minimal (physical exam, venipuncture, X ray) informed consent is assumed by the patient's gesture of acceptance. However, for invasive procedures or research participation, a discussion of risks, benefits, and burdens is conducted and documented with the patient's signature. For elaborate procedures such as heart transplant the consent process may be carried out over several days by a multidisciplinary team and involve family members as well as the patient. The quality (personal relevance) of the information provided for consent and the process of informing the patient are more important than the completeness of the consent form. The patient's signature on the consent form is just the accepted standard of proof that the consent process occurred and successfully engaged the patient. However, it may not indicate that the patient had the capacity to provide genuinely informed consent. Questions of capacity cannot always be resolved before the consent process begins, but they must be resolved before the process ends. The educational component inherent in the consent process should offer the potential of better protecting the patient.

Delegated or Negotiated Autonomy

Procedures and care plans that are burdensome to the patient will likely be burdensome to the family. Thus when a treatment is burdensome and dependent on persons beyond the patient to be put in effect, those persons' moral and personal interests are also at stake. For example, hospitalized older adults whose nursing care needs (colostomy care, indwelling catheter, total assistance with activities of daily living) will persist after discharge may prefer that family provide for all aspects of care once they return home. Many families gladly learn the necessary techniques and shoulder the routine without complaint. Others may feel overwhelmed and prefer the assistance of a visiting nurse or home health aides. The patient has no inherent right to force the family or the physician to accept the burden of ongoing care or the responsibilities of delegated decision making. With regard to purely medical decisions, patient autonomy is central. In decisions that involve the rights and interests of others, accommodation rather than autonomy is the relevant principle (Callopy, 1995)

As an example, with persons whose dementia has progressed to the point that constant supervision is necessary for safe care, the patient may prefer not to have strangers in the home and may decline a home health aide or attendance at a day-care center, leaving the spouse seemingly trapped. The alternative may be nursing home admission. The autonomy of both the patient and the dementia caregiver are at stake (Kane, 1993). In these examples it is reasonable to ask patients to negotiate their preferences in line with the preferences of those on whom they rely. Autonomy implies responsibility as well as capacity. When independence is compromised, autonomy may need to be negotiated.

ASSESSMENT OF DECISION MAKING: COMPETENCE OR CAPACITY?

Determining when and why a person's decisional capacity is impaired is a common problem in geriatric care. The approach to the assessment of decisional capacity is one of common sense rather than diagnosis and is informed by the patient's functioning both in the present and past. Often the consultant will not be able to resist pressure to render a "competent or not" opinion. In the majority of instances, the status of the patient's capacity is obvious. Some obviously impaired patients have family members who make their decisions, who act as *de facto* guardians (surrogate decision makers). However, guardians whether court appointed or otherwise may not always act in the patient's best interest or defer in instances in which the patient may be capable of expressing an informed opinion. Similarly, the person is more likely considered capable when he or she assents rather than when he or she refuses the physician's recommendation. It is presumed that the physician is operating in the patient's best interest, particularly when the risk-to-benefit ratio of the proposed treatment seems highly favorable. It is in the gray zone, where either capacity or the desirability of an intervention is uncertain, where formal assessment procedures are needed. When a person's competence is called into question, a number of principals can guide the practitioner to a more nuanced determination of decisional capacity, as summarized in Table 14.1.

Competence is a legal term for the societal presumption that an adult is able to enter into a contract, make a last will and testament, or participate in his or her defense during civil or criminal proceedings (Roca, 1994). Incompetence may be *de jure* (i.e., formally declared by judicial proceeding) or *de facto* (obvious or suspected given the circumstance). Competence and capacity are used interchangeably in clinical settings, but it is capacity that is the issue in health decisions. Unlike the more categorical legal concept of competence, capacity may fluctuate over time depending on the moment-to-moment health and aware-

TABLE 14.1. Principles of Decisional Capacity Assessment

- Competence and capacity are used interchangeably, but it is capacity that is the issue in clinical settings.
- Capacity may fluctuate but still be adequate.
- Decisional capacity is specific to the circumstance.
- The adequacy of capacity depends on the risks, benefits, and burdens of proposed intervention and the consequences of the specific choice.
- Decisionally capable persons should be able to:
  1. Understand they are being asked to make a choice and express the choice consistently.
  2. Appreciate the nature of their condition including diagnosis, prognosis, and possible treatments.
  3. Balance the risks, benefits, and burdens of various choices.
  4. Apply a relatively stable set of values to the choice of available options.
  5. Communicate the rationale behind the choices.
- The exercise of poor judgment is not synonymous with impaired capacity.
- Decisionally capable persons who are aware of the consequences of their choices are allowed to assume the resultant risks.
- A psychiatric evaluation is advisable when decisional capacity is in question.
- When patients lack capacity, they should be protected from the consequences of impaired decisions.
- When capacity is indeterminate, other factors external to the patient are given consideration (e.g., caregivers, family).
- When the patient has capacity but makes an unwise decision, there may yet be areas of agreement that support a collaborative, albeit less than optimal, plan of care with the providers.

ness of the patient. Capacity also resides along a sliding scale relative to the magnitude of the decision at hand (see Table 14.2). It is decision specific. A simple decision such as the appointment of a health care proxy requires less capacity than a decision to choose chemotherapy over surgery for a malignancy. As a result, the adequacy of capacity varies based on the potential risk, benefits, and burdens of treatment as well as the patient's current mental state.

To understand decisional impairment it is helpful to review the attributes of decisionally capable persons. Several groups (Appelbaum & Grisson, 1992; Marson et al., 1995; Roth et al., 1977) have proposed ideal criteria which are summarized as follows: Decisionally capable persons understand they are being asked to make a choice and can express their decision consistently. They appreciate the nature of their condition including diagnosis, prognosis, and possible treatments. They are able to balance the risks, benefits, and burdens of various

TABLE 14.2. Examples of Decision-Specific Capacity Assessments

Designation of a health care proxy, durable power of attorney
Property management
Testamentary capacity
Place of residence (refusal of admission to nursing home)
Invasive or disfiguring medical or surgical procedures
Undergoing heroic or exceptionally burdensome procedures (vital organ
    transplantation, peritoneal or hemodialysis)
Discontinuation or refusal of
    Intubation or ventilators
    Cardiac massage and cardioversion
    Food and fluids delivered by artificial means
    Hospitalization
    Antibiotics
Involuntary admission to a mental health facility
Administration of psychotherapeutic medications over objection

choices. They apply a relatively stable set of values to the choice of available options. And they are able to communicate the rationale behind the choices. Although this hierarchy of attributes appears theoretical, it has been subjected to empirical validation. And the methods of validation, whether or not one chooses to use the specific evaluation tools, provide directions through the capacity interview.

Semistructured Capacity Interviews

The MacArthur Competency Assessment Tool—Treatment (MacCAT-T) is a manualized, semistructured 15- to 20-minute interview which provides a sequence of information and inquiry designed to quantify patient capacity to consent to treatment (Grisso et al., 1997). Specific criteria with written examples are provided to assess the quality of patient responses as adequate, partially adequate, or inadequate. However, each area is not assigned equivalent weight. Reasoning receives a score of 0–8; understanding, 0–6; appreciation, 0–4; and expression, 0–2. No attempt is made to establish a threshold or criterion score for incapacity. Rather, the extent of capacity (higher scores imply greater capacity) is based on the clinical context to arrive at a judgment for the individual.

The interview begins with a review of the patient's condition and proceeds to a disclosure of recommended treatment, risks, and benefits. The patient's capacities to understand, appreciate, reason, and conclude with a clearly expressed choice are assessed in the process. Asking the patients to paraphrase or describe their condition, proposed treatment, risks, and benefits assesses understanding. Errors in understanding prompt the assessor to repeat the initial review and inquiry before assigning a score. Asking patients whether the disclosed information applies to them as individuals and whether the proposed treatment offers at least some chance of benefit assesses appreciation. Delusion, distorted perceptions or denial, but not simple differences of opinion must be present to consider appreciation deficient. Choice is assessed simply by evidence of the patient's expressed preference. Finally, reasoning is assessed by asking patients to reflect on the potential consequences of their choices as well as alternatives. The score is based on whether or not the patients' choices follow logically from their expressed understanding and the extent to which they generate potential consequences not explicitly disclosed by the interviewer.

Empirical Evidence for Levels of Capacity

Grisso et al. (1997) compared MacCAT-T scored capacity to consent for medication between recently hospitalized patients with psychosis and mentally healthy community residents matched for age, gender, race, education, and occupational status. Of note, 12% of the hospitalized potential participants were judged too impaired by primary care staff to participate. Based on their MacCAT-T scores, 68% of the psychotics evidenced adequate to partially adequate understanding, 53% adequate to partially adequate reasoning, and 78% adequate appreciation. Among community residents, 95% evidenced adequate to partially adequate understanding and 70% adequate to partially adequate reasoning. Thus patients who participated in the study (most could not or would not) gave adequate to partially adequate evidence of understanding, reasoning, and appreciation. However, only a minority of healthy community residents of similar age, gender, race, educational, and occupation status showed perfectly adequate reasoning.

Using similar procedures, Marson et al. (1996) also found little difference between control and demented subjects on the ability to state a nonrandom choice. And at the higher level of difficulty of capacity (i.e., "understand the treatment situation and choices") not all controls were capable of stating fully competent recitals from test vignettes. However, multiple cognitive functions underlay decisional capacity. Once dementia has advanced to the point where receptive aphasia and severe dysnomia are present, few patients will be capable of reliably expressing a treatment choice. Executive dysfunction interferes with the capacity to identify the consequences of a treatment choice. Deficits in conceptualization, semantic memory, and verbal recall interfere with capacity to understand treatment situation and choices.

The majority of persons with Alzheimer's disease could evidence a reasonable choice, appreciate the consequences, and provide rational reasons if their Mini-Mental Status Exam score was 19 or above (Marson et al., 1995). Obviously these findings reflect the research setting in which the individual is isolated from the influence and support of family. Also, the outcomes are derived from a single session rather than repeated passes at the problem that would occur in a more clinical situation. On the other hand, the participants were asked to examine hypothetical rather than personal scenarios in which they would be less emotionally threatened and presumably more rational. In summary, the proposed ideal attributes of persons with decisional capacity seem relatively valid as demonstrated by empirical studies of capacity interviews.

Capacity Enhancement: Adding Relevance to the Capacity Interview

Ultimately the question of capacity is one of relative rather than absolute adequacy to the task (Levenson, 1990). It is neither realistic nor desirable to seek a "capacimeter" which might serve as a universal metric of decisional capacity (Kapp & Mossman, 1996). Yet there are formal elements of the mental status exam in a capacity assessment which should be made explicit, as shown in Table 14.3 and which will reinforce the principles of assessment listed in Table 14.1. First, was the quality of rapport and trust sufficient for genuine communication? Did the patient evince adequate executive function and the capacity to plan and anticipate outcomes? Are judgment and insight relatively intact? Is the patient aware of the consequences of consent or refusal? What is the level of cognitive impairment? If the patient was able to complete a Mini-Mental Status Exam, the score may add weight to the examiner's determination. However, a level of impairment must often be inferred from observation. Finally, is the patient free of or able to overcome distortions in beliefs and perceptions? Persons with persistent psychosis or fluctuating consciousness may be able to reason in a convincing, consistent fashion regarding the specific treatment decision despite distortions in other areas of awareness.

Assessment of capacity should also identify obstacles to the patient's decisional ability (Table 14.4). Although the adequacy of capacity is an ad hoc, commonsense judgment, there is a defined role for psychiatric and medical assessments. The practitioner's knowledge of medical procedures, diagnosis, prognosis, and recognition of reversible causes of incapacity is essential (Jonsen et al., 1992). The person performing the capacity assessment should also be alert for reversible, transient, or predictably recurrent obstacles to capacity. Is there a mis-

TABLE 14.3. Elements of Mental Status Exam Critical to the Assessment of Decisional Capacity

Quality of rapport and trust (adequate for genuine communication)

Executive capacity (ability to plan, anticipate outcomes)

Judgment/insight (aware of the outcome if they refuse)

Level of cognitive impairment

Freedom from, or the ability to overcome distorted beliefs and perceptions

match in communication style between patient and the practitioner recommending the intervention? Do cultural differences between the patient and practitioner need to be addressed? Is the practitioner unaccustomed to the hearing impairment and slowed information processing evident in some persons of advanced age? Is the patient educationally disadvantaged or developmentally disabled? Are there iatrogenic factors such as polypharmacy which cloud the patient's thinking? Has prolonged hospitalization traumatized the patient and made for a hopeless perspective? Has sleep deprivation in the ICU or emergency room impaired the patient's consciousness?

Is an unrecognized and presumably reversible delirium present? If not reversible, are there sufficient moments of clarity when the person can be informed and exercise adequate judgment? If family were present to buffer anxiety and assist in communication, could the patient approach a genuinely informed decision? Conversely, is the patient so enmeshed with a dysfunctional family that the source of inca-

TABLE 14.4. Factors That May Be Reversible or Recurring Obstacles to Capacity

Patient–provider mismatch

Iatrogenic and institutional factors (polypharmacy, lengthy confinement)

Phobic avoidance of medical procedures

Waxing and waning of cognition (delirium, fluctuating capacity)

Environmentally induced distress ("CCU psychosis," sleep deprivation)

Lack of familiarity with terms, procedures, or care staff (stranger anxiety)

Major mental illness

Delusional distrust or despair, grandiose or exaggerated self-regard

Overwhelming situational anxiety, exposure to dying or disfigured peers

Bereavement

Enmeshment with dysfunctional family

Personality disorder, posttraumatic stress disorder

pacity is more the family than the patient? Is a major mental illness distorting judgment through delusional distrust or despair, grandiose unfounded optimism, or exaggerated self-regard? Is the patient's capacity overwhelmed by situational anxiety and exposure to dying or disfigured peers? Is a posttraumatic stress disorder from prior hospitalization of the patient or a family member present? Does the impairment emanate from a personality disorder that keeps relations between the patient and the care team volatile and adversarial?

Identifying malleable obstacles to decisional ability may sufficiently reverse impairment without eliminating it and allow for an informed choice. Even when the informed choice is unwise, there may yet be areas of agreement that support a collaborative plan of care. Patients will often accept psychotropic medication to alleviate sleep deprivation, reduce anxiety, and manage depression or psychosis, which will allow them the comfort required to consider treatment options. The person performing the capacity assessment may also suggest a mediator to enhance communication or reduce conflict between the patient and practitioner proposing the intervention (Lo, 1995b). A family meeting with members of the treatment team often will resolve the impasse. Even when the treating physician declines to participate, the meeting, if handled with skill (see Chapter 8), may be beneficial, provided the person conducting the meeting is well informed of the risks, burdens, benefits, and therapeutic alternatives.

When capacity is indeterminate or beyond the influence of the practitioner, sources beyond the patient may be given consideration. Obviously a court order may be requested when the practitioner is uncertain and fears abandoning the patient to an impaired decision. More often consent from family will be sought as the naturally occurring surrogates. Table 14.5 provides the hierarchy of decision makers for incapacitated patients. When advanced directives or a durable power of

---

TABLE 14.5. Hierarchy of Decision Makers for the Incapacitated Patient

1. Advanced directives, documented while the patient is competent, prevail over family preferences.

2. Without advanced directives, an in-family discussion of treatment options is indicated. The family becomes a *de facto* guardian (spouse, children, siblings, others).

3. If the family cannot resolve conflicts over treatment decisions, petition the court to appoint a guardian to decide for the patient.

4. When there is no one to speak for the patient, the health care providers become *de facto* guardians.

Note. Adapted from Malloy et al. (1991). Copyright 1991 by Lippincott Williams & Wilkins. Adapted by permission.

attorney (proxy) for health care are not available family become *de facto* guardians. When there is no family or concerned party, the physician will become *de facto* guardian. Table 14.6 indicates the procedure to follow when family conflict arises and results in a therapeutic impasse. On occasion it will be necessary to reframe the request for a capacity determination (once an initial determination has been attempted) into a request for a bioethics consultation (Dubler & Marcus, 1994). This will expand the problem to its true dimensions and make explicit the competing viewpoints of the involved parties.

Assessment for Involuntary Psychiatric Treatment

When the decision is involuntary admission to a psychiatric facility, two components must be satisfied. To treat the person involuntarily, a

TABLE 14.6. Dealing with Family Conflicts over Treatment Decisions for Incompetent Patients

1. Establish consensus regarding medical facts within the health care team before meeting the family.
2. Convene a meeting of all family members and health care providers who will contribute to the decision-making process. Be particularly aware of individuals who hold strong preferences but do not attend. Do not hesitate to ask for the services of a consultant.
3. Use everyday language to describe the patient's condition, treatment, and prognosis. Take care to be consistent; differing portrayals of the case will arouse needless conflict.
4. Outline the areas in which decisions are required with realistic examples.
   a. Reversible life-threatening events (e.g., cardiac arrest)
   b. Reversible life-threatening illness (e.g., pneumonia)
   c. Treatable but disabling events or illness (e.g., stroke)
   d. Nutrition (e.g., nasogastric and gastrostomy tubes and parenteral nutrition)
   e. Range of procedures from least to most invasive (blood work to surgery)
5. Avoid power struggles and conflicts over control by acknowledging the family's authority. Make the health care providers' preferences explicit before indicating alternatives, advantages, and disadvantages. Advise the family members of their responsibility to reach consensus and provide the team with a final decision.
6. Nominate one family member and one team member to be the focus of communication.
7. Give the family a deadline to provide a decision but formally arrange one or more follow-up meetings for further information and support.
8. If the family cannot reach consensus, identify the differences in perceptions and preferences. If further information does not resolve the differences, follow the legal priority.

Note. Adapted from Malloy et al. (1991). Copyright 1991 by Lippincott Williams & Wilkins. Adapted by permission.

third element must be shown. First, a mental illness must substantially imperil the safety of the person or others. Second, the patient's judgment must be impaired as a direct result of the mental illness. Third, other than in an emergency, to medicate such persons over their objections requires a separate judicial proceeding. The psychiatrist must demonstrate that despite confinement to hospital, both danger and impaired judgment will persist without treatment. The linkage of genuine danger and substantial impairment is key to the practitioner's argument for any intervention, not just medication, over the patient's objection. A sample affidavit from my practice is provided at the end of this chapter. Although the issue addressed was surgery over the objection of a delusional patient, the outline can be adapted for applications for a guardian as well.

Assessment for the Appointment of a Guardian

State and county courts have specialized divisions that focus on legal matters involving persons alleged to be incapacitated. These divisions are called "probate courts" or "surrogates' divisions" (Buchanan, 1998). Individuals presiding over these divisions may be judges or persons with little legal training or medical background who are appointed to serve. Because probate court rarely involves the presentation of evidence before a jury, the judge's opinion is definitive. Hence the testimony of the individual who assessed the allegedly incapacitated person's abilities carries considerable weight (Richards & Rathbun, 1993). Mental health law varies from state to state, but the principles of documenting the findings are as follows: If there is a question about what to include, consult the client's attorney. The law may require a notarized signature making the document an affidavit. If a notary is not required, the document is an affirmation.

Following the practitioner's name, address, credentialing statement, and dates when the patient was examined, a thorough description of the mental disorder and prognosis is recorded. Next list the medications, doses, target signs, or symptoms and effects on mood, behavior, cognition, and judgment. Describe the prognosis of the mental disorder. Describe physical disorders, effects of treatment, and prognosis. Next provide a functional assessment that will be used to specify the powers granted to the guardian. Depending on the question at hand, the assessment may describe the alleged incapacitated person's ability to manage (1) property and finances, (2) personal needs and medical care, and (3) activities of daily living. Cognitive function should be quantified with an instrument such as the Mini-Mental Status Exam. The practitioner should also describe any specific behavioral inadequacies, as well as the alleged incapacitated person's understanding and appreciation of the character and consequences of impaired abilities and behavior. Next, provide examples that demonstrate how the person will suffer harm from the inability to manage personal needs or carry out activities of daily living. Also, describe financial transactions or events if any, which demonstrate damage done to the person as a result of impaired capacity to manage property and finances or make health care decisions. Following the objective details of the incapacity, provide a statement that the demands for personal needs and/or financial affairs and health care decisions are substantial, extensive, and exceed the person's capacity. Assume that the alleged incapacitated person will attend the hearing. If attendance will serve no useful purposes (e.g., the person is nonresponsive), or will be detrimental (e.g., displace an agitated person with dementia from familiar surroundings), state why in detail. Finally, specify the duration of the guardian's appointment. It may be indefinite or limited to an event such as a financial transaction (placement in nursing home, payment of home care services) or medical intervention. A sample document from my practice, a glossary of legal terms, and a list of sources of information and referral appear at the end of this chapter.

Capacity to Make a Last Will and Testament

The frequency with which older adults remarry after the loss of a spouse will only increase as the population ages. And the complexity of financial relations will also increase as members of the new family lay claim to their legacy. As a result, conflict among potential beneficiaries will result in challenges to the validity of the deceased person's (the principal's) will and any codicils (additions). The ability to make a valid will, known as testamentary capacity, hinges on two elements. First, the principal is aware that a will is being composed, knows the extent and varieties of property to be bequeathed, and can identify potential beneficiaries. Second, is the legal notion that a valid will is not the result of exploitation through the use of "undue influence." Undue influence results when a party violates the trust or fiduciary relationship on which the principal depends. Undue influence implies vulnerability on the principal's part combined with suspicious circumstances suggesting that a beneficiary has been deprived of legitimate inheritance by a manipulator. Both competence and undue influence are judgments for the court. However, the evaluator may document evidence of capacity and the nature of the relationship as displayed or portrayed by the principal during assessment. With some impaired persons there will be a sufficiently lucid interval to demonstrate capacity to make a valid will despite transient or intermittent cognitive deficits. Serial assessments with notation as to medications, time of day, or other circumstances associated with reversible or surmountable deficits should be documented. A score in the unimpaired range on a cognitive screening instrument such as the Mini-Mental Status Exam or the lengthier Mattis Dementia does not define capacity to make a will. But it will be objective evidence of a level of impairment on which inferences about capacity can be drawn. When conflict between beneficiaries is likely, some elder lawyers will recommend a cognitive assessment at the time of the will to protect the estate against challenge (Baker et al., 1985; Charatan, 1987).

Capacity to Consent to Research

Capacity to consent to research, particularly studies of mental health, must be considered a special category (Marwick, 1997). For example, with the rapid advances in treatment of dementia there is a growing interest in research participation. Procedures and processes to provide for the ethical participation of decisionally incapacitated patients will become increasingly important. Dukoff and Sunderland (1997) reported their experience in obtaining durable power of attorney for research participation among persons with dementia admitted to the National Institute of Mental Health study unit. Cognitive impairment scores ranged from unimpaired to moderate impairment (Mini-Mental Status Exam 27–16) and most participants were only moderately disabled in the area of personal care (Global Deterioration Scale score less than 5). Using questions such as those listed in Table 14.7, they concluded that early- to midstage dementia does not preclude appointing a durable power of attorney for research and that the likelihood of appointed proxies not being informed of the patient's wishes is small.

Grisso et al. (1997) provide a hierarchy of attributes of informed research participants. Informed research participants are able to do the following:

1. Evidence a choice (i.e., not a random, meaningless assent).
2. Manifest an understanding of relevant information.
3. Appreciate how the information applies to their situation.
4. Rationally manipulate the communicated information, consider consequences.

By overlaying situations that entail progressively greater decisional demands, a hierarchy or sliding scale of decisional capacity (from least to greatest) emerges as follows:

TABLE 14.7. Questions Suitable to Assess Capacity to Appoint a Durable Power of Attorney for Research

1. "If you were asked to enter a [description purposefully left blank] research study but were unable to decide for yourself, would you want someone else to decide whether or not you should participate?"
2. "If the research could help but could also harm you, would you still want to participate?"
3. "Who do you choose to make research decisions for you when you are no longer capable?"
4. "About what, do you want that person to decide?"
5. "What are consequences of your participation; what might happen?"

Note. Adapted from Dukoff and Sunderland (1997). Copyright 1997 by the American Psychiatric Association. Adapted by permission.

1. Appoint a research surrogate or durable power of attorney authorized to provide permission for research participation.
2. Consent to research in which therapeutic benefit is possible and the risk/benefit is highly favorable.
3. Consent to research in which therapeutic benefit is possible but the risk/benefit is less than highly favorable.
4. Consent to research in which therapeutic benefit is unlikely and the risk/benefit ratio is less than highly favorable.

Application of the hierarchy results in the following: First, persons not able to express a reliable, consistent choice are all incapable of giving informed consent even for the appointment of a surrogate for research. Second, those persons who are unable to appreciate how the information applies to their situation for consent to research in which therapeutic benefit is possible but the risk/benefit ratio is highly favorable, are incapacitated. For example, the potential participant who is not able to consistently distinguish research participation from receipt of treatment may have adequate capacity when the possible risks are minimal and the benefits high but not when the risks are high.

Third, persons who are unable to appreciate how the information applies to their situation for consent to research in which therapeutic benefit is possible but the risk/benefit ratio is less than highly favorable are incapacitated. For example, incapacitated potential participants would be unable to consistently describe the research as offering a chance of *both* improving their condition ("my memory problem") and causing harm ("might make me nauseated").

Fourth, those persons who are unable to rationally manipulate the communicated information are unlikely to be capable of consenting to research in which therapeutic benefit is unlikely and the risk/benefit ratio is less than highly favorable. For example, an incapacitated potential participant would not be able to consistently describe all three elements of the research as "can't help me, probably will not harm me, but might help others." These examples should prove useful in efforts to meet the standards proposed by the National Bioethics Advisory Commission.

Recommendations of the National Bioethics Advisory Commission

In 1998, the National Bioethics Advisory Commission (NBAC) recommended the following for research among persons with any mental disorder. Research that "would enroll subjects who lack decision-making capacity in protocols that a reasonable, competent person would decline to enter" should not be approved. For research protocols that present a greater than minimal risk to a potential subject with a mental disorder, a qualified professional should assess the person's capacity for informed consent. A person found to lack capacity should be informed of the determination before permission may be sought from the person's legally authorized representative to enroll the subject in the study. Incapacitated persons may not be enrolled in any study over their objections. For research involving greater than minimal risk with prospects of direct medical benefit to the subjects, their legally authorized representative may enroll incapacitated persons. The legally authorized representative may be a friend or family member and may be the subject's health care proxy or surrogate but must be available enough to monitor the subject's welfare during the study. Advanced directives in which competent persons document the circumstances (specific risks or procedures) under which they might participate in research prior to the loss of capacity are termed "prospective authorization." Prospective authorization appoints a legally authorized representative to make decisions regarding research enrollment. For research of greater than minimal risk but no prospect of direct medical benefit to the subject, the NBAC recommends that a federal-level special standing panel assess the appropriateness of the study in addition to the local institutional review board. To be ethically permissible, greater danger to the subject should be accompanied by more explicit acceptance of risk in the prospective authorization. Although the assertion that anyone with a mental illness may be decisionally impaired is controversial, declaring proxy consent for research and prospective authorization of the incapacitated person acceptable represents major advances for research ethics.

OTHER BIOETHICAL ISSUES OF CONCERN

Designation of a Proxy Decision Maker

By law, persons admitted to any hospital or nursing home are to be presented the option of appointing a proxy for health care decisions and the opportunity to specify advanced health care directives (Patient Self-Determination Act, Omnibus Budget Reconciliation Act of 1990). The law is meant to protect persons from unwanted end-of-life care at a time of diminished capacity. Unfortunately, the time of admission to a facility is the least desirable time to make these decisions (Silverman et al., 1995). Nursing homes are accidental communities (Macklin, 1990) and vary widely in their capacity to formulate advanced care plans. In 1990, prior to enactment of the Patient Self-Determination Act, 32% of residents had do-not-resuscitate (DNR) orders, 2% do-not-hospitalize orders, and 5% living wills. By 1993, 51% had DNR orders, 4% had do-not-hospitalize orders, and 14% had living wills. Staffing rather than designation of the responsibility seemed the major determinant of higher rates of advanced plans for care (Castle & Mor, 1998). Hence, primary care providers in the community are more likely to put the protective intent of the law into effect provided they are knowledgeable of the procedures and aware of the implications. In addition to preserving the individual's dignity, the cost of unwanted care could be considerably reduced if the intent of the Patient Self-Determination Act were fully realized. Patients with severe cognitive impairment are able to reliably appoint a health care proxy (Mezey et al., 2000).

How to Work with the Heath Care Proxy or Surrogate

Crises in care decisions can often be avoided by requesting that the patient appoint a health care proxy if a period of incapacity is anticipated (Zelezuik et al., 1999). In the absence of a proxy, the practitioner should determine who might serve as a surrogate if capacity is lost (see Table 14.5).

1. Ensure that documents appointing the proxy are in the medical record and in possession of both the patient and proxy.
2. Ask patients to discuss preferences with their proxies and include them or the surrogate in discussions in the event of an emergency or hospitalization.
3. If the patient becomes incapacitated, provide the proxy or surrogate the same information you would have given the patient.

4. Be aware that deciding for others is often more difficult than deciding for oneself.
5. Avoid "false choices" such as presenting transfer to the ICU as a choice for the proxy when in reality the intensive care physicians will decide.
6. Explain that a DNR order does not imply "do not treat."
7. Reassure the proxy that the patient will not be abandoned.
8. Explore palliative care options when the goal is no longer cure.
9. Advise the proxy or surrogate of institutional resources such as patient advocates, social services, translators, chaplainry, or the availability of bioethics consultation.

When there is confusion, uncertainties or conflict over a decision a bioethics consultation will be particularly helpful (Dubler et al., 1999).

Advanced Health Directives

Advanced directives specify the circumstances under which life-prolonging interventions may be withheld or withdrawn or research participation accepted once the patient is no longer capable of exercising autonomy. These circumstances include terminal conditions from which the patient is unlikely to recover and in which the specific therapeutic procedures may temporarily reverse an intervening acute illness but will have no impact on the underlying terminal condition. Such therapeutic procedures typically include the use of cardiopulmonary resuscitation, intubation, use of a ventilator, and dialysis. However, some persons will choose to forego antibiotics, food, and fluids by artificial means (intravenous fluids, tube feedings) in the event that their capacity is lost and their condition terminal.

Persons who designate a health care proxy usually choose a spouse or other family member to make decisions regarding medical treatment in the event that the patient is either temporarily of permanently incapable of making decisions. The treating physician may not be appointed as proxy. However, another physician, including the physician who formerly cared for the person before hospital or nursing home admission, may be appointed provided that person is not an employee of the facility. In the abstract, a health care proxy has no formal role until the patient is incapacitated so that the person's autonomy should be respected for all decisions. However, when loss of capacity, whether temporary or permanent, is reasonably foreseeable or the person's condition may be terminal, early involvement of the proxy is highly desired. Not involving the proxy beforehand may convert a critical juncture in the patient's course into a prolonged crisis in decision making. Asking that a proxy be appointed and involved is particularly important when the physician lacks a longer-term relationship with the patient and family which might have informed all parties as to the patient's preferences. Similarly, appointment of a health care proxy and discussion of advanced directives should occur early in the course of dementia before the patient's capacity is substantially degraded.

Caring for a Colleague's Parent

Being asked to care for a colleague's or influential person's parent is flattering. Yet caring for the aged VIP (very imperiled person) places an added burden on the practitioner that should be recognized from the outset. Self-examination will not avoid all errors but will lessen the extent of well-meant but off-the-mark efforts. The confidential advice of a trusted consultant is another means of keeping true to the patient's needs rather than acceding to other unavoidable social or political concerns. Knowledgeable practitioners frequently prescribe episodic treatment for their parents, but the practice should be discouraged and kept to a minimum. The colleague should be relieved of the burden of professional care and asked to act as a family member with all the implications. Because colleagues will be knowledgeable and to some extent enmeshed in the agencies and institutions that provide for their parent's care, the practitioner should attempt to consolidate the network of communications to one individual. Confidentiality will be a problem for the practitioner, patient, and family. Legitimate access to the medical record during a hospital admission is broadly based and not policed. Modern health care providers operate as a team and teams cannot work in secret. Practitioners should assume that their patient and his or her family will read their entries. Thus the practitioners' record keeping should reflect the perspective of patient and family and reflect their own viewpoints with diplomacy. Speculations and sensitive personal material are best omitted. If important, they may be conveyed verbally to the team. The temptation to delegate care tasks to the family member should be resisted. This protects the colleague as well as preserving one's clinical objectivity and the emotional distance that will prove so important during a crisis. Team dynamics are also important. Staff caring for other patients who do not receive the "special" attention will experience envy and resentment, which is understandable and at times justified but cannot be allowed to interfere with best care.

MEDICAL FUTILITY: WHO DECIDES, WHO DEFINES?

There is no ethical imperative for providing futile treatment (Brett & McCullough, 1986). However, the definition of futility is often not as straightforward as it seems. Decisions about life-sustaining interventions revolve around who makes the decision as well as the facts of the medical situation. Indeed, 80% of DNR orders are written for patients who lack the capacity to make the decision. Lo (1995a) cites four strict definitions of futility. First, there is no pathophysiological rationale for the intervention. Second, the patient is receiving maximal treatment and the intervention is failing. For example, cardiopulmonary resuscitation (CPR) for the patient in septic shock who remains hypotensive despite maximum vasopressors will not restore circulation. Any additional intervention beyond the present maximum will provide no added benefit. Third, the intervention has already failed the patient. After 30 minutes of CPR, the patient remains in asystole. The intervention, CPR that has already failed, need not be continued. Fourth, the intervention will not achieve the goals of care. Here Lo (1995a) uses the example of an obtunded hospital patient with advanced, metastatic cancer of the lung who has clearly stated that no further treatment is acceptable unless it has a chance of returning him to home. If the patient arrests, CPR may restore circulation and respiration. However, only a miracle is likely to return the patient to home care status. Indeed, few metastatic cancer patients survive the resuscitation attempt and next to none survive free of mechanical ventilation. Although the fatality rate is not 100%, the overwhelming odds are against the patient's returning home. Physicians are not ethically obligated to operate with 100% certainty, nor are they expected to wait for miracles. Indeed, offering the false hope of a miracle is ethically objectionable.

Difficulties arise when loosely defined definitions of futility are applied. Again, Lo (1995a) cites four examples. First, the likelihood of success, although not minuscule, is highly unlikely. Yet interpretations of highly unlikely may be perceived as arbitrary or unfair. An intervention with a 1% survival rate may make success seem remote. But if the survival rate were 2% or 5%, would the patient or family consider success "highly" unlikely? Different probabilities might be acceptable (i.e., less than highly unlikely) depending on the risks and potential benefits of the intervention. Second, physicians may believe an intervention is futile when they do not expect to achieve a worthwhile goal of care. Obviously, what is worthwhile is a judgment and open to differences in preferences and values. Providing CPR for the terminally ill hospital patient will not reverse the outcome of the terminal illness.

But it may buy time for distant family to make a final visit. Here, there is no ethical obligation to provide CPR, yet for reasons of compassion, the physician may agree to hold the DNR order. Prolonging life is worthwhile to the family, even though it has little intrinsic value to the patient. Third, physicians may judge an intervention futile because the result of therapeutic success will not provide the patient an acceptable quality of life. For example, an out-of-hospital resuscitation of a person with dementia will leave the survivor with more severe deficits and objectively less quality of life. Yet quality of life is inherently subjective, and it is the patient not the physician who is the subject. Thus it is the patient's values and preferences that should be used when making a quality-of-life decision. Granted, physicians will be more knowledgeable about the outcome of an intervention and the prognosis of the patient's condition. Beyond an awareness of those probabilities, the physician has no special expertise in quality of life. Without knowledge of the patient's perspective, arguments about quality of life risk characterizing viewpoints other than the physician's as irrational (Lo, 1995a). Finally, the futility argument may be raised when the potential benefits of an intervention seem not to justify the expenditures. Patients, regardless of age, who develop combined multiple organ system failure (renal, hepatic, cardiac) might survive longer in the intensive care unit. In this sense ICU care is not futile in that it will prolong life, yet it is unlikely in the extreme to improve the patient's chances of leaving the hospital alive. In a busy hospital, ICU beds are a scarce resource and such a patient will likely be triaged to less intensive care. In this example it is cost and allocation of resources rather than futility that is at stake. Masking the cost argument as medical futility hides the sad but necessary social decisions of whose life is worth saving and how much are we willing to spend on one another's care.

The Fair Approach to Futility

There are additional problems with the concept of medical futility. First the physician's assessment of futility may be mistaken. It may be based on anecdotal experience (biased sample), outdated training, or ignorance of recent advances. Second, futility decisions may be inconsistent, determined by the physician's personal preference or the culture of care within the facility. Third, futility may be represented as scientifically based or objective and mask a value judgment inherent in any life-and-death decision. Such judgments are "ethical, political, and social choices" as well as medical (Lo, 1995a). This is not to say that the practitioner's medical values are not important or necessarily at odds with patient and family preferences. Rather, safeguards are needed to ensure that the practitioner's unilateral decision is appropriate as opposed to being arbitrary.

An awareness of the problems with unilateral futility arguments leads to safeguards that will protect the practitioner from technical errors as well as the appearance of being unfair. It will also protect patients and families from the suffering of false hope and unwanted care that arises out of lack of information and support. Lo (1995a) suggests three steps to safeguard the decision about the futility of an intervention. First, obtain a second opinion. If in agreement, the second opinion provides reassurance to the physician and other involved parties. If not, the second opinion will help clarify goals and options. Second, inform the patient and family or surrogate decision maker of the judgment. If a demand for a futile intervention is made ask for more discussion. What are the expectations of the intervention? Are there factual errors of understanding? Is the decision to withhold an intervention being interpreted as a decision to withhold care or abandon the patient? Are there family needs or previous undisclosed patient preferences that might alter the physicians' perception of futility? Finally, establish guidelines, end points, to determine the futility of the intervention. A time-limited trial of the intervention may answer the question of futility for all parties. For example, in the patient emaciated by dementia, will a monthlong trial of improved nutrition via feeding tube restore a degree of independence or improve cognition? In some instances professional societies have published directives (Hastings Center, 1987; Council on Ethical and Judicial Affairs of the American Medical Association, 1992). In other instances the patient's advanced directives may clarify the goals. In any event, the practitioner who involves others in the decision-making process without abdicating responsibility for the ultimate recommendation will be least likely to encounter difficulties.

PHYSICIAN-ASSISTED SUICIDE

Views on physician-assisted suicide have become polarized between civil libertarians who champion the individual's right of self-determination, and moralists who fear an irrevocable coarsening of medical ethics and social values (Lee et al., 1996). The professions have grave reservations, but the public is much more accepting and indictments for physicians assisting suicide are rare and convictions are almost unheard of (Schwartz & Watson, 1998). Although the Supreme Court refused to recognize a constitutional right to suicide (*Vacco v. Quill,* 1997) the arguments for and against continue. The example of the

Netherlands, where health care has been universal since the end of World War II and where physician-assisted suicide is accepted practice, is frequently cited with approval (Hendin, 1995). However, the lack of equity in access to health care resources, economic disparities and perceived injustices in the United States are arguments against physician-assisted suicide (Coleman & Miller, 1995; Garland, 1992). The inadequate treatment of pain, depression, and anxiety and lack of palliative care, which characterizes much of medical practice in the United States, should also raise the threshold under which assisted suicide is considered (Post et al., 1996; Support Principal Investigators, 1995). And there are other arguments against physician-assisted suicide. If an individual desires suicide, what right has that person to ask another to participate in the act? And what standards apply that will keep suicide limited to those with imminently terminal or intractably painful conditions rather than expanded to include the disabled or those with chronic mental illness and intractable emotional pain? How can safeguards be defined much less regulated? If family history is a major predictor of suicide, what legacy is being passed on to subsequent generations? Will financial incentives for the managed care physician or the family members who see their legacy evaporating in the cauldron of long-term care tip the balance toward hurrying death?

Proponents of assisted suicide argue that respect for the patient's right to discontinue ventilator and nutritional support has not resulted in widespread expansion of treatment withdrawal. Patients, families, and physicians have not fallen down the slippery slope to encourage either the poor or disabled to die. Regarding lack of equitable access to health care, refusing access to assisted suicide only compounds the injustice. Through the "doctrine of double effect," death secondary to sedation (respiratory arrest) is not deemed objectionable if the primary effect sought was the alleviation of pain. The double-effect doctrine is part of Catholic theology and has been adopted by the American Medical Association (Council on Ethical and Judicial Affairs, 1992) and the courts as common law (Compassion in Dying v. Washington, 1996). For some, the distinction between death due to double effect and physician-assisted suicide is insubstantial. There is also the perception that a "don't ask, don't tell" rule has taken effect in which the practice of physician-assisted suicide is widespread but little talked about and never prosecuted (Schwartz & Watson, 1998). In effect, the law against mercy killing remains but is ignored. Here the argument is that professional secrecy is superior to legal consensus.

The first report from the Oregon Death with Dignity Act countered many of the fears expressed by the professions and moralists

(Chin et al., 1999). Physicians are required to report the issuance of a prescription for suicide (usually a rapid-acting barbiturate with an antiemetic). Patients must be decisionally capable adult residents of Oregon and have a prognosis of 6 months of survival or less. They are required to provide their physician with one written and two oral requests separated by 15 days. Oregon ranks third among the states in the rate of admissions to hospice care such that terminally ill patients have access to palliative care. Of the 23 persons who received a legal prescription from their physician for suicide, 15 died as a direct result, 6 died of other causes, and 2 did not carry through. The patients cited feared loss of autonomy and body function rather than intractable pain or financial concerns as the reason for suicide. Level of education and health insurance coverage were not associated with the choice. Most physicians who wrote the prescriptions found the experience emotionally taxing or were uncomfortable sharing their feelings with colleagues out of feared stigmatization.

A subsequent survey of 65% (n = 2,649) of all Oregon physicians by Ganzini et al (2000) extended these initial findings. Between October of 1997 and August 1998, there were 221 requests to physicians for lethal prescriptions and 165 requests in which there were reliable outcome data. The mean age of the patients was 68. Loss of independence was the leading reason for the request followed by poor quality of life, being "ready to die," and need to control the circumstances of death. Less than half the patients cited pain or other physical symptoms as reasons. Being a financial burden to others or lack of social support was cited by 11% or less. Twenty percent of the total had significant symptoms of depression, and none of these were prescribed a lethal drug. In 68 patients the physicians instituted at least one palliative care effort such as pain control or hospice referral. Close to half of these patients withdrew their request for assisted suicide. Of a total of 29 patients who received a lethal prescription, 17 committed suicide with the drug. In summary, Oregon physicians granted 1 in 6 requests for a lethal prescription, but only 1 in 10 requests were followed by assisted suicide. Fears that physicians would act with impunity to force suicide on poor or underinsured or terminally ill patients and their families were not realized. How the practice will evolve in coming years is a matter of intense interest.

Data from the Netherlands provides an unsettling but inevitable contrast to the preliminary experience in Oregon. In the Netherlands both euthanasia and assisted suicide have been accepted since the Royal Dutch Association of Pharmacy issued prescribing guidelines in 1987. In 24 months there were 114 recorded cases of intended physician-assisted suicide recorded, of which 16% were complicated by prolonged time to death and failure to induce or sustain coma. Some patients either vomited the drugs or could not otherwise consume the total prescribed dose. Two awoke from coma. The physicians converted 21 of these to euthanasia by administering lethal injections. (Groenewoud et al., 2000).

In the United States, public acceptance of physician-assisted suicide will likely grow as a result of the Oregon report. Practitioners will not be able to avoid the issue but can choose their approach to the discussion. Familiarity with end-of-life and palliative care principles (see Chapter 13) will provide alternatives to abandoning the patient to a suicidal impulse.

HOW TO CONDUCT A BIOETHICS CONSULTATION

Risk managers are an everyday part of hospital practice, but bioethics consultants are less readily available. As a result, the practitioner needs to know what to expect from a bioethics consultant. And the scarcity of bioethics in most locales means that the practitioner may need to conduct the consultation. Although a request for an ethics consultation may be an academic exercise meant to clarify the ethical bases of the care plan, more often a conflict has arisen in which the consultant is asked to intervene. In some instances a statement of the practical realities and applicable ethical principals will suffice. However, the consultant rarely is authorized by administration or risk management to arbitrate conflicts by fiat. The more likely outcome is an effort to mediate conflict between competing interests.

The goal of a bioethics consultation is the resolution of ethical dilemmas in care through the support and protection of patients to make health care decisions. However, the rights and concerns of interested parties, including the family, facility, service agencies, and health care providers, must be acknowledged when patients depend on others to put their preferences into effect or to achieve their needs. If the patient cannot reach or is too impaired to approach a decision, the decision is made by a surrogate to promote the best interest of the patient.

A bioethics consultation will focus on the balance of interests, responsibilities, and rights of the patient, family, facility, and providers as they apply to the treatment decision. The principles of fairness, honesty, compassion, confidentiality, and respect for privacy apply to all aspects of the process including disclosure of information and acquisition of informed consent. The resulting analysis is framed in terms of ethical principles including autonomy, beneficence, nonmalfeasance, and justice. When ethical principles are in conflict or are perceived to compete for primacy, patient autonomy should be looked to in order to resolve the dilemma.

The request for a bioethics consultation usually arises out of a crisis whether real or perceived. However, not every crisis is a life-and-death matter. Thus a rapid response is necessary but the completed product may be acceptably delayed. There is usually time to assemble the interested parties and to collect information on which to make an analysis and recommendation. Shortcuts will prove regrettable. Truly emergent requests may exceed the consultant's capacity and an acknowledgment of one's limitations is always appropriate.

First, the consultant should discuss the context of the case with the requesting party. The manifest reason for the request may be less important that the underlying factors. The consultant's task is to recognize the stated problem and to help make explicit other factors motivating the request. Next, the consultant should contact the interested parties to establish the facts of the case and if appropriate convene a meeting. If necessary, the consultant should request the assistance of other consultants in law, ethics, medical specialty, social service, clergy, or the facility's risk management staff. A preliminary meeting among team members is important to clarify their understanding of options and preferences. A larger meeting will follow to generate consensus, develop the analysis, and resolve the dilemma or conflict. Once a consensus on the facts has been achieved and the consultant has summarized it to the group's satisfaction, he or she should proceed to a discussion of the care plan options.

To develop the ethical analysis of treatment decisions, the consultant must first determine the adequacy of the patient's decisional capacity. If the patient is not capable of making the decision under consideration and there are no reversible obstacles to decisional capacity, the consultant must look to a living will or health care proxy. Is there convincing evidence from prior behavior or discussions that might be used to project the person's wishes to the present? Did the patient have a parent, child, sibling, or friend who experienced a similar problem? Did the patient express an opinion as to the desirability of the options? Even if a surrogate decision maker is required, presumed preferences in addition to best interests will add weight to the final decision. Although family is the natural surrogate in most states, they too are not always free of conflict. Table 14.6 provides an example of conflict management in which family members cannot initially decide on course of treatment for their impaired relative.

The consultant must make sure the patient and family are aware of the medical facts, diagnosis, prognosis, and treatment options. Everyday language is used to convey a clear and unitary picture of the patient's condition, proposed interventions, and prognosis. The consultant should specify the decision that needs to be made and the team's recommendations. He or she should prioritize what the team sees as in the patient's best interests rather than providing a menu of options. The consultant should be aware that the medical facts are more often an expression of probabilities than certainties. Will additional consultations, time, or information from other sources reduce uncertainty? Have all reasonable options been considered? With the factual background in hand, it is useful to identify the chief ethical dilemma. The dilemma will be an expression of interests and concerns of the patient, family, health care professionals, or the facility. The input from all concerned parties is crucial to the ultimate perception of fairness. Conflicts of interests and purely self-serving agendas are more often potential than real, but they should be made explicit nonetheless. Once the facts of the case and the interests of the involved parties are clear, the consultant should identify the relevant ethical and legal principles that apply. These principles are then used to inform rather than foreclose the subsequent discussion with the goal being a principled solution. Having made recommendations, the consultant should proceed to acknowledge the family's authority given the situation and advise them of their responsibility to make a decision. He or she should ask that they appoint one member to communicate with one member of the team. It is advisable to give a deadline for the decision and set a follow-up meeting, which will precede the intervention. In the follow-up meeting, the consultant should review the plan and, if no decision has been made, elicit differences in perceptions and preferences to establish agreement.

Whatever the principled solution may be, the involved parties must understand who the appropriate and authorized decision maker is. Determining who decides manages but does not eliminate conflict or uncertainty. The choices and probable consequences of each decision should be stated clearly and simply in terms of burden and benefits to the patient. If the family or patient needs additional support or information to decide, the consultant should provide the necessary liaison to other sources. A second opinion, contact with clergy and discussion with an advocacy or peer support group may be helpful but the needy party will require assistance in identifying the source. A deadline for the decision should be established, otherwise ambivalence and procrastination rather than information gathering may result. Once an agreed-on solution is identified, the consultant should review the principles on which it is based and the consequences that will likely follow. The solution may not meet everyone's ideal yet may still be principled. Consensus rather than conformity is the goal. The consultant should determine the means of implementing the solution, including a timetable and plans for follow-through. In outline form, the consultant should document the names of participating parties, the options discussed, and the agreed-on plan. The consultant must follow through to ensure that conflicts are managed and that marginal obstacles do not become major impediments. If there is no progress, the consultant should acknowledge the impasse and inform the family that a judicial decision will be required. A legal petition will often mobilize the family but on occasion will need to proceed to conclusion. The adversarial nature of the proceeding need not force an adversarial stance upon the interim care of the patient. An agreement to disagree and let the court decide may allow an interim therapeutic alliance to develop.

SUMMARY

The promise of biomedical advances cannot be realized without improvements in the practitioner's understanding of bioethics. And the need to contain costs and achieve equitable access to the benefits of care are competing social imperatives, not temporary conflicts. Conflict is inevitable but need not be destructive if managed with skill, fairness, and transparency. With experience and assistance from consultants, the generalist practitioner can achieve ethically principled outcomes despite numerous obstacles. Achieving a realistic balance between personal autonomy and protective care is the defining challenge of social policy for impaired persons.

APPENDIX

Sources of Legal Information for the Practitioner, Patients, and Their Families

For information regarding the laws in your state:
American Bar Association Commission on Legal Problems of the Elderly
740 15th Street, NW
Washington, DC 20005

National Senior Citizens Law Center
1815 H Street, NW, Suite 700
Washington, DC 20006

To locate a lawyer with expertise in the legal problems of older persons:
The National Academy of Elder Law Attorneys, Inc.
655 North Alvernon Way, #108
Tucson, AZ 85711

Legal Services for the Elderly
130 West 42nd Street, 17th Floor
New York, NY 10036
212-391-0120

Sample Physician's Affidavit, Application
for the Appointment of a Guardian

SUPREME COURT OF THE STATE OF NEW YORK
COUNTY OF BRONX
In the Matter of the Application for the Appointment of a Guardian for L.B., a
patient at Bronx Psychiatric Center

AFFIDAVIT OF PHYSICIAN

Gary J. Kennedy, MD, affirms the following under the penalties of perjury:

1. I am a physician duly licensed to practice medicine in the State of New
    York and on the staff of the above captioned psychiatric center. I am a
    Board Certified Psychiatrist with Added Qualifications in Geriatrics.
2. I have examined the alleged incapacitated person, Ms. L.B., on the 1st
    and 7th days of June 1996 at the above-captioned psychiatric center
    and found her to be suffering from schizoaffective disorder, bipolar
    type, with paranoid delusions resulting in substantial impairment in
    judgment and insight, more specifically the necessity for treatment of
    both mental and physical illness.
3. That the aforesaid patient had a mental disorder and the prognosis
    for said disorder is poor. There are no additional medical examina-
    tions or procedures that might detect reversible causes of her impair-
    ment. Furthermore, L.B.'s capacity to understand the risks, benefits,
    and burdens of diagnostic and therapeutic procedures to address the
    carcinoma of her colon is severely degraded as a direct result of her
    mental disorder. Her capacity to appreciate the consequences of re-
    fusing diagnostic and therapeutic procedures is also severely im-
    paired.
4. That the medications that the aforementioned patient is taking and
    the desired therapeutic benefit of said medications for the patient's
    behavior, cognition, and judgment are as follows:

Medication	Desired effect
Risperidone, 6 mg daily	Contain delusions that others intend to harm her and reduce aggressive

	impulses such that she will accept necessary personal care, hygiene, and health maintenance procedures which she failed to accomplish in the community
Carbamazepine, 800 mg daily	Stabilize emotional extremes to minimize unprovoked outbursts
Lorazepam, 2 mg daily	Control anxiety and lessen agitation

5. The patient has the following physical illness and prognosis: infiltrating carcinoma of the ascending colon diagnosed by biopsy without evidence of metastatic spread. Without surgery and lymph node dissection the carcinoma will result in death through either secondary infection or invasion and destruction of vital organs (liver, lung, brain). The probability of survival beyond 5 years is rare in the extreme. With surgery, combined with either chemotherapy or radiation or both, the likelihood of a bowel obstruction is substantially reduced and the chances of survival are considerably increased. Without preparatory diagnostic procedures (chest X ray, liver scan, bone scan, CT scan of the brain) to determine the extent of metastases, the benefits of radiation or chemotherapy to extend her survival would be significantly reduced.

6. That the patient's functional level may be described as follows:
   a. Ability to conduct property management: grossly impaired.
   b. Ability to manage personal needs: moderately to grossly impaired (see item d below).
   c. Ability to manage activities of daily living: moderately impaired. She is unable to attend to personal hygiene, grooming, and clean clothes without daily reminders from staff. She requires considerable urging to accept routine health maintenance procedures such as annual physical exam, vaccinations to prevent communicable disease. She denies the need for both physical and mental health services despite demonstrated inability to care for herself.
   d. Cognition and behavior: She is suspicious and volatile without provocation and isolates herself from others. She also clings to the delusions that others seek only to harm her and that if left to her own devices she would be perfectly healthy. She initially refused colonoscopy and biopsy of the colonic mass, relenting only after some months of coaxing by staff and family. She steadfastly refuses follow-up appointments with the clinic to discuss either her condition or proposed treatment. Despite grossly impaired judgment her cognition is otherwise unimpaired as evidenced by

as score of 28 correct out of a possible 30 answers from the Mini-Mental Status Examination.

 e. Understanding and appreciation of the consequences of refusing diagnostic and therapeutic procedures to address her cancer: grossly impaired. She alternates between denying the biopsy findings ("it was not cancer") and stating that the "surgery [biopsy] cured it" despite being informed that it did not. Neither will she allow attempts to more fully inform her of the risks, benefits, and burdens of accepting or rejecting cancer treament despite numerous efforts by physicians, nurses, and family members.

7. I further recommend that the Court find L.B. to be an Incapacitated Person and that the appointment of a Guardian is necessary for medical decision making to preserve her personal safety which is threatened by cancer. The expected duration of need for a Guardian is the period of time required for preparation and completion of the surgery and ancillary treatment that is expected to last no less than 6 months. I further recommend that the Guardian be empowered to consent on L.B.'s behalf and over her objection if need be to all diagnostic and therapeutic procedures including surgery, radiotherapy, chemotherapy related to the cancer, and any additional measures necessary to insure L.B.'s well-being, including attention to any complications related to her illness or treatment for 6 months following surgery.

8. Despite L.B.'s mental disorder, I recommend her presence at the hearing to facilitate her awareness of the gravity of the situation and to state her preferences and rationale directly. Nonetheless, the likelihood that she will be traumatized by the proceedings, which she will have difficulty accepting and participating in, cannot be ignored.

Gary J. Kennedy, MD

---

sworn to me on this date 24 June 1996
[Signature and seal, Notary Public, State of New York]

Glossary of Terms

Legal terminology varies from state to state such that the definitions listed below are an approximation for terms of art used in judicial proceedings.

Advanced directives   Choices specified by a competent person to direct future care should incapacity arise. Includes medical durable power of attorney, health care proxy, and living will.

Agent   The person to whom a durable power of attorney is assigned. Also called a surrogate or attorney-in-fact.

Alleged incapacitated person   A person whose ability to make decisions has been formally questioned.

Durable power of attorney   A legal document signed by a competent person that appoints a surrogate to make financial decisions on the person's behalf. Is "durable" in the sense that it remains in effect in the event of the person's incapacity. It may be "general" (broad) or "limited" (specific). May be assigned to one or more agents to act "jointly" or "severally" (alone without the signature of other agents). It may not be used to make or revoke a last will and testament.

Guardian or conservator   Court appointed (*de jure*) person who is empowered to manage the ward's financial affairs. May be authorized by the court order to make medical decisions as well. Authority to involuntarily admit the ward to a psychiatric facility is excluded from the powers in all 50 states.

Health care proxy   A legal document which assigns the power to make medical decisions to one or more agents (alternates) should the principal become incapacitated. Takes effect only during the period of incapacity. Family members or intimate companions are considered de facto health care proxies (legal surrogate) in most but not all states.

Living will   Written instructions provided by a competent person stipulating the circumstances under which life support procedures (cardiopulmonary resuscitation, use of respirator, artificial food and fluids) should be withheld or withdrawn. May also include directives for the use of antibiotics, surgery, or hospitalization. Usually applies to terminal conditions, vegetative state, or conditions in which the person is unlikely to recover the ability to recognize or relate to family and friends.

Medical durable power of attorney   A legal document signed by a competent person which appoints another to make decisions regarding consent to and refusal of medical treatments on the principal's behalf in the event of future incapacity. Authority to involuntarily admit the principal to a psychiatric facility is excluded from the powers in all 50 states.

Principal   The person who assigns a durable power of attorney.

Surrogate   A person whose authority to make decisions for someone else is based on state statute or case law (legal surrogate) or who is asked by the medical team (informal surrogate) to make decisions because no one has been appointed by the patient or court to do so.

Ward   Person assigned a guardian or conservator.

REFERENCES

Alpers, A., Lo, B. (1999). Avoiding family feuds: Responding to surrogate demands for life-sustaining interventions. *Journal of Law Medicine and Ethics, 27,* 74–80.

Appelbaum, P. S., Grisso, T. (1992). Assessing patients' capacities to consent to treatment. *New England Journal of Medicine, 319,* 1635–1638.

Baker, F. M., Perr, I. N., Yesavage, J. A. (1985). *An overview of legal issues in geriatric psychiatry.* Washington, DC: American Psychiatric Association.

Brett, A. S., McCullough, L. B. (1986). When patients request specific interventions: Defining the limits of the physician's obligation. *New England Journal of Medicine, 315,* 1347–1351.

Brock, D. W., Wartman, S. A. (1990). When competent patients make irrational choices. *New England Journal of Medicine, 322,* 1595–1599.

Buchanan, S. F. (1998). The medico-legal connection: The role of laws, courts, and lawyers. *Clinical Geriatrics, 6,* 72–74.

Callopy, B. J. (1995). Power, paternalism, and the ambiguities of autonomy. In L. M. Gamroth, J. Semradek, & E. M. Tourquiest (Eds.), *Enhancing autonomy in long-term care: Concepts and strategies* (pp. 165–180). New York: Springer.

Castle, N. G., Mor, V. (1998). Advance care planning in nursing homes: Pre- and post Patient Self-determination Act. *Health Services Research, 33,* 101–124.

Charatan, F. B. (1987). Geriatric psychiatry: Legal and forensic issues. In R. Rosner & H. I. Schwartz (Eds.), *Geriatric psychiatry and the law* (pp. 3–16). New York: Plenum.

Chin, A. E., Hedberg, K., Higginson, G. K., et al. (1999). Legalized physician-assisted suicide in Oregon—The first year's experience. *New England Journal of Medicine, 340,* 577–583.

Coleman, C. H., Miller, T. E. (1995). Stemming the tide: Assisted suicide and the constitution. *Journal of Law, Medicine, and Ethics, 23,* 389–397.

Compassion in Dying v. Washington, 79 F. 3d 790, 858 (9th Cir. 1996).

Council on Ethical and Judicial Affairs of the American Medical Association. (1992). Decisions near the end of life. *Journal of the American Medical Association, 267,* 229–233.

Dubler, N. N. (1998). Mediation and managed care. *Journal of the American Geriatrics Society, 46,* 359–364.

Dubler, N. N., Blustein, J., Post, L. F. (1999). *Making health care decisions for others: A guide to being a health care proxy.* New York: Division of Bioethics, Montefiore Medical Center, Albert Einstein College of Medicine.

Dubler, N. N., Marcus, L. J. (1994). *Mediating bioethical disputes: A practical guide.* New York: United Hospital Fund of New York.

Dubler, N. N., Nimmons, D. (1992). *Ethics on call.* New York: Harmony Books.

Dukoff, R., Sunderland, T. (1997). Durable power of attorney and informed consent with Alzheimer's disease patients: A clinical study. *American Journal of Psychiatry, 154,* 1070–1075.

Finns, J. J. (1999). Commentary: From contracts to covenant in advanced care planning. *Journal of Law, Medicine and Ethics, 27,* 46–51.

Ganzini, L., Nelson, H. D., Schmidt, T. A., et al. (2000). Physician's experiences with the Oregon Death with Dignity Act. *New England Journal of Medicine, 342,* 557–563.

Garland, M. J. (1992, Spring–Summer). Justice, politics, and community: Expanding access and rationing health services in Oregon. *Law, Medicine, and Health Care, 20,* 67–81.

Grisso, T., Applebaum, P. S., Hill-Fotouhi, C. (1997). The MacCAT-T: Clinical tool to assess patient's capacity to make treatment decisions. *Psychiatric Services, 48,* 1415–1419.

Groenewoud, J. H., van der Heide A., Onwuteaka-Philipsen, B. D., et al. (2000). Clinical problems with the performance of euthanasia and physician-assisted suicide in the Netherlands. *New England Journal of Medicine, 342,* 551–556.

Hastings Center. (1987). *Guidelines on the termination of life-sustaining treatment and the care of the dying.* Briarcliff Manor, NY: Author.

Hendin, H. (1995). Assisted suicide, euthanasia, and suicide prevention: The implications of the Dutch experience. *Suicide and Life-Threatening Behavior, 25,* 193–203.

Jonsen, A. R., Siegler, M., Winsdale, W. J. (1992). *Clinical ethics* (3rd ed.). New York: McGraw-Hill.

Kane, R. A. (1993). Ethical and legal issues in long-term care: Food for futuristic thought. *Journal of Long Term Care Administration, 21,* 66–74.

Kapp, M. B. (1992). *Geriatrics and the law: Patient rights and professional responsibilities* (2nd ed.). New York: Springer.

Kapp, M. B., Mossman, D. (1996). Measuring decisional capacity: Cautions on the construction of a "capacimeter." *Psychology, Public Policy and the Law, 2,* 73–95.

La Puma, J., Scheidermayer, D. (1996). Ethical issues in managed care. *American Journal of Managed Care, 2,* 167–171.

Lee, M. A., Nelson, H. D., Tilden, V. P., et al. (1996). Legalizing assisted suicide: Views of physicians in Oregon. *New England Journal of Medicine, 334,* 310–315.

Levenson, S. A. (1990, Winter). Evaluating competence and decision-making capacity in impaired older patients. *The Older Patient,* pp. 11–15.

Lo, B. (1995a). Futile interventions. In *Resolving ethical dilemmas* (pp. 73–81). Baltimore: Williams & Wilkins.

Lo, B. (1995b). Decision-making capacity. In *Resolving ethical dilemmas* (pp. 82–94). Baltimore: Williams & Wilkins.

Macklin, R. (1990). Good citizen, bad citizen. In R. A. Kane & R. L. Kane (Eds.), *Everyday bioethics: Resolving dilemmas in nursing home life* (pp. 77–92). New York: Springer.

Malloy et al. (1991). The daughter from California syndrome. *Journal of the American Geriatrics Society, 39,* 396–399.

Marson, D. C., Chatterjee, A., Ingram, K. K., et al. (1996). Toward a neurologic model of competency: Cognitive predictors of capacity to consent in Alzheimer's disease using three different legal standards. *Neurology, 46,* 1–7.

Marson, D. C., Ingram, K. K., Cody H. A., et al. (1995). Assessing the competency of patients with Alzheimer's disease under different legal standards. *Archives of Neurology, 52,* 949–954.

Marwick C. (1997). Medical news and perspectives, "Bioethics commission examines informed consent from the subjects who are 'decisionally incapable.' " *Journal of the American Medical Association, 278,* 618–619.

Mezey, M., Teresi, J., Ramsey, G., et al. (2000). Decision-making capacity to execute a health care proxy: Development and testing of guidelines. *Journal of the American Geriatrics Society, 48,* 179–187.

National Bioethics Advisory Commission. (1998). Research involving persons with mental disorders that may affect decision making capacity. *http/ bioethics. gov/capacity/TOC. htm.*

Omnibus Budget Reconciliation Act of 1990, Public Law No. 101–508, §§ 4206 and 4751.

Post, F. L., Bluestein, J., Gordon, E., et al. (1996). Pain: Ethics, culture, and informed consent to relief. *Journal of Law, Medicine, and Ethics, 24,* 285–300.

Richards, E. R., Rathbun, K. C. (1993). *Law and the physician: A practical guide.* Boston: Little Brown.

Roca, R. P (1994, March). Determining decisional capacity: A medical perspective. *Fordham Law Review, 62,* 1177–1196.

Roth, L. H., Meisel, A., Lidz, C. (1977). Tests of competency to consent to treatment. *American Journal of Psychiatry, 134,* 279–284.

Sachs, G. A., Cassel, C. K. (Eds.). (1994). Clinical ethics. *Clinical Geriatric Medicine, 10,* 403–553.

Schwartz, R., Watson, K. (1998). Physician-assisted suicide. *Annals of Long Term Care, 6,* 71–74.

Shuster, E. (1997). Fifty years later: The significance of the Nuremberg code. *New England Journal of Medicine, 337,* 1426–1440.

Siegler, M. (1985). The progression of medicine: From physician paternalism to patient autonomy to bureaucratic parsimony. *Archives of Internal Medicine, 145,* 713–718.

Silverman, H. J., Tuma, P., Schaeffer, M. H., et al. (1995). Implementation of the patient self-determination act in a hospital setting: An initial evaluation. *Archives of Internal Medicine, 155,* 502–510.

SUPPORT Principal Investigators. (1995). A controlled trial to improve care for seriously ill hospitalized patients. *Journal of the American Medical Association, 274,* 1591–1598.

Sorum, P. C. (1996). Ethical decision making in managed care. *Archives of Internal Medicine, 136,* 2041–2045.

Vacco v. Quill 117 S. Ct. 606 (1997).

Zeleznik, M., Post, L. F., Mulvihill, M., et al. (1999). The doctor–proxy relationship: Perception and communication. *Journal of Law, Medicine and Ethics, 27,* 13–19.

15

Advice on Exercise and Nutrition

A clinical/educational approach that will help patients and their families develop better nutritional and exercise habits can play a pivotal role in reducing the morbidity and mortality of the most common chronic illnesses in the United States. However, changes in diet and activity habits are difficult to achieve (U.S. Department of Health and Human Services, 1996). How successfully the person ages is, to an important extent, the result of how hard he or she works at it (Rowe & Kahn, 1998). Maintaining a high level of physical and mental function supported by a highly connected social fabric spells success, even when the person has not been able to avoid illness. Commonsense suggestions and a few surprises promise to preserve the function and quality of life of older patients without overburdening the clinician.

NUTRITION AND EXERCISE AS PRIMARY AND SECONDARY PREVENTION

Obesity and diets high in fat and salt and low in fiber are associated with a higher prevalence of cardiovascular disease, diabetes, arthritis, or malignancy. Illnesses associated with dietary excess include coronary heart disease, hypertension, diabetes, and stroke (White, 1997). Large waist circumference and elevated body mass index are also associated with impaired quality of life and disability in activities of daily living (Han et al., 1998). Diseases associated with dietary imbalance or excess are among the major contributors to death and disability in the United States. Insufficient intake of nutrients plays a direct role in osteoporosis, constipation, degraded oral hygiene, and protein–calorie malnutrition (U.S. Preventive Services Task Force, 1996). Cost-effectiveness estimates in terms of dollars saved as a result of focused nutritional care following trauma, hip fracture, cardiovascular disease, pulmonary and renal infections, and endocrine and metabolic disorders range from $147 million (Barents Group, 1996) to $1.3 billion over 7 years (Lewin Group, 1997).

Lack of even modest physical exercise is associated with excess mortality from all causes, particularly heart disease (Judge, 1996; Williams, 1998). Improvements in body weight, diet, and exercise may lessen if not eliminate the need for antiarthritic, antidiabetic, antiangina, and antihypertensive medications. Although the burden of the most common chronic illnesses in the United States could be reduced by changes in diet and exercise, these reductions depend on altered social behaviors and are not easily achieved. However, modest improvements that are far from heroic have meaningful benefits for health and well-being. Even in late life, loss of endurance and strength can be recovered through a modest exercise program.

Some older persons may seek to eliminate medications through diet and exercise. For mild hyperglycemia, hypertension, and angina they may be able to achieve a reduction in dose or frequency and in some instances drop the medication altogether. However, dose reduction is a more achievable goal than attaining drug-free status. Similarly, the elimination of forbidden treats (sweets, savory items, holiday or festival foods) is unrealistic, but reduction in frequency or amounts is not. With foods, nothing is forbidden but all things should be taken in moderation.

DIETARY INTERVENTION

Diet and exercise are important adjuncts to treatment and may be preventive in some instances. However, the primary care clinician is most often caring for someone with illness already present. Thus the prescription should be carefully tailored to social reinforcers and realistic expectations. For the majority of Americans, weight increases until age 60 or 70. Thus once the increase has leveled off, modest changes in behavior, diet, and exercise may be quite effective. Long-term, sustained modest gains are the goal rather than immediate, dramatic benefits. Loss of weight and change in nutritional habits are best achieved by a global, incremental approach that incorporates changes in food selection, preparation, exercise, and social reinforcers. This will make it possible to formulate a treatment plan for realistic, sustainable changes in nutritional and exercise habits. The ability to educate patients and their families regarding desirable body weight, healthy proportions from the food groups, and a modest, no-cost exercise program such as brisk walking is reasonable for all practitioners.

First the clinician needs to elicit a diet and exercise history that takes into account medical conditions, culture, preferences, work, and leisure activity. Who prepares the meals? What is ordered from the menu when the family dines out? Are highly glycemic refined "white foods" (bread, pasta, potatoes, rice) the major source of carbohydrates? Are "box or bag foods" with high fat and sodium (mixes, chips, sweets) a common indulgence? Are soft foods preferred due to dental problems? A diet free of cooking oils, nuts, fatty foods, and animal products, with the exception of nonfat dairy items, is ideal for patients with coronary atherosclerosis. Yet a more realistic program that emphasizes the social importance of dining and the recreational aspects of exercise will lead to more lasting changes than an abstemious regimen. Changes in behavior should focus on ensuring that breakfast is never skipped and is followed by two to four small meals. Skipping meals will only escalate the portion size and calorie count.

Most hospitalized patients will not follow a calorie-, salt-, or fat-reduced hospital diet once they are discharged. Neither the meals nor the ambience of the hospital are conducive to learning new and rewarding nutritional habits in the community where access to favored foods and reinforcers of bad habits are the norm. A posthospital visit to educate the patient and the household cook is more important than the initial hospital dietary counseling.

Table 15.1 outlines the general principles of good nutrition. Adding more fruits and vegetables (frozen contains more vitamins than fresh) will improve vitamin, water, and fiber content of the diet and displace the more problematic items which are higher in fat and lower in fiber. Substituting low-fat daily products fortified with vitamin D for meats will increase calcium as well as reduce fat intake. Portion size should be controlled to approach 300 calories per entrée. Table 15.2 lists Rowe and Kahn's (1998) advice regarding specific nutrients. These include adding calcium and vitamin D through either low-fat dairy products or supplements. Additional folic acid may best be achieved with supplements. Supplementation with selenium and vitamins E, B_{12}, and B_6 may be beneficial in moderate doses, but the benefits are less clear. Although roughly 10% of Americans go beyond these accepted measures to embrace alternative nutritional strategies, there is little compelling evidence to argue the beneficial outcomes of extreme nutritional interventions (Cassileth & Chipman, 1996).

There is suggestive evidence that the diet-derived antioxidants

TABLE 15.1. General Principles of Good Nutrition

- Maintain body weight to body mass index (BMI) of 22–27 (above 29 = obese) (BMI = body weight in pounds × 703 ÷ height in inches squared).
- Take the majority of foods from plant rather than animal sources.
- Restrict the intake of high-fat foods, particularly animal fats.
- Maintain the consumption of dietary fiber between 20 and 35 grams per day.
- Moderate or eliminate alcohol (two drinks or less for men, one or less for women).
- Restrict the use of smoked, salt-cured, or salt-pickled foods.

Note. Data from U.S. Preventive Services Task Force Report (1996).

ascorbate and beta-carotene are associated with better memory function (Perrig et al., 1997). Nutritional supplementation with alpha-tocopherol (Sano et al., 1997) has also slowed the disability of Alzheimer's disease. Persons with either Alzheimer's disease or vascular dementia may have disturbed antioxidant balance (Sinclair et al., 1998). However, the role of antioxidants in disease prevention remains con-

TABLE 15.2. Specific Nutrient Guidelines Advocated by Rowe and Kahn for Successful Aging

Nutrient	Daily amount	Sources
Protein	12% of total calories	Lean meat, fish, poultry, eggs, low-fat dairy products, legumes combined with cereals
Fat	30% or less of total calories	Eggs, vegetable oils, avocados, preferred over saturated oils and animal fats (butter, lard)
Carbohydrates	60% of total calories	Fruits, vegetables, legumes, cereals
Fiber	20–35 g	Fruits, legumes, cereals
Vitamin B_6	2 mg	Chicken, fish, liver, unmilled cereals, peanuts, walnuts
Folic acid	400 µg[a]	Leafy vegetables, liver, yeast, fruits
Vitamin B_{12}	1 mg	Red and organ meats
Vitamin D	700 IU[a]	Fortified milk, seafood, eggs
Vitamin E	200 mg[a]	Vegetable oils, green leafy vegetables, nuts, wheat germ
Selenium	200 µg[a]	Tuna, asparagus, Brazil nuts, meat, poultry, bread, vegetables
Calcium	1,200 mg[a]	Dairy products, broccoli, kale, collards

Note. Data from Rowe and Kahn (1998).
[a]May require supplement to reach suggested level.

troversial, with conflicting findings from well-done studies (Rowe & Kahn, 1998). Because vitamin A is so broadly available and so readily absorbed, Rowe and Kahn (1998) do not advise supplementing the dietary intake.

The more compelling evidence of nutrition's capacity to prevent disease and extend the lifespan comes for calorie-restriction studies of laboratory animals. Calorie-restriction augments DNA repair, regulates insulin dynamics, reduces oxidative stress, and preserves immune function. Rats whose caloric intake is reduced to near starvation levels experience a 40% increase in lifespan. However, they are so hungry they will kill and eat cage mates and cannot reproduce. Ongoing studies of primates offer a less stark comparison. Monkeys whose caloric intake is restricted to 70% of ad-lib-fed control animals keep their body weight at young adult levels. The restricted animals also receive vitamin and mineral enhancements. They exhibit lower blood pressure and serum lipids, greater insulin sensitivity, and less diabetes. Less spinal arthritis and cancer are also observed. Mortality rates among the test animals are lower in the early stage of the study. Of note, although the restricted animals are obviously hungry (they eat ravenously), they are no more aggressive and no less energetic than the ad-lib-fed group (Couzin, 1998).

In summary, maintaining body weight at young adult levels through regular exercise and the replacement of fats with more fruits and vegetables rich in vitamins A, C, E, and beta-carotene may be the best and simplest recommendation. A therapeutic vitamin (numerous brands) can be added without complicating the regimen or escalating the costs or risking toxicity from the fat-soluble vitamins.

GAINING WEIGHT

Patients with cancer experience loss of weight and appetite due to the catabolic process of their disease and the gastrointestinal effects of chemo- and radiation therapy. Their need for narcotic analgesics further impairs their nutritional status via constipation. Megestrol acetate, dronabinol, and prednisone are appetite stimulants which may be required but have a number of side effects. Homemade or commercial nutritional supplements may also be required but can provoke diarrhea due to lactose intolerance and may lack palatability. Alternatively, changing to a more calorie-dense choice of offerings and adding scheduled snacks between meals should be suggested. Patients should experiment with the schedule of meals and snacks so that appetite is not suppressed. Calorie-dense foods are typically higher in fat. Their addition to meals in moderation can have a significant impact. Similarly, purposefully selecting snacks with higher fat or protein content will make every meal count. Full-fat cheeses, yogurt, and avocado can be added to sandwiches. Milk can be substituted for water in soups, savory dishes, and beverages (White, 1997). Finger foods (sandwiches, cookies, cakes) can be made continuously available to persons with dementia to facilitate slow but sure intake.

TREATMENT OF OVERWEIGHT AND OBESITY

Risk stratification by body mass index (BMI) and the presence of at least one medical condition identifies patients who should reduce weight for health reasons. BMI is calculated by multiplying body weight in pounds by 703 and dividing the result by height in inches squared. At 5 feet 7 inches and 159 pounds, the person's BMI is 25. At the same height but with a weight of 191, the BMI is 30. A person with a BMI between 25 and 29 is considered at low but not least risk for medical comorbidities. However, those with diabetes (FBS > 126 mg/ dl), hypertension (systolic > 140, diastolic > 90), or hypercholesterolemia (HDL < 35 mg/dl for men, < 45 for women) should consider treatment for being overweight. Patients with a BMI greater than 29 are considered obese and in need of treatment whether or not a comorbid condition is present (National Heart Lung and Blood Institute, 1998). Obesity is best conceptualized as a chronic illness that like diabetes or hypertension may be controlled but rarely cured. Thus the realistic goal of treatment is sustained weight reduction by 5 to 15% rather than return to lean body mass of early adult years. The goal is better function and risk reduction rather than better appearance (Bray, 1999).

Changes in diet and behavior as listed previously, and exercises are essential to success. For persons at highest risk—those with BMI above 30—appetite suppressant medication may also be considered. Appetite suppression may be useful to initiate treatment and to help patients who relapse. However, long-term safety data are limited. Sibutramine is the only appetite suppressant approved by the FDA for long-term use, meaning up to 12 months. Its side effects include dry mouth, asthenia, insomnia, constipation, and mild elevations in heart rate and blood pressure. It may not be appropriate for persons with recent stroke, myocardial infarction, and congestive heart failure. It should not be prescribed in conjunction with other serotonergic medications or monoamine oxidase inhibitors.

Orlistat is an intestinal lipase blocker that increases the fecal elimination of fat and achieves a 10% weight reduction after 1 year among persons who limit fat intake to 30%. It is FDA approved. Side effects include bloating, loose stools, and anal leaking, which become less troublesome as patients learn to use the medication with reduced fat intake (Bray, 1999).

CONSTIPATION

Constipation is a frequent complaint among seniors, particularly those who have unrealistic bowel expectations, consume little dietary fiber, take inadequate amounts of liquid, require narcotic analgesics, or do not exercise. Obviously, physical activity and more fluid and fiber are the primary interventions. Simply increasing the amounts of fruits and vegetables will increase both fluid and fiber content. Adding one to three tablespoons of dietary fiber from psyllium will more than meet the recommendations. Bloating and cramping are less likely if the psyllium is introduced gradually. Many inexpensive preparations are available in a variety of flavors and consistencies. Patients also need to be aware that daily elimination is not the goal of good bowel hygiene.

HEALTHY EXERCISE FOR SENIORS

The importance of physical exercise in late life cannot be overestimated (Kelley, 1998; Toole, 1997). And the need to emphasize the social and motivational aspects of exercise should not be neglected. An exercise history and review of present opportunities for activity begin the assessment. Was the person an athlete when younger? Were group sports the only exercise outlet? Are safe, easily accessed areas conducive to walking available? Is there an air-conditioned mall nearby to escape the heat or avoid the cold? Is there a partner available to reinforce the effort? Simple maneuvers such as recommending that the older couple exercise together provides an important reinforcement. A morning program of exercise is more often sustained than one carried out in the afternoon or evening. However, a morning routine may require a much longer warm-up period. Exercise has an alerting effect that may interfere with sleep. Reinforcing the older adult's sense of self-efficacy ("I can do it") and providing emotional support ("Yes, you can") may sound catchy but proves to be a substantial contributor to physical activity and functional independence (Seeman et al., 1994). Measures that improve physical health and well-being have important benefits to the older adult's mental health. Physical activity at all levels of intensity has been linked to improvements in perceived stress, anxiety, and well-being (Department of Health and Human Services, 1996). Benefits are achieved through a reduction in physical debility and through improved self-image, sense of efficacy, and simple pleasure in functioning. Exercise also lowers blood sugar by increasing insulin sensitivity (Mayer-Davis et al., 1998).

Manson et al. (1999) reviewed exercise guidelines from the Centers for Disease Control and Prevention in a report on heart disease reduction associated with walking and vigorous exercise. The exercise guidelines suggested 30 minutes of vigorous exercise daily, 7 days a week. Manson et al.'s study concurred but added that 3 hours of brisk walking weekly conferred similar benefits to more vigorous exercise. Women who began exercising only in midlife also achieved benefits. The benefits amounted to a 30 to 40% reduction in coronary events among a cohort of 72,488 women ages 40 to 65 years followed for 8 years. The benefits remained substantial even after correcting for age, illness, and lifestyle differences in the participants. King et al. (2000) found significant reductions in physical pain among both endurance-strengthening (fit and firm) and stretching-flexibility (stretch and flex) exercising elders. Because most older adults get less than the recommend level of exercise, the percentage of coronary events that are potentially preventable if the exercise guidelines were universally applied approaches 50%.

The traditional three components to effective exercise are flexibility, strength and endurance. As shown in Table 15.3, I add balance, injury prevention, persistence, and reinforcement to round out the physiological, anatomic, and motivational components for an optimal program. The exercise prescription form is provided in Figure 15.1 but must be tailored from the outset to the patient's interests, motivation, and fitness potential (Swinburn et al., 1998). For seniors who are not overly ambitious but want a simple routine, a 20-minute walk three times a week may be sufficient to begin. They can add the first three steps of Tai Chi—"sun rising," "step right," "step left"—which incorporate the postural awareness, balance, and quadriceps strengthening of the long form but are easier to learn. Tai Chi will also increase the person's upper extremity motor control (Yan, 1999). Instructions for pain-free stretching and range-of-motion exercises can be found in most exercise books and magazines. It is important to emphasize that

TABLE 15.3. Physiological, Anatomic, and Motivational Principles of Exercise Programs for Older Persons

Component	Methods	Goal	Functional or physiological benefits	Target illness or condition
Flexibility	Daily graduated stretching without pain, warm up first	Increased range of motion	Lessened disability, pain reduction, contracture prevention, improved gait, improved sexual performance	Arthritis, pain, immobility, falls and gait disturbance, stroke rehabilitation
Strength	Weight bearing exercise, Tai Chi, mechanized resistance training	Increased muscle strength and mass	Fewer falls, better cardiovascular performance, reduced medications for diabetes. Better ambulation	Diabetes, rehabilitation post myocardial infarction or stroke, Parkinson's disease, gait disturbance, falls, osteoporosis
Endurance	Walking, swimming, cycling, running, tennis, basketball	Greater stamina at all levels of functioning	Weight loss, better cardiovascular and sexual performance, reduced medications for diabetes, angina, hypertension	Diabetes, angina, obesity, hypertension, anxiety, panic, depression, myocardial infarction or stroke rehabilitation, chronic lung disease
Injury prevention	Warm-up, moderation, regularity, progressive increase in duration and effort, proper clothing, footwear, equipment	Preservation of exercise routine, prevention of pain and disability, resiliency	All of the above	Arthritis, podiatric conditions
Balance	Postural awareness, Tai Chi, dance or movement therapy	Safer exercise and activities of daily living	Reduced risk of falls	Stroke, Parkinson's disease, gait disturbance
Persistence	Daily routine, variety, cross training, group training	Stretching and endurance training daily, strengthening and balance every other day, fatigue without pain	All of the above	All of the above
Reinforcement	Recreational rather than therapeutic attitude, group training, convenience, low cost, fashionable attire, written prescription, follow-up	Fun, socialization, motivation, pride in one's appearance, maintenance of gains and goals	All of the above	All of the above

Purpose	Type of physical activity	Duration, intensity, baseline	Duration, intensity, week 1	Duration, intensity, week 2	Duration, intensity, week 3	Duration, intensity, week 4	Duration, intensity, week 12
To establish your routine level of physical activity	Walking, housekeeping, gardening, sports						
To warm up, prevent injury, improve balance and posture	Slow walking or range-of-motion exercises, postural awareness, Tai Chi (first three steps)						
To increase endurance	Brisk walking, sports						
To increase strength	Stair climbing, chair squats, biceps curls, triceps extensions, sit-ups, resistance training, Tai Chi long form						
To relax, cool down, increase flexibility	Slow walking followed by gentle stretching, range-of-motion exercises						

FIGURE 15.1. The exercise prescription. The general rules are: (1) Start easy, even a little exercise counts; (2) go slow, give yourself 12 weeks to get in shape; (3) if an exercise hurts, trade it for one that doesn't; (4) keep track of your progress; (5) have fun; a little exercise you enjoy is better than a heavy routine you hate; (6) don't quit, you're only old once! How to use this chart: (1) Record your present level of physical activity in an average week; this is your baseline; for example, write the minutes you spent walking or in sports, or the number of stair flights you climbed, or the weight of packages you carried; (2) then underline the type of physical activities and exercises we agreed are safe for you to perform; (3) begin by exercising every other day, doing each chosen activity at a relaxed effort; at the end of the first week record the minutes or amount of exercise you accomplished; (4) for the second week you can exert a little more effort but not increase the amount; (5) in week 3 begin exercising 5 days a week but do not increase the effort; (6) from weeks 4 to 6 increase the days per week of exercise to 7, add effort only if you feel like it; (7) by the end of the 12th week you should be spending a half hour in your exercise routine for 5 to 7 days per week; and it's time to see me again to review your progress and future goals.

stretching should come after the exercise rather than before. Stretching must also be introduced gradually to tissues that have lost their elasticity with age and inactivity. For optimal benefit, a daily routine incorporating 30 to 45 minutes of endurance exercise and including resistance (weight) training will be needed (Williamson & Kirwan, 1997). Dumbbells can be used to strengthen the upper extremities with curls for the biceps, standing military press for the deltoids, and supine (bench) press for triceps. Rising from the edge of a chair repeatedly while holding the dumbbells and keeping the back straight will strengthen the quadriceps (Welle, 1998). Hypertension is not a contraindication to strength training. Indeed, diastolic pressures will decrease (2–3mmHg) over a 4-week period of three sessions per week (Brandon et al., 1997). Walking 30 minutes on most days of the week should be sufficient to achieve substantial health benefits (Stofan et al., 1998). The goal is to expend 150 calories a day or 1,000 per week (Rowe & Kahn, 1998).

Highly motivated individuals and those with an athletic background may seek to return to their sport but will need considerable time and effort to regain reasonable fitness and avoid injury. Structured exercise through a health club or exercise group may be preferred for the solitary senior or one whose spouse or family is a negative reinforcer. The probability that only half of structured exercise participants will continue for 15 months should not be a deterrent. Increases in strength and coordination will decline but remain above baseline measures (Boyette et al., 1997) Among nursing home residents, weight training with eight repetitions, three times a week for eight weeks more than doubled strength and increased walking speed by 50%. These gains were sustained afterward with only one weight workout per week (Fiatarone, 1995). Programs incorporating strength, flexibility, balance, and endurance can be administered to groups including frail, demented, or incontinent residents and are more likely to preserve physical function than simple range-of-motion exercise (Darien-Alexis et al., 1999). In summary, some form of exercise from range of motion to competitive sports will be beneficial for nearly every senior.

SUMMARY

Simple, commonsense improvements in diet and exercise can have major effects on the health and well-being of older Americans, both in preventing disease and in modifying the severity of illness after onset. These improvements include reducing the intake of fats and animal products; increasing quantities of fruits, vegetables, fiber, and water; adding calcium and vitamin D either through low fat dairy products or supplementation; supplementing the diet with folic acid; and walking 30 minutes a day (augmented with stretching and resistance training if manageable). Body weight should approach that of lean young adulthood. Supplementation with selenium and vitamins E, B_{12}, and B_6 may be beneficial in moderate doses but the benefits are less clear. The clinician's attention to social reinforcers and proper technique can increase the long-term adherence to healthy behavior by ensuring that meals are satisfying and workouts are fun. This means making a healthful diet a family affair, keeping expectations realistic and long-term oriented, and urging that exercise be a social rather than solitary pursuit. That better diet and physical activity mean better health will hardly strike the average senior as novel. However, seniors will be pleasantly surprised to find their practitioner knowledgeable and optimistic about nutrition and exercise.

BOOKS ON EXERCISE AND NUTRITION
FOR THE GENERAL READER

Rowe, J. W., Kahn, R. L. (1998) *Successful Aging*. New York: Pantheon Books.
Exercise: A Guide from the National Institute on Aging. Public Information Office, National Institute on Aging; National Institutes of Health Publication No. NIH 99-4258. *http://www.nih.gov/nia*.

REFERENCES

Barents Group. (1996). *The clinical and cost-effectiveness of medical nutrition therapy: Evidence and estimates of potential Medicare savings from the use of selected nutrition interventions*. Washington, DC: Nutrition Screening Initiative.

Boyette, L. W., Sharon, B. F., Brandon, J. (1997). A follow-up study on the effect of strength training in aging. *Journal of Nutrition, Health and Aging, 1*, 109–113.

Brandon, J., Sharon, B. F., Boyete, L. W. (1997). Effects of a training program on blood pressure in aging. *Journal of Nutrition, Health and Aging, 1*, 98–102.

Bray, G. A. (1999). Treatment of obesity in the elderly. *Clinical Geriatrics, 7*, 41–58.

Cassileth, B. R., Chapman, C. C. (1996). Alternative and complimentary cancer therapies. *Cancer, 77*, 1026–1034.

Couzin, J. (1998). Low-calorie diets may slow monkey's aging. *Science, 282*, 1018.

Darien-Alexis, L., Ecclestone, N. A., Myers, A. M., et al. (1999). A randomized outcome evaluation of group exercise programs in long-term care institutions. *Journal of Gerontology: Medical Sciences, 54A*, M621–M628.

Fiatarone, M. A. (1995). Editorial: Fitness and function at the end of life. *Journal of the American Geriatrics Society, 43*, 1439–1440.

Han, T. S., Tijhuis, M. A. R., Lean, E. J., et al. (1998). Quality of life in relation to overweight and body fat distribution. *American Journal of Public Health, 88,* 1814–1820.

Judge, J. O. (1996). Exercise. In D. B. Reuben, T. T. Yoshikawa, & R. W. Besdine (Eds.), *Geriatric review syllabus* (3rd ed., pp. 87–92). Dubuque, IA: Kendall/ Hunt.

Kelley, G. (1998). Aerobic exercise and lumbar spine bone density in postmenopausal women: A meta-analysis. *Journal of the American Geriatrics Society, 46,* 143–152.

King, A. C., Pruitt, L. A., Phillips, W., et al. (2000). Comparative effects of two physical activity programs on measured and perceived physical functioning and other health-related quality of life outcomes in older adults. *Journal of Gerontology: Medical Sciences, 55A,* M74–M83.

Lewin Group. (1997, May). Significant Medicare savings with medical nutrition therapy. RDs improve heath care and reduce costs. *ADA Courier,* 15–16.

Manson, J. E., Hu, F. B., Rich-Edwards, J. W., et al. (1999). A prospective study of walking as compared with vigorous exercise in the prevention of coronary heart disease in women. *New England Journal of Medicine, 341,* 650–658.

Mayer-Davis, E. J., D'Agostino, R., Jr., Karter, A. J., et al. (1998). Intensity and amount of physical activity in relation to insulin sensitivity: The Insulin Resistance Atherosclerosis Study. *Journal of the American Medical Association, 279,* 669–674.

National Heart, Lung and Blood Institute. (1998). Clinical guidelines on the identification, evaluation, and treatment of overweight and obesity in adults— The evidence report. National Institutes of Health. *Obesity Research, 6,* 51S–209S.

O'Toole, M. L. (1997). Do older individuals need more than usual physical activities to maintain strength and function? *Journal of the American Geriatrics Society, 45,* 1534–1535.

Perrig, W. J., Perrig, P., Stähelin, H. B. (1997). The relation between antioxidants and memory performance in the old and very old. *Journal of the American Geriatrics Society, 45,* 718–724.

Rowe, J. W., Kahn, R. L. (1998). *Successful aging.* New York: Pantheon Books.

Sano, M., Ernesto, C., Thomas, R. G., et al. (1997). A controlled trial of selegeline and alpha-tocopherol, or both as treatment for Alzheimer's disease. *New England Journal of Medicine, 336,* 2177–2183.

Seeman, T. E., Charpentier, P. A., Berkma, L. F. (1994). Predicting changes in physical performance in a high-functioning elderly cohort: MacArthur studies of successful aging. *Journal of Gerontology: Medical Sciences, 49A,* M97–M108.

Sinclair, A., Bayer, A. J., Johnston, J., et al. (1998). Altered plasma antioxidant status in subjects with Alzheimer's disease and vascular dementia. *International Journal of Geriatric Psychiatry, 13,* 840–845.

Stofan, J. R., DiPietro, L., Davis, D., et al. (1998). Physical activity patterns associated with cardiorespiratory fitness and reduced mortality: The Aerobics Fitness Center Longitudinal Study. *American Journal of Public Health, 88,* 1807–1813.

Swinburn, B. A., Walter, L. G., Arroll, B., et al. (1998). The green prescription study: A randomized controlled trial of written exercise advice provided by general practitioners. *American Journal of Public Health, 88,* 288–291.

Welle, S. (1998). Resistance training in older persons. *Clinical Geriatrics, 6,* 48–59.

White, J. W. (Ed.). (1997). *The role of nutrition in chronic disease care.* Washington, DC: Nutrition Screening Initiative.

Williams, P. T. (1998). Coronary heart disease risk factors of vigorously active sexagenarians and septuagenarians. *Journal of the American Geriatrics Society, 46,* 134–142.

Williamson, D. L., Kirwan, J. P. (1997). A single bout of concentric resistance exercise increases basal metabolic rate 48 hours after exercise in healthy 59–77-year-old men. *Journal of Gerontology: Medical Sciences, 52A,* M352–M355.

U. S. Department of Health and Human Services. (1996). *Physical activity and public health: A report from the Surgeon General.* Atlanta: National Center for Chronic Disease Prevention and Health Promotion.

U. S. Preventive Services Task Force Report. (1966). *Guide to clinical preventive services* (2nd ed.). Baltimore: Williams & Wilkins.

Yan, J. H. (1999). Tai Chi practice reduces movement force variability for seniors. *Journal of Gerontology: Medical Sciences, 54A,* M629–M634.

Index